AF624871

FLUOROSCOPY REDUCTION TECHNIQUES

for Catheter Ablation of Cardiac Arrhythmias

ONLINE ACCESS

The purchase of a new copy of this book entitles the first retail purchaser to free personal online access to a digital version of this edition.

Please send a copy of your purchase receipt to info@cardiotext.com with subject ZEROFLUORO EBOOK, and we will email you a redemption code along with instructions on how to access the digital file.

FLUOROSCOPY REDUCTION TECHNIQUES

for Catheter Ablation of Cardiac Arrhythmias

Editors:
MANSOUR RAZMINIA, MD
PAUL C. ZEI, MD, PhD

cardiotext
PUBLISHING
Minneapolis, Minnesota

© 2019 Mansour Razminia, Paul C. Zei

Cardiotext Publishing, LLC
3405 W. 44th Street
Minneapolis, Minnesota 55410
USA

https://cardiotextpublishing.com

Any updates to this book may be found at: https://bit.ly/zerofluoro

Comments, inquiries, and requests for bulk sales can be directed to the publisher at: info@cardiotextpublishing.com.

All rights reserved. No part of this book may be reproduced in any form or by any means without the prior permission of the publisher.

All trademarks, service marks, and trade names used herein are the property of their respective owners and are used only to identify the products or services of those owners.

This book is intended for educational purposes and to further general scientific and medical knowledge, research, and understanding of the conditions and associated treatments discussed herein. This book is not intended to serve as and should not be relied upon as recommending or promoting any specific diagnosis or method of treatment for a particular condition or a particular patient. It is the reader's responsibility to determine the proper steps for diagnosis and the proper course of treatment for any condition or patient, including suitable and appropriate tests, medications or medical devices to be used for or in conjunction with any diagnosis or treatment.

Due to ongoing research, discoveries, modifications to medicines, equipment and devices, and changes in government regulations, the information contained in this book may not reflect the latest standards, developments, guidelines, regulations, products or devices in the field. Readers are responsible for keeping up to date with the latest developments and are urged to review the latest instructions and warnings for any medicine, equipment or medical device. Readers should consult with a specialist or contact the vendor of any medicine or medical device where appropriate.

Except for the publisher's website associated with this work, the publisher is not affiliated with and does not sponsor or endorse any websites, organizations or other sources of information referred to herein.

The publisher and the authors specifically disclaim any damage, liability, or loss incurred, directly or indirectly, from the use or application of any of the contents of this book.

Unless otherwise stated, all figures and tables in this book are used courtesy of the authors.

Library of Congress Control Number: 2019937130

ISBN: 978-1-942909-30-9

eISBN: 978-1-942909-35-4

Printed in the United States of America

2 3 4 5 6 7 24 23 22 21 20 19

Dedication

To my parents, to my wife Soraya, and my children, Hana & Daniel, without whose love and support nothing would be possible.

To Dr. Richard F. Kehoe, my mentor and cherished friend, who not only taught me the art of electrophysiology, but also helped me become a better person.

—Mansour Razminia

This book and all the work I do would not be possible without the support and love of my wife Eva, and my daughters Clementine, Maja, and Violet. I thank my parents who gave me every opportunity for success in life. And, my deepest gratitude goes to Bill Stevenson, who still inspires me as an electrophysiologist and as a gentleman.

—Paul C. Zei

Contents

Contributors

Editors

Mansour Razminia, MD
Director, Cardiac Electrophysiology, Amita St. Joseph Hospital, Elgin, Illinois

Paul C. Zei, MD, PhD
Director, Comprehensive Atrial Fibrillation Program, Cardiac Arrhythmia Service, Brigham and Women's Hospital, Harvard Medical School, Boston, Massachusetts

Contributors

Amin Al-Ahmad, MD, FACC, FHRS, CCDS
Cardiac Electrophysiologist, Texas Cardiac Arrhythmia Institute, St. David's Medical Center, Austin, Texas

Dan Alyesh, MD, FACC
Electrophysiology Section, South Denver Cardiology, Littleton, Colorado

Martin Borlich, MD
Department of Cardiology, Heart Center, Segeberger Kliniken; Academic Teaching Hospital of the Universities of Kiel, Lübeck and Hamburg, Bad Segeberg, Germany

Kristen Breedlove, MPAS, PA-C
Physician Assistant, Heart Center at Akron Children's Hospital, Akron, Ohio

Jim W. Cheung, MD, FACC, FHRS
Division of Cardiology, Associate Professor of Medicine, Weill Cornell Medicine—New York Presbyterian Hospital, New York, New York

John Clark, MD
Director, Arrhythmia Center, The Heart Center at Akron Children's Hospital, Akron, Ohio

Nicholas J. Costa, MD
Cardiac Electrophysiology, Weill Cornell Medicine—New York Presbyterian Hospital, New York, New York

Hany Demo, MD, FACC, FHRS
Director of Cardiac Electrophysiology, Swedish Covenant Hospital, Chicago, Illinois

Oliver D'Silva, MD
Cardiac Electrophysiology, Advocate Illinois Masonic Medical Center, Chicago, Illinois

Jason T. Engel, CVT
Texas Cardiac Arrhythmia Institute, St. David's Medical Center, Austin, Texas

John D. Ferguson, MBChB, MD, FACC, FHRS
Associate Professor, Cardiovascular Medicine, University of Virginia, Department of Medicine, Charlottesville, Virginia

Carola Gianni, MD
Texas Cardiac Arrhythmia Institute, St. David's Medical Center, Austin, Texas;

Rodney P. Horton, MD
Texas Cardiac Arrhythmia Institute, St. David's Medical Center, Austin, Texas

Christopher I. Jones, MD
The University of Chicago Medicine, Center for Arrhythmia Care, Heart and Vascular Center, Pritzker School of Medicine, Chicago, Illinois

Ian H. Law, MD, FACC, FHRS
Department of Pediatrics, Division of Pediatric Cardiology, University of Iowa Stead Family Children's Hospital, Iowa City, Iowa

Raman L. Mitra, MD, PhD, FACC, FHRS
Medical Director, Cardiology, Beacon Advanced Cardiovascular Specialists-South Bend, Beacon Health System, South Bend, Indiana

Carlos Monreal, CVT
Texas Cardiac Arrhythmia Institute, St. David's Medical Center, Austin, Texas

Gustavo X. Morales, MD
Cardiac Electrophysiology, Grandview Medical Center, Birmingham, Alabama

Andrea Natale, MD, FACC, FHRS, FESC
Texas Cardiac Arrhythmia Institute, St. David's Medical Center, Austin, Texas; Interventional Electrophysiology, Scripps Clinic, La Jolla, California; Electrophysiology, Los Robles Cardiac and Cardiovascular Center, Thousand Oaks, California; Department of Internal Medicine, Dell Medical School, Austin, Texas

José Osorio, MD
Director, Cardiac Electrophysiology, Grandview Medical Center, Birmingham, Alabama

Clayton Robison, CVT
Texas Cardiac Arrhythmia Institute, St. David's Medical Center, Austin, Texas

Zachary J. Rosenblatt, CVT
Arrhythmia Services, California Pacific Medical Center, San Francisco, California

José Mauricio Sánchez, MD, FHRS, FACC
Cardiac Electrophysiology, The Heart Health Center, St. Luke's Hospital, St. Louis, Missouri

Saurabh Shah, MD, FHRS
Cardiac Electrophysiology, Advocate Illinois Masonic Medical Center, Chicago, Illinois

Robin Singh, MD
Cardiac Electrophysiology, Harvard Medical School, Brigham and Women's Hospital, Boston, Massachusetts

Philipp Sommer, MD, FHRS, FESC, FEHRA
Department of Electrophysiology, Heart and Diabetes Center NRW, University Hospital of Ruhr University Bochum, Bad Oeynhausen, Germany

Sri Sundaram, MD, FHRS
Electrophysiolgy Section, South Denver Cardiology, Littleton, Colorado

Amit Thosani, MD, FHRS
Director, Cardiac Electrophysiology, Allegheny General Hospital, Allegheny Health Network, Pittsburgh, Pennsylvania

Roderick Tung, MD, FACC, FHRS
Associate Professor of Medicine; Director, Cardiac Electrophysiology & EP Laboratories, The University of Chicago Medicine Center for Arrhythmia Care—Heart and Vascular Center, Chicago, Illinois

Nicholas H. Von Bergen, MD
Department of Pediatrics, Division of Pediatric Cardiology, The University of Wisconsin School of Medicine and Public Health, Madison, Wisconsin

Theodore Wang, MD
Cardiac Electrophysiology, Advocate Illinois Masonic Medical Center, Chicago, Illinois

Cameron Willoughby, DO
Department of Electrophysiology, Electrophysiology Director, McLaren Macomb Medical Center, Mount Clemens, Michigan

Foreword

Clinical cardiac electrophysiologists must keep up with the rapid advances in the scientific and technical aspects of care for arrhythmia patients. As a procedural specialty, the tools and techniques used to deliver therapy are critical to the success of the practicing electrophysiologist. Advancements in the technical aspects of catheter ablation have increased the ability of electrophysiologists to improve the procedure's efficiency and safety. In particular, electroanatomic mapping and imaging using intracardiac ultrasound have enabled more complex procedures and led to improved understanding of the anatomy and electrophysiology of ablation targets.

Not long ago, the majority of ablation procedures would involve exposing both the patient and the operators to high doses of radiation. Commonly, biplane fluoroscopy was utilized, and the operator would position catheters based on locations identified using multiple angles of fluoroscopy. Current tools have allowed significant reductions in fluoroscopy exposure to both the patients and the operators. For patients, this means reducing the risks associated with radiation exposure, such as malignancy and skin burns. For operators, it means reducing both the risk from exposure to radiation as well as the risk of orthopedic problems related to wearing leaded protective gear.

Procedural techniques have been developed to optimize workflow safety and efficacy in a minimal- or zero-fluoroscopy environment. What was once thought to be impossible or unsafe can now be performed safely. Operators have learned to position catheters using intracardiac ultrasound imaging, with the assistance of catheter mapping systems that record positional data for the catheter in 3D space.

In *Fluoroscopy Reduction Techniques for Catheter Ablation of Cardiac Arrhythmias*, Drs. Razminia and Zei bring together multiple experts who share techniques and practical advice that allow for avoiding pitfalls while performing a safe and effective procedure in a low- or zero-fluoroscopy environment. It is clear that electrophysiologists must embrace a better understanding of fluoroscopy reduction techniques for the sake of our patients as well as our personal health.

In *Fluoroscopy Reduction Techniques for Catheter Ablation of Cardiac Arrhythmias*, the reader will find the tools not only to potentially reduce fluoroscopy, but in some cases completely eliminate it—without compromising safety or efficacy.

Fluoroscopy Reduction Techniques for Catheter Ablation of Cardiac Arrhythmias is an important text for all electrophysiologists, replete with crucial advice on the optimal use of non-fluoroscopic tools for better ablation safety and efficacy. I congratulate Drs. Razminia and Zei on this important contribution and am confident that it will be a welcome source of information in moving to a future of fluoroscopy reduction.

—Amin Al-Ahmad, MD
Cardiac Electrophysiologist,
Texas Cardiac Arrhythmia Institute,
St. David's Medical Center,
Austin, Texas

Foreword

The past three decades have seen tremendous progress in cardiac electrophysiology. Interventional electrophysiology has grown from a few procedures offered to a limited number of patients with refractory arrhythmias to being a mainstay of therapy for a wide variety of arrhythmias, ranging from supraventricular tachycardias and symptomatic premature beats to atrial fibrillation and life-threatening ventricular tachycardia—and even some types of ventricular fibrillation. Advances were made by many dedicated clinicians, scientists, and engineers who contributed to the development of our present methods. Critically, the understanding of cardiac anatomy and its relation to arrhythmias progressed as better and better tools were developed to define and correlate anatomy with electrophysiology. Throughout this period, fluoroscopic imaging has been of critical importance as the major means of relating the location of electrophysiologic catheters and device leads to the cardiac anatomy. Imaging with ionizing radiation, however, comes with its own risks, well known to all, including the potential for tissue damage, risk of malignancy, and injury to the electrophysiologist and laboratory personnel as a consequence of the protective lead garments required. Maintaining the radiation dose as low as possible has long been an important goal for all electrophysiology laboratories. Fortunately, we have now reached the point where non-fluoroscopic imaging methods can potentially allow the majority of catheter ablation procedures to be performed with minimal or no fluoroscopic imaging.

Approaches to reducing fluoroscopy are built on the use of electroanatomic mapping systems and advanced skills with ultrasound imaging. Adapting these methods to achieve the goals of mapping and ablation without increasing the risks associated with manipulating catheters and sheaths in the vascular system has been a goal that has been substantially achieved by many. The use of force-sensing catheters also likely helps prevent inadvertent cardiac perforation and vascular injury. Although these methods are increasingly used, they are not yet widely disseminated throughout the electrophysiology community. Acquiring the necessary skills while maintaining patient safety is critically important.

In *Fluoroscopy Reduction Techniques for Catheter Ablation of Cardiac Arrhythmias*, Drs. Razminia and Zei and their coauthors bring a wealth of experience and information together into an accessible, practical, well-illustrated text. The book is particularly timely. It provides methods to reduce fluoroscopy through every stage of an ablation procedure, such that operators can gradually apply methods to aspects that are applicable to their individual skill sets. The methods described are of benefit to all practitioners, and many are applicable to parts of procedures for which fluoroscopy cannot yet be replaced (such as epicardial access and ablation adjacent to coronary arteries).

I congratulate Drs. Razminia and Zei on a wonderful contribution to the electrophysiology literature that will foster continued advances in the field to improve safety and outcomes. Every practitioner is interested in safely implementing methods to further reduce fluoroscopic imaging during their procedures. This book is a wonderful source of guidance toward that goal.

—William G. Stevenson, MD
Vanderbilt University Medical Center,
Nashville, Tennessee

Preface

Dear Readers,

We are excited and delighted to present to you what we hope is a comprehensive, state-of-the-art, yet practical overview of the rationale, methodology, and **"hands-on" tips and tricks for reduction or elimination of fluoroscopy during mapping and catheter ablation of cardiac arrhythmias.** We intend this text to address the entire spectrum of commonly (and less commonly) performed procedures. We envision a hands-on guide that will assist the electrophysiologist and their team in the electrophysiology laboratory to safely and effectively work toward significant reduction in fluoroscopy utilization.

At the time of this writing, it is quite clear to most every electrophysiologist that **reducing radiation exposure to the patient, physician, and EP lab staff is a critical goal for multiple reasons.** If we consider the "As Low as Reasonably Achievable (ALARA)" tenet for radiation exposure and risk, **the ultimate goal should be the complete elimination of fluoroscopy exposure,** and hence associated risk. Indeed, even very low exposure is still too much exposure if the alternative is zero radiation exposure, so long this alternative remains safe and can allow the electrophysiologist to achieve successful outcomes no worse than otherwise. One of the many pleasant surprises to which most every author in this text and we can attest is an observation that **procedural safety has likely improved significantly after adoption of these techniques.** It turns out that having a more realistic, real-time visualization of catheter vs. tissue relationships improves the operator's understanding of catheter location and hence lowers risks of perforation or other traumatic complications. These observations are beginning to be borne out in the ever-growing literature evaluating fluoroscopy-free or minimal fluoroscopy catheter ablation.

There is an inherent challenge to writing a text on this subject at this time in our field. It is fair to say that there has yet to be widespread adoption of the techniques outlined in this text. Moreover, the technological tools available to assist all of us in this process continue to evolve, improve, and mature. As a result, providing the most up-to-date advances, data, and recommendations is critical to ensuring the reader has a useful reference that can be utilized for quite some time. We believe the combination of a host of expert and experienced authors and a **rich library of videos** accompanying this text serves that goal.

There are a few bookkeeping points we would like to make. The first is terminology. Nearly every author in this text has fully adopted a completely fluoroscopy-free approach to their procedures. Keep in mind that at the time of this writing, this approach is an off-label use of most of the tools and technologies described in our text. However, as our authors have relayed over and over again throughout our text, both the available published data and their vast personal experiences have demonstrated safety and efficacy of this approach. Second, a completely non-fluoroscopic procedure is an easily defined entity, as zero radiation is zero radiation. But, how do we define *reduced* fluoroscopy? Reduced in relation to what standard? Numerous references report "typical" fluoroscopy utilization during common ablation procedures, so is an EP physician's average fluoroscopy use below those reported numbers considered reduced? Or should the standard be something else? We argue that in the context of our text, fluoroscopy reduction should be seen as a notable reduction in fluoroscopy reliance in the reader's personal usage in most cases. **Fluoroscopy should be viewed as generally unnecessary, or at best a modality needed in a very narrow range of situations**. There will always be challenging cases where fluoroscopy may have a role, but an overall significant reduction should be at least the initial goal.

As you read through each chapter, you will notice several things. First, there is clearly diversity in some details on how to perform aspects of each particular procedure. That is inherent to our field in general, and there is by no means a need to alter one's entire workflow to accommodate fluoroscopy reduction or elimination. On the other hand, there are several important common themes you will notice. The importance of both ICE and EA mapping goes without saying. **Core**

competencies that should absolutely be mastered in a fluoroscopy-free approach include ultrasound-based vascular access (Chapter 5), ICE-guided transseptal puncture (Chapter 6), familiarity (if not expertise) in ICE manipulation and views (Chapter 2), and a thorough understanding of the underlying principles, capabilities, and limitation of mapping systems. In the latter regard, your local clinical specialist for your mapping system can prove to be an invaluable resource.

Speaking of mapping systems, we want to also emphasize some additional important points. One critical theme in this text is that we charged the authors, when possible, to provide information that is agnostic to the specific mapping system or ICE system. You will see that each author clearly has more experience with one system or another, and so the expertise they convey will be focused on that system. **However, we have ensured that the general principles discussed are applicable across platforms, and if indeed there are features or limitations specific to one system or another, those are addressed appropriately.**

We would also like to point out some interesting observations that we have made during our journey through this process. As implied earlier, we have all noticed anecdotally, now more and more corroborated by published data, that **a fluoroscopy-free approach appears to be associated with improved safety, i.e., fewer complications.** We postulate several factors. Vascular access guided by ultrasound allows direct visualization of the vascular structures and their relationships. This is a vast improvement to either an approach based on physical landmarks or fluoroscopy, as neither of these traditional approaches can visualize these relationships. Second, **some of the simplest and most straightforward ablation procedures we perform have potentially been significantly improved.** When ICE is utilized during typical CTI ablation, for instance, commonly as an adjunct to PVI when clinically indicated, we have acquired a significantly improved understanding of the local anatomy, as structures that cannot be otherwise easily visualized are seen on ICE, including prominent Eustachian ridges, CS ostia, trabeculations, and so on. Indeed, on many occasions, it is specifically these anatomic variants that have hindered successful ablation, and visualization has helped to identify the issue at hand. This principle also applies to many, if not most of the other commonly performed ablation procedures. Moreover, aside from whether or not one utilizes contact force sensors during catheter ablation, **the ability to see in real-time catheter vs. myocardial relationships is vastly improved over fluoroscopic imaging.** This very likely improves both safety and efficacy.

At the time of this publication, we realize that areas of need for further fluoroscopic reduction include primarily epicardial access-based procedures and device implantation. As of this writing, there are operators out there working towards these goals, and we expect new chapters to be added on these and other topics in future editions of this text.

Some final words of advice. The fluoroscopy reduction journey, of course, involves a learning curve. We suggest breaking down each procedure into individual sub-steps and working on fluoroscopy reduction for each step. For instance, for PVI, start with adaptation of ultrasound-guided vascular access, then once mastered, perhaps work on catheter placement, then move on to left atrial mapping and ablation, including esophageal monitoring, and finally work on transseptal puncture. During this process, please feel free to reach out to any of the authors in this text. One of the wonderful aspects of our field is that it is populated with generous and humble individuals, and we are all explicitly available if you would like to contact us with further questions or if you would even like to visit our EP labs to observe procedures. In fact, several of us have been hosting visitors for quite some time already.

Again, thank you for your interest in this topic, and we wish you all the success in achieving your goals.

—Mansour Razminia
Chicago, IL
raz1@hotmail.com

—Paul C. Zei
Boston, MA
pzei@bwh.harvard.edu

Abbreviations

3D	three-dimensional
aAFL	atypical atrial flutter
ABL	ablation catheter
ACT	activated clotting time
AF	atrial fibrillation
AFL	atrial flutter
AI	ablation index
ALARA	"as low as reasonably achievable"
ALPM	anterolateral papillary muscle
AMC	aortomitral continuity
AoV	aortic valve
APCs	atrial premature contractions
ARVC	arrhythmogenic right ventricular cardiomyopathy
ASV	aortic sinus of Valsalva
AV	atrioventricular
AVN	atrioventricular node
AVNRT	atrioventricular nodal reentrant tachycardia
AVRT	atrioventricular reentry tachycardia
BEIR	Biological Effects of Ionizing Radiation
CCW	counterclockwise
CF	contact force sensing
CFAE	complex fractionated atrial electrograms
CHD	congenital heart disease
CPR	cardiopulmonary resuscitation
CS	coronary sinus
CT	computed tomography
CTI	cavotricuspid isthmus
CW	clockwise
DOAC	direct oral anticoagulant
EAM	electroanatomic mapping
ECG	electrocardiogram
ECMO	extracorporeal membrane oxygenation
EGM	electrogram
EP	electrophysiology
EPS	electrophysiologic study
EV	Eustachian valve
FP	fast pathway
HB	His bundle
IART	intra-atrial reentrant tachycardia
IAS	intra-atrial septum
ICDs	implantable cardioverter defibrillators
ICE	intracardiac echocardiography
IVC	inferior vena cava
LA	left atrium/left atrial
LAA	left atrial appendage
LAD	left anterior descending
LAO	left anterior oblique
LBBB	left bundle branch block
LCC	left coronary cusp
LIE	left inferior extension
LILE	left inferior lateral area
LIS	left inferior septal extension
LMCA	left main coronary artery
LSPV	left superior pulmonary vein
LV	left ventricle
LVAD	left ventricular assist device
LVOT	left ventricular outflow tract
MRI	magnetic resonance imaging
MSP	multisensor self-expandable probe
MV	mitral valve
NCC	non-coronary cusp
NFCV	non-fluoroscopic catheter visualization system
NIPS	noninvasive programmed stimulation
os	ostium
PMPM	posteromedial papillary muscle
PMVF	polymorphic ventricular fibrillation

PMVT polymorphic ventricular tachycardia
PV pulmonary vein
PVCs premature ventricular complexes
PVI pulmonary vein isolation
RA right atrium/right atrial
RAO right anterior oblique
RCC right coronary cusp
RF radiofrequency
RIE right inferior extension
RIPV right inferior pulmonary vein
RMN remote magnetic navigation
RSPV right superior pulmonary vein
RV right ventricle
RVOT right ventricular outflow tract
SSP single-sensor probe
SVC superior vena cava
SVT supraventricular tachycardia
TEE transesophageal echocardiography
TK triangle of Koch
TT tendon of Todaro
TTE transthoracic echocardiographic
TV tricuspid valve
TVA tricuspid valve annulus
US ultrasound
VA ventricular arrhythmia
VT ventricular tachycardia
WACA wide area circumferential ablation
WPW Wolff-Parkinson-White

Video Descriptions

Chapter 2: How to Use Intracardiac Echocardiography to Reduce Fluoroscopy

Video 2.1 Home view. ICE catheter in the neutral position. RA is on the upper half of the screen. Tricuspid valve and RV on the lower half. The long-axis AV at 2 o'clock and RVOT at 4–5 o'clock. [00:06]

Video 2.2 Right ventricle view. The ICE catheter in the home view anterior tilt is applied with slight CW and CCW rotation continuously maintain the opening and closing of the tricuspid valve leaflets in view. The catheter is advanced, once across, returned to neutral. The catheter is rotated CW to scan though the RV, interventricular septum, LV and LA. [00:30]

Video 2.3 Septal view. CW rotation of ICE from home view until the IAS comes into view. [00:06]

Video 2.4 Left atrium from septal view. MV seen first at 6 o'clock. With CW rotation, the PV come into view as follows: left superior PV at 4 o'clock, followed by left inferior PV at 5 o'clock, followed by right inferior PV at 6 o'clock, and finally right superior PV at 5 o'clock. The esophagus is seen along the posterior wall between the left and right PV. Note left tilt was not needed to visualize the right PV in this case. [00:15]

Video 2.5 Left atrium from right ventricle view. CW rotation from the right ventricle view to scan through the left atrium. Left PV at 5 o'clock. AV at 11–12 o'clock. Right coronary cusp is at the top, non-coronary cusp along the IAS, and left coronary cusp near the MV. Note the left main coronary artery in the left coronary cusp. [00:15]

Video 2.6 Left ventricle from right ventricle view. Note the image has been flipped left to right. CW rotation from the right ventricle view, the posteromedial papillary muscle comes into view first with an ablation catheter adjacent to it. With further CW rotation the anterolateral papillary muscle then LV outflow tract comes into view. [00:10]

Video 2S Chapter summary and step-by-step procedures by Mansour Razminia. [19:00]

Chapter 4: How to Use Technologies such as MediGuide and CARTOUNIVU to Reduce Fluoroscopy During Catheter Ablation

Video 4.1 Ablation of atypical atrial flutter using Precision as the 3D mapping system and MediGuide for non-fluoroscopic catheter visualization. Mapping with a circular mapping catheter reveals counterclockwise perimitral flutter in LAT and sparkle map (TCL 211 ms). Ablation of anterior isthmus line prolongs TCL to 237 ms. New map shows localized septal reentry with a PPI = TCL at the septal annulus. Ablation here terminates the tachycardia. LAT map during SR proves the complete block of the septal line with a delay over the line of >150 ms. Final fluoroscopy time of the procedure is 0.3 min; radiation dose is 191 $\mu Gy \cdot m^2$. [3:11]

Chapter 6: How to Perform Transseptal Puncture Without Fluoroscopy

Video 6.1 The transseptal needle is advance into the long sheath. [00:03]

Video 6.2 The long sheath is then slowly brought down from the SVC under ICE visualization until the sheath and needle are located at the intra-atrial septum. [00:03]

Video 6.3 ICE imaging of transseptal puncture across intraatrial septum. [00:03]

Video 6.4 The sheath is advanced over the wire into the LA visualized under ICE guidance. [00:03]

Video 6S Chapter summary and step-by-step procedures by Mansour Razminia. [10:49]

Chapter 8 How to Monitor Esophageal Temperature Without Fluoroscopy

Video 8S Chapter summary and step-by-step procedures by Mansour Razminia. [7:17]

Chapter 9: How to Ablate Atrioventricular Nodal Reentrant Tachycardia Using No Fluoroscopy

Video 9.1 A step by step video tutorial for AVNRT ablation utilizing voltage and propagation wave collision mapping. [7:43]

Chapter 10: How to Ablate Accessory Pathways Using No Fluoroscopy

Video 10.1 Placement of a duodecapolar catheter in the coronary sinus. [00:29]

Video 10.2 Yellow dots show His cloud and the His catheter is orange at the RA (red) right ventricle (green) junction. The decapolar catheter (blue) is shown in the CS (yellow). What appears to be a second CS catheter was a saved image of the original CS placement to make sure that the CS has not moved during the case. The real time CS catheter shows an inferior deflection at electrodes 7-8 due to pacing electrode selection, which is seen with EnSite. A 4-mm cryocatheter (Medtronic, Minneapolis Inc., MN) was used for ablation due to the proximity to the compact AV node. The red dot was used to mark the most proximal region of His bundle recording. The blue dots represent the ablation points. Note the use of transparency and color to delineate structures, catheters and key electrogram sites. The pathway was ablated without affecting AV nodal conduction despite a very small intermittent His bundle deflection on the second beat seen on the ablation catheter electrogram. Note the larger A to V ratio on the ablation catheter compared to the His bundle catheter. [00:40]

Video 10.3A ICE image and sound map of the left atrium. [00:02]

Video 10.3B Using SmartTouch catheter in the IVC to create volumetric map of the IVC, RA, SVC, and CS. The red dots represent the mitral annulus recorded on ICE. The pulmonary veins (blue and green are shown coming off the LA. The ablation catheter starts at the IVC and is advanced under force guidance and curved and swept in the RA to create the volumetric map. The esophagus can be seen behind the LA in brown. [01:17]

Video 10.3C Transseptal site on ICE, marked in blue on RA septum with integrated ICE and EAM. [00:37]

Video 10.3D Placing of CS catheter. [1:19]

Video 10.3E RAO and clipping plane and LAO with contact force SmartTouch catheter entering CS os with 4 g of force. Illustrates how the contact force is used to safely navigate the catheter to the distal CS and create the CS volumetric map. [00:14]

Video 10.3F Non-fluoroscopic technique for retrograde aortic access. LV (meshed grey) and ascending aorta (meshed pink), which is then merged with catheter map of the descending aorta and arch as the catheter is advanced. The catheter is then prolapsed into the left ventricle. [2:02]

Chapter 11: How to Ablate Typical Atrial Flutter Using No Fluoroscopy

Video 11S Chapter summary and step-by-step procedures by Mansour Razminia. [5:35]

Chapter 12: How to Ablate Atrial Tachycardia and Atypical Flutter Using No Fluoroscopy

Video 12S Chapter summary and step-by-step procedures by Mansour Razminia. [3:55]

Chapter 13: How to Perform Radiofrequency Ablation of Atrial Fibrillation Using No Fluoroscopy

Video 13.1 ICE images of the left atrium showing a PentaRay and ablation catheter in the chamber, demonstrating the ability to visualize catheters in the left atrium in real time during mapping and ablation. [00:05]

Video 13.2 ICE images of the left atrium showing a PentaRay exiting the transseptal sheath into the left atrium, demonstrating the ability to track catheter movement and relationship to the left atrium continuously in real time. [00:42]

Chapter 14: How to Perform Cryoballoon Ablation of Atrial Fibrillation Using No Fluoroscopy

Video 14S Chapter summary and step-by-step procedures by Mansour Razminia. [33:42]

Chapter 15: How to Perform PVC Ablation Originating From the RV and RVOT Using No Fluoroscopy

Video 15S Chapter summary and step-by-step procedures by Mansour Razminia. [6:28]

Chapter 16: How to Perform Ablation in the Coronary Cusps Using No Fluoroscopy

Video 16.1 Phased-array ICE used view and aid in ablation catheter navigating up the femoral artery and into the iliac and aorta retrograde through the arterial system. [00:03]

Video 16.2 ICE advanced within the venous system to visualize the ablation catheter. [00:03]

Video 16.3 ICE advanced within the venous system to visualize the ablation catheter. [00:03]

Video 16.4 The ICE catheter is placed into the SVC and directed toward the ascending aorta and follow the ablation catheter back down toward the cusps. [00:03]

Video 16.5 Rotation of the phased-array ICE catheter counter clock wise or rightward will bring the NCC and RCC into view. [00:02]

Video 16.6 The left coronary cusp will be located to the left of the RCC. Clockwise rotation of the ICE catheter will bring the LCC into view. [00:03]

Video 16.7 Color Doppler on ICE can be used to determine the location of ostium of the major coronary arteries in order to avoid injury to these structures. [00:03]

Video 16S Chapter summary and step-by-step procedures by Mansour Razminia. [5:29]

Chapter 18: How to Perform Papillary Muscle PVC Ablation Using No Fluoroscopy

Video 18S Chapter summary and step-by-step procedures by Mansour Razminia. [16:02]

Chapter 19: How to Perform Ablation of Ischemic and Non-Ischemic Ventricular Tachycardia Using No Fluoroscopy

Video 19.1A Zero-fluoroscopy method for crossing the ICE catheter across the tricuspid valve. [00:16]

Video 19.1B LV ICE survey. [00:31]

Video 19.3A Tracing the open aortic valve with ICE to guide retrograde access. [00:12]

Video 19.3B Crossing the aortic valve without fluoroscopy. [00:08]

Video 19.3C Crossing the aortic valve using a multipolar diagnostic catheter without fluoroscopy. [00:15]

Video 19.4A Use of the ablation catheter to position a sheath at the preferred site of transeptal crossing. [00:13]

Video 19.4B Advancement of needle and dilator into the sheath at the site of transeptal crossing. [00:04]

Video 19.4C RF energy applied to the needle to cross the interatrial septum. [00:04]

Video 19.4D J-wire is advanced into the left superior pulmonary vein under ICE guidance. [00:04]

Video 19.5A EA LV map in a congenital cardiomyopathy patient. [00:07]

Video 19.5C Activation mapping during VT using a multielectrode catheter. [00:28]

Video 19.5D RF ablation with contact force sensing at site of VT termination. [00:07]

Section 1

Basis of Imaging in the Electrophysiology Lab

1

Radiation Safety in the Electrophysiology Lab

Kristen Breedlove, MPAS, PA-C; John Clark, MD

Introduction

Present-day fluoroscopy has its roots in the late 19th century. The risks of radiation were not known at the outset. In the subsequent 120 years, we have learned much about both the benefits of medical radiation, as well as the risks. This chapter will outline some of the history of the radiation risks, as well as protective measures that can be used to keep both the patient and the staff safe.

The 2 people primarily responsible for the birth of the modern day cath lab are Wilhelm Roentgen and Thomas Edison. In November 1895, Roentgen discovered x-rays while experimenting with various elements within electrified vacuum tubes. He observed that barium platinocyanide, painted on a piece of cardboard, would fluoresce when the cathode tube was electrified with an aluminum window in it. He called the new rays "x" rays, x being the mathematical symbol for "unknown." While positioning various elements between the cathode ray tube and the fluorescent screen, he noticed that when his hands came between the 2, he could see the bones in his hands. Two weeks later, still experimenting with the new form of radiation, he took the first human radiograph of his wife Bertha's hand (**Figure 1.1**).

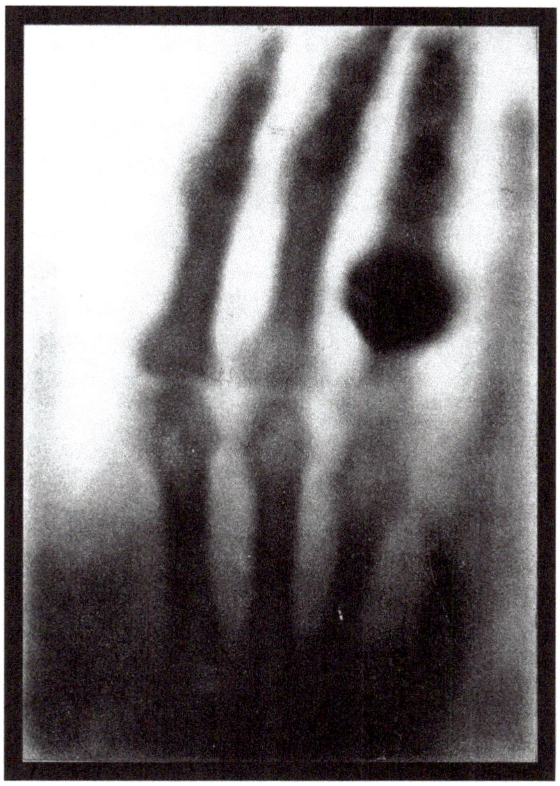

Figure 1.1 The first human radiograph: Bertha Roentgen's hand.

When Bertha saw the bones of her hand and wedding ring, she is reported to have exclaimed, "I have seen my death!" If the quote is in fact true, then it was prescient, because she did later succumb to radiation-induced sarcoma.

Fluoroscopy Reduction Techniques for Catheter Ablation of Cardiac Arrhythmias. © 2019 Mansour Razminia, Paul C. Zei, eds.
Cardiotext Publishing, ISBN: 978-1-942909-30-9.

Very soon after Roentgen discovered x-rays, Thomas Edison began his own experiments. By painting barium platinocyanide on the inside of a cardboard box built to fit over his eyes and block out any ambient light, he was able to visualize human bones in real time (**Figure 1.2**). His system was extremely simple and quite elegant. It is very much like a popular virtual reality system of today (**Figure 1.3**).

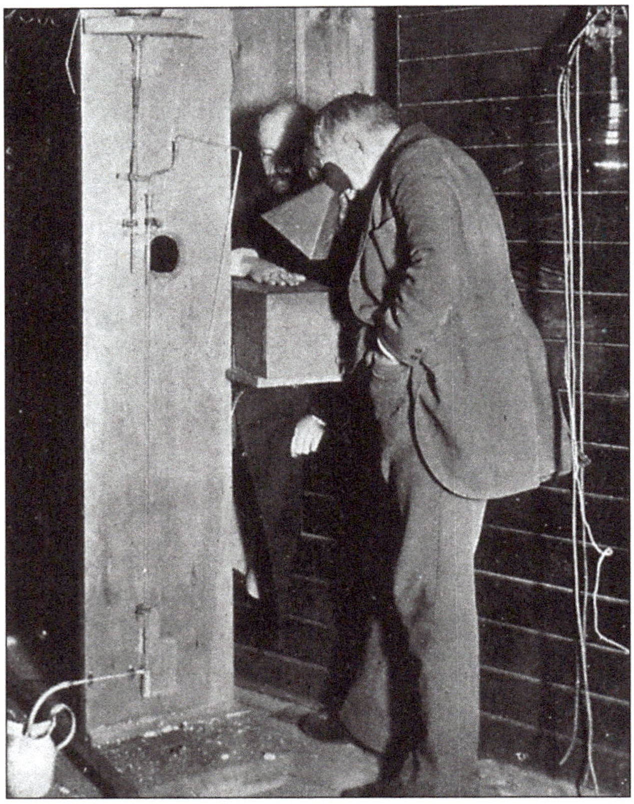

Figure 1.2 Thomas Edison viewing Clarence Dally's hand through an early fluoroscope.

Edison was one of the first to recognize the danger of x-rays. He himself suffered cataracts, which impaired his vision, and his lab assistant, Clarence Dally, suffered radiation dermatitis, which progressed to a fatal malignancy. Many of the early workers in x-ray research labs would later develop fatal malignancies. This group of workers became known as "x-ray martyrs." In the late 1890s, the risk of an x-ray worker becoming an x-ray martyr was as high as 25%.[1] By the early 1900s, the risk had dropped to about 1% to 2%.

Radiation-Associated Risks

Today, we recognize 2 types of radiation risk: deterministic and stochastic. Deterministic risks are dose-dependent. Below a threshold dose, the effect is not seen. Above the threshold, the severity is dose dependent, with higher doses resulting in worse injury. Deterministic risks include dermatitis, hair loss, and cataracts. Stochastic effects have no threshold level for occurrence. A greater dose will confer a greater risk, but any dose conveys some risk. While the odds of the complication occurring are dose dependent, the severity of the complication is independent of dose. Ionizing radiation causes creation of hydroxyl radicals within cells. The hydroxyl radicals can then ionize DNA base pairs, which lead to DNA strand breaks. Stochastic effects are related to this DNA damage. The DNA base pairs are usually repaired at the molecular level. If the damage is not repaired, the long-term risks of malignancy or birth defects may be seen. The risk is cumulative and lifelong. Young patients, since they have a longer remaining lifespan and greater chance of further radiation exposure, are at greater risk of stochastic effects. For the same dose of exposure, a child's risk can be as much as 4 times greater than an adult's.[2]

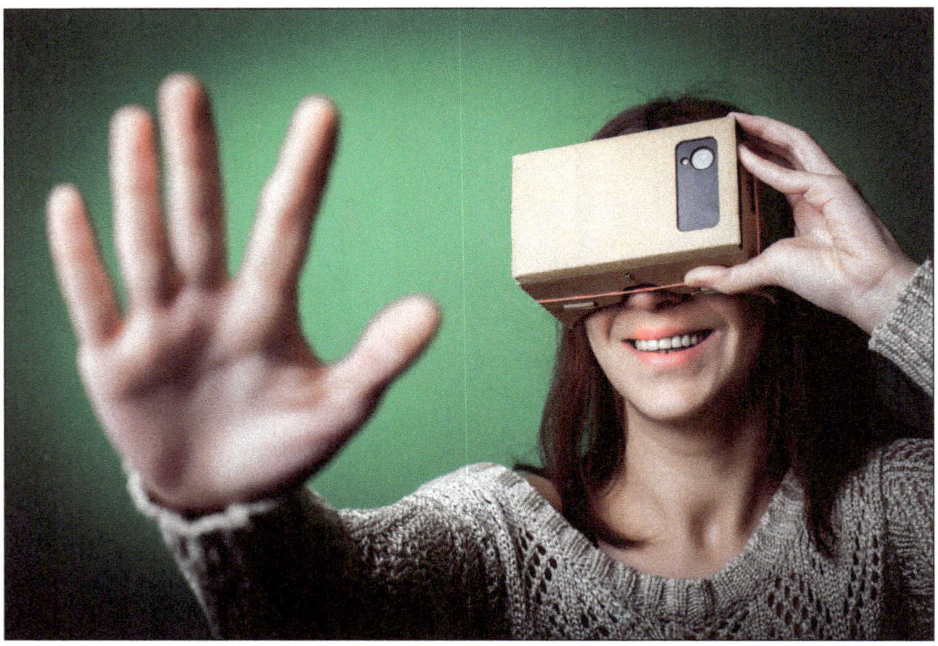

Figure 1.3 Girl viewing her hand in a virtual reality system.

Malignancy Risk

The risk of malignancy from a single ablation procedure is small, but not zero. Many studies over the years have attempted to quantify it. Kovoor et al. measured radiation doses using thermoluminescence dosimeters in 9 adult females undergoing supraventricular tachycardia (SVT) ablation.[3] From the radiation doses measured, they estimated a lifetime added risk of fatal malignancy of 0.03% for every 60 minutes of fluoroscopy. Perisinakis, using similar methods, estimated a risk of 0.065% malignancy from 60 minutes of fluoroscopy, and a risk of genetic defects of 1:1,000,000.[4] Lickfett et al. reported a malignancy risk of 0.07% for women, and 0.1% for men for 60 minutes of fluoroscopy in their lab.[5] So the realistic risk is likely to lie somewhere in the range of 1:1,000 to 1:5,000 for routine SVT ablations.

Deterministic Risks

The most common deterministic risks are cataracts, hair loss, and radiation-induced dermatitis. For the patient, the most likely deterministic risk is dermatitis. Given the technology of today's fluoroscopy equipment, one might expect that radiation dermatitis never occurs. Surprisingly, there are many case reports in the literature, even as recently as 2018.[6-10] The diagnostic clues to radiation dermatitis are a geometric rash, usually round or rectangular, arising 1 to 8 weeks after a radiologic procedure. **Figure 1.4** shows a typical example.

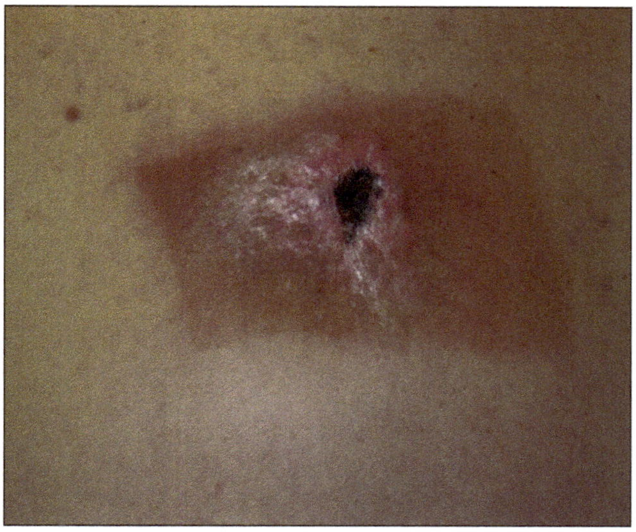

Figure 1.4 Radiation dermatitis.

Findings typically seen on histology include epidermal atrophy, dermal sclerosis, dilated superficial blood vessels, and atypical stellate fibroblasts. Malignant transformation into squamous cell or basal cell carcinoma can be seen. The threshold for development of dermatitis is about 5 Gy. If a patient receives a total dose >10 Gy, they should have follow-up to screen for dermatitis. If found, they should have close follow-up and possible surgical intervention due to the risk of malignant transformation. Biopsy is not usually indicated due to poor healing of the affected area.

Indirect Exposure Risks

While patients are at risk from direct exposure to radiation, the staff is at risk from scatter radiation. Scatter radiation results in staff exposure doses of about 1/1000 of the patient dose. Electrophysiology lab staff are therefore at risk for deterministic and stochastic radiation effects. The most common deterministic effect is cataracts. Multiple studies have looked at the incidence of lens opacities in cardiologists and cath lab staff.[11-14] The incidence of posterior lens opacities ranges from 17 to 52%, which is about 3 times greater than control populations. Similar to the patient data, stochastic effects among EP lab staff are uncommon, but not rare. Venneri reviewed the radiation exposure records of 15 staff members in interventional cardiology who had records available for at least 10 years. Based on their exposure records, the estimated lifetime risk of malignancy was 1/192.[15] Picano estimated in 2014 that a busy electrophysiologist working for 20 years has a 1% additional lifetime risk of malignancy.[16]

Documenting Medical Radiation Exposures

Medical radiation exposure in the United States increased more than 7-fold between the early 1980s and 2006.[17] There is currently a movement to document all radiation exposure for all patients undergoing radiologic testing.[18] Electronic medical records (EMRs) should facilitate the tracking of patients' lifetime exposure. That record will likely also lead to better decision making as to the type of test needed. The goal for all patients should be the right test, at the right time, with the right dose of radiation.[19]

While our exposure to medical radiation has been steadily increasing, our awareness of the increase, and its risks, has not kept pace. Correia surveyed 100 cardiologists in 2004 to gauge their awareness of radiation exposure and risk.[20] Almost 90% of cardiologists believed that medical radiation accounted for <10% of the total radiation exposure of U.S. citizens, and 67% believed it was <1%. Those are unsettling statistics, given that the actual amount is much closer to 50%. While many are unaware of the degree of exposure of radiation in the United States, we may also be underestimating the degree of risk.

Beels et al. reported a very elegant study in which the radiation dose to children undergoing cardiac cath procedures was measured. Also measured was the number of DNA breaks found in peripheral blood cells before and after the procedure, using gamma-H2AX. Using the Committee on the Biological Effects of Ionizing Radiation

(BEIR) principles, they were able to estimate the lifetime added risk of cancer, and the number of expected DNA breaks that should be observed. They found that there was a 4-fold greater number of DNA breaks counted than the BEIR method had predicted.[21]

Another sobering finding was published by Roguin in 2013.[22] They were able to find 26 cases of brain tumors in physicians whose primary area of practice was in the cath lab or radiology lab. Of the 26 patients in whom the location of the tumor was identified in the chart, 23 of them were left-sided. That study does not prove causation, but it does raise some concerning possibilities. Since the performing physician stands on the patient's right side, the left side of the physician will be closest to the x-ray generator. Therefore, the left brain should receive a greater radiation dose than the right brain. It could therefore be possible that brain tumors would be more likely in the left hemisphere.

Populations at Greater Risk

There are particular clinical scenarios that deserve specific attention related to radiation dose: pregnancy, small children, congenital heart disease, and obese patients. Please refer to chapters in this text focused on the pregnant and pediatric populations for additional information.

Exposures in Pregnant Women

Pregnancy is a special concern because there are 2 patients who can potentially be injured by radiation, and the fetus is more sensitive to deleterious effects from exposure. The available data supports a linear, no threshold relationship of risk to the fetus from radiation exposure.[23] Damilakis estimated the risk of lifetime cancer to a fetus after a routine SVT ablation in the mother is 1:18,000.[24] Multiple reports have demonstrated the feasibility of ablation without fluoroscopy in the pregnant female.[25–32] Given all the complicating factors of arrhythmias during pregnancy, ablation without fluoroscopy will likely become the preferred therapy.

Exposures in Young Children

As previously stated, radiation in small children carries significantly higher risk than the same dose in an adult. This is because their cells are more rapidly dividing, and because they have a longer time frame over which malignant transformation can occur. Children with congenital heart disease have the additional concern of potentially needing multiple diagnostic and interventional procedures in subsequent years. The amount of radiation exposure in this population can be quite large, and it occurs at a young age.[33]

Exposures in Obese Patients

Obese patients will require more radiation to penetrate through their tissue to allow acceptable visualization. The obese patient will typically receive twice the radiation dose of a non-obese patient.[34] Each of these scenarios must be kept in mind and planned for when an electrophysiology procedure is undertaken.

Reducing Overall Exposure

Given all of the above information, one can readily see the importance of minimizing radiation exposure. The 1998 American College of Cardiology expert consensus document on radiation safety in the practice of cardiology recommends radiation doses "as low as reasonably achievable" (ALARA).[35] There are 2 ways to accomplish that goal: first, minimize radiation; and second, maximize protection. The best way to minimize radiation dose is to routinely employ electroanatomic mapping systems (EAMS). Since there are helpful instructions toward that goal in every chapter of this book, they will not be restated here. **Figure 1.5** is a good graphic representation of how much radiation exposure can be reduced by implementing electroanatomic mapping. The image shows radiation badge readings over a 10-year period encompassing a transition to EAMS.

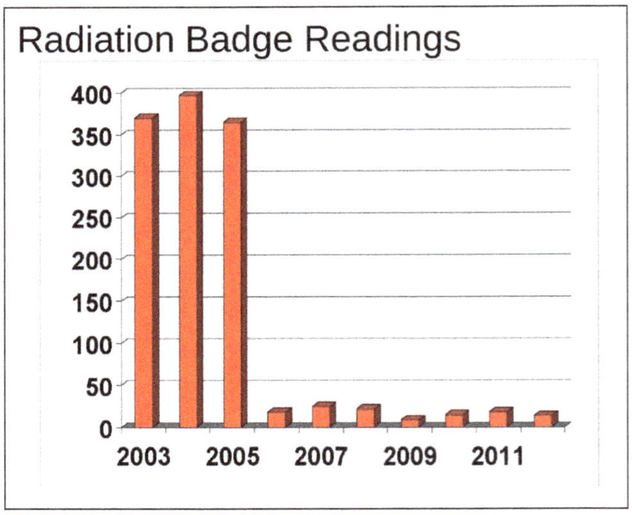

Figure 1.5 Ten-year graphic display of the author's radiation badge readings. The abrupt decline of exposure in 2006 coincides with the year in which the facility made the transition to electroanatomic mapping.

When fluoroscopy must be used, there are many additional ways of decreasing the dose delivered. Foremost among these is simply being aware of how much fluoroscopy is being used. When one pays attention to the fluoroscopy time, it is much easier to find ways to cut it down. Other means of minimizing exposure are to optimize projection angle, minimize magnification, avoid using cine mode if stored fluoroscopy will suffice, keep the detector close to the patient, collimate as much as possible, minimize the frame rate, and optimize auto-adjustment settings to allow for a grainier image when possible.[36]

As an example of how effective this can be, consider the results of just minimizing the frame rate. Fluoroscopy screens refresh at a rate of 30 Hz (30 frames/second). This was, therefore, the standard imaging rate of the x-ray generator. However, catheter manipulation can be adequately accomplished with frame rates much slower than 30/second. A frame rate of 7.5/second will decrease the radiation exposure to 25% the amount of a standard frame rate. Some labs decrease the frame rate to as low as 1/second. While this does much to decrease radiation exposure, there is probably a lower limit to frame rate, below which may increase the complication rate or total procedure time. Adjunctive tools can also be employed, including intracardiac echocardiogram, transesophageal echocardiogram, and magnetic resonance imaging.[37-43] By utilizing all of these methods, patient and staff radiation exposure should approach zero.

Injuries from Protective Shielding

Thus far, we have only discussed the risks of radiation. We have not considered the risks of radiation protection. Orthopedic complications related to wearing lead-lined garments for long periods of time are well recognized. Ross et al. surveyed 346 physicians who routinely required lead protection at work, and 371 physicians whose jobs did not require lead shielding. Those physicians who routinely wore lead aprons were 3 times more likely to have cervical spine symptoms.[44] Goldstein noted that the incidence of spinal symptoms increased as a function of caseload and number of years in practice.[45] In a survey of 1500 employees, Orme noted work-related pain symptoms in 54% of radiology-based employees, compared to 44% of non-radiology employees ($P = 0.001$).[46] Because of the orthopedic problems associated with wearing lead, there are some alternatives to lead aprons being developed.[47-49] Also, there is a suspended lead apron available that can take the weight off the wearer's back.[50]

Conclusion

Today's fluoroscopy equipment is quite safe. However, although the risks of radiation exposure are small, they are measurable and real. The only way to truly eliminate those risks is to eliminate radiation exposure. Electroanatomic mapping systems hold great promise for reducing radiation exposure to zero. Within the pages of this book are many excellent tips from operators experienced in this area. It is this author's hope that anyone considering adopting a zero-fluoroscopy approach in the cath lab would visit the lab of any one of the authors in this book. Bring a lab staff member with you. When they see procedures being performed without the need for lead aprons, you will get full buy-in from your staff. Radiation protection for both the patient and staff are of primary importance. But the comfort of an unleaded workplace will bring years of satisfaction.

References

1. Kemerink GJ, van Engelshoven JMA, Simon KJ, Kütterer G, Wildberger JE. Early X-ray workers: An effort to assess their numbers, risk, and most common (skin) affliction. *Insights Imaging.* 2016;7(2):275–282. doi:10.1007/s13244-015-0457-2
2. Johnson JN, Hornik CP, Li JS, et al. Cumulative radiation exposure and cancer risk estimation in children with heart disease. *Circulation.* 2014;130(2):161–167. doi:10.1161/CIRCULATIONAHA.113.005425
3. Kovoor P, Ricciardello M, Collins L, Uther JB, Ross DL. Risk to patients from radiation associated with radiofrequency ablation for supraventricular tachycardia. *Circulation.* 1998;98(15):1534–1540. doi:10.1161/01.CIR.98.15.1534
4. Perisinakis K, Damilakis J, Theocharopoulos N, Manios E, Vardas P, Gourtsoyiannis N. Accurate assessment of patient effective radiation dose and associated detriment risk from radiofrequency catheter ablation procedures. *Circulation.* 2001;104:58–62.
5. Lickfett L, Mahesh M, Vasamreddy C, et al. Radiation exposure during catheter ablation of atrial fibrillation. *Circulation.* 2004;110(19):3003–3010. doi:10.1161/01.CIR.0000146952.49223.11
6. Spiker A, Zinn Z, Carter WH, Powers R, Kovach R. Fluoroscopy-induced chronic radiation dermatitis. *Am J Cardiol.* 2012;110(12):1861–1863. doi:10.1016/j.amjcard.2012.08.023
7. Srimahachota S, Udayachalerm W, Kupharang T, Sukwijit K, Krisanachinda A, Rehani M. Radiation skin injury caused by percutaneous coronary intervention, report of 3 cases. *Int J Cardiol.* 2012;154(2):e31–e33. doi:10.1016/j.ijcard.2011.05.016
8. Boncher J, Bergfeld WF. Fluoroscopy-induced chronic radiation dermatitis: A report of two additional cases and a brief review of the literature. *J Cutaneous Pathol.* 2012;39(1):63–67. doi:10.1111/j.1600-0560.2011.01754.x
9. Reichman EF. Fluoroscopy-induced radiation dermatitis. *J Emerg Med.* 2014;47(5):e117–e119. doi:10.1016/j.jemermed.2014.06.054
10. Batrani M, Kubba A, Sundharam J. Fluoroscopy-induced chronic radiation dermatitis masquerading as morphea: A diagnostic pitfall. *Indian J Pathol Microbiol.* 2018;61(3):393. doi:10.4103/IJPM.IJPM_566_17
11. Ciraj-Bjelac O, Rehani MM, Sim KH, Liew HB, Vano E, Kleiman NJ. Risk for radiation-induced cataract for staff in interventional cardiology: Is there reason for concern? *Cath Cardiovasc Interv.* 2010;76(6):826–834. doi:10.1002/ccd.22670
12. Ciraj-Bjelac O, Rehani M, Minamoto A, Sim KH, Liew HB, Vano E. Radiation-induced eye lens changes and risk for cataract in interventional cardiology. *Cardiology.* 2012;123(3):168–171. doi:10.1159/000342458

13. Jacob S, Boveda S, Bar O, et al. Interventional cardiologists and risk of radiation-induced cataract: Results of a French multicenter observational study. *Int J Cardiol.* 2013;167(5):1843–1847. doi:10.1016/j.ijcard.2012.04.124
14. Elmaraezy A, Ebraheem Morra M, Tarek Mohammed A, et al. Risk of cataract among interventional cardiologists and catheterization lab staff: A systematic review and meta-analysis: Risk of cataract among in IC's. *Cath Cardiovasc Interv.* 2017;90(1):1–9. doi:10.1002/ccd.27114
15. Venneri L, Rossi F, Botto N, et al. Cancer risk from professional exposure in staff working in cardiac catheterization laboratory: Insights from the National Research Council's Biological Effects of Ionizing Radiation VII Report. *Am Heart J.* 2009;157(1):118–124. doi:10.1016/j.ahj.2008.08.009
16. Picano E, Piccaluga E, Padovani R, Antonio Traino C, Grazia Andreassi M, Guagliumi G. Risks related to fluoroscopy radiation associated with electrophysiology procedures. *J Atr Fibrillation.* 2014;7(2):1044. doi:10.4022/jafib.1044
17. Schauer DA, Linton OW. National Council on Radiation Protection and Measurements Report shows substantial medical exposure increase. *Radiology.* 2009;253(2):293–296. doi:10.1148/radiol.2532090494
18. Miller DL, Balter S, Dixon RG, et al. Quality improvement guidelines for recording patient radiation dose in the medical record for fluoroscopically guided procedures. *J Vasc Interv Radiol.* 2012;23(1):11–18. doi:10.1016/j.jvir.2011.09.004
19. Picano E, Vano E, Rehani MM, et al. The appropriate and justified use of medical radiation in cardiovascular imaging: A position document of the ESC Associations of Cardiovascular Imaging, Percutaneous Cardiovascular Interventions and Electrophysiology. *Eur Heart J.* 2014;35(10):665–672. doi:10.1093/eurheartj/eht394
20. Correia MJ, Hellies A, Andreassi MG, Ghelarducci B, Picano E. Lack of radiological awareness among physicians working in a tertiary-care cardiological centre. *Int J Cardiol.* 2005;103(3):307–311. doi:10.1016/j.ijcard.2004.08.070
21. Beels L, Bacher K, De Wolf D, Werbrouck J, Thierens H. γ-H2AX foci as a biomarker for patient x-ray exposure in pediatric cardiac catheterization: Are we underestimating radiation risks? *Circulation.* 2009;120(19):1903–1909. doi:10.1161/CIRCULATIONAHA.109.880385
22. Roguin A, Goldstein J, Bar O, Goldstein JA. Brain and neck tumors among physicians performing interventional procedures. *Am J Cardiol.* 2013;111(9):1368–1372. doi:10.1016/j.amjcard.2012.12.060
23. Doll R, Wakeford R. Risk of childhood cancer from fetal irradiation. *Br J Radiol.* 1997;70:130–139. doi:10.1259/bjr.70.830.9135438
24. Damilakis J, Theocharopoulos N, Perisinakis K, et al. Conceptus radiation dose and risk from cardiac catheter ablation procedures. *Circulation.* 2001;104(8):893–897.
25. Manjaly Z-R, Sachdev B, Webb T, Rajappan K. Ablation of arrhythmia in pregnancy can be done safely when necessary. *Eur J Obstet Gynecol Reprod Biol.* 2011;157(1):116–117. doi:10.1016/j.ejogrb.2011.01.019
26. Wu H, Ling L-H, Lee G, Kistler PM. Successful catheter ablation of incessant atrial tachycardia in pregnancy using three-dimensional electroanatomical mapping with minimal radiation: Brief Communication. *Intern Med J.* 2012;42(6):709–712.doi:10.1111/j.1445-5994.2012.02812.x
27. Ferguson JD, Helms A, Mangrum JM, DiMarco JP. Ablation of incessant left atrial tachycardia without fluoroscopy in a pregnant woman. *J Cardiovasc Electrophysiol.* 2011;22(3):346–349. doi:10.1111/j.1540-8167.2010.01847.x
28. Stec S, Krynski T, Baran J, Kulakowski P. "Rescue" ablation of electrical storm in arrhythmogenic right ventricular cardiomyopathy in pregnancy. *BMC Cardiovasc Disord.* 2013;13(1). doi:10.1186/1471-2261-13-58
29. Leiria TLL, Pires LM, Kruse ML, de Lima GG. Supraventricular tachycardia and syncope during pregnancy: A case for catheter ablation without fluoroscopy. *Rev Portug Cardiol.* 2014;33(12):805.e1–805.e5. doi:10.1016/j.repce.2014.07.003
30. Zuberi Z, Silberbauer J, Murgatroyd F. Successful non-fluoroscopic radiofrequency ablation of incessant atrial tachycardia in a high risk twin pregnancy. *Indian Pacing Electrophysiol J.* 2014;14(1):26–31.
31. Hogarth AJ, Graham LN. Normal heart ventricular tachycardia associated with pregnancy: Successful treatment with catheter ablation. *Indian Pacing Electrophysiol J.* 2014;14(2):79–82.
32. Bigelow AM, Crane SS, Khoury FR, Clark JM. Catheter ablation of supraventricular tachycardia without fluoroscopy during pregnancy. *Obstet Gynecol.* 2015;125(6):1338–1341. doi:10.1097/AOG.0000000000000601
33. Ait-Ali L, Andreassi MG, Foffa I, Spadoni I, Vano E, Picano E. Cumulative patient effective dose and acute radiation-induced chromosomal DNA damage in children with congenital heart disease. *Heart.* 2010;96(4):269–274. doi:10.1136/hrt.2008.160309
34. Ector J, Dragusin O, Adriaenssens B, et al. Obesity is a major determinant of radiation dose in patients undergoing pulmonary vein isolation for atrial fibrillation. *J Am Coll Cardiol.* 2007;50(3):234–242. doi:10.1016/j.jacc.2007.03.040
35. Limacher MC, Douglas PS, Germano G, et al. ACC Expert Consensus Document. Radiation safety in the practice of cardiology. American College of Cardiology. *J Am Coll Cardiol.* 1998;31(4):892–913.
36. Heidbuchel H, Wittkampf FHM, Vano E, et al. Practical ways to reduce radiation dose for patients and staff during device implantations and electrophysiological procedures. *EP Europace.* 2014;16(7):946–964. doi:10.1093/europace/eut409
37. Reddy VY, Morales G, Ahmed H, et al. Catheter ablation of atrial fibrillation without the use of fluoroscopy. *Heart Rhythm.* 2010;7(11):1644–1653. doi:10.1016/j.hrthm.2010.07.011
38. Razminia M, Willoughby MC, Demo H, et al. Fluoroless catheter ablation of cardiac arrhythmias: a 5-year experience. *Pacing Clin Electrophysiol.* 2017;40(4):425–433. doi:10.1111/pace.13038
39. Lerman BB, Markowitz SM, Liu CF, Thomas G, Ip JE, Cheung JW. Fluoroless catheter ablation of atrial fibrillation. *Heart Rhythm.* 2017;14(6):928–934. doi:10.1016/j.hrthm.2017.02.016
40. Nedios S, Sommer P, Bollmann A, Hindricks G. Advanced mapping systems to guide atrial fibrillation ablation: Electrical information that matters. *J Atrial Fibrillation.* 2016;8(6):1337. doi:10.4022/jafib.1337

41. Caponi D, Corleto A, Scaglione M, et al. Ablation of atrial fibrillation: Does the addition of three-dimensional magnetic resonance imaging of the left atrium to electroanatomic mapping improve the clinical outcome?: A randomized comparison of CARTO-MERGE vs. CARTO-XP three-dimensional mapping ablation in patients with paroxysmal and persistent atrial fibrillation. *Europace.* 2010;12(8):1098–1104. doi:10.1093/europace/euq107
42. Clark J, Bockoven JR, Lane J, Patel CR, Smith G. Use of three-dimensional catheter guidance and trans-esophageal echocardiography to eliminate fluoroscopy in catheter ablation of left-sided accessory pathways. *Pacing Clin Electrophysiol.* 2008;31(3):283–289. doi:10.1111/j.1540-8159.2008.00987.x
43. Regoli F, Faletra FF, Scaglione M, Nucifora G, Moccetti T, Auricchio A. Pulmonary vein isolation guided by real-time three-dimensional transesophageal echocardiography: Real-time three-dimensional echocardiography and pulmonary vein isolation. *Pacing Clin Electrophysiol.* 2012;35(3):e76–e79. doi:10.1111/j.1540-8159.2011.03029.x
44. Ross AM, Segal J, Borenstein D, Jenkins E, Cho S. Prevalence of spinal disc disease among interventional cardiologists. *Am J Cardiol.* 1997;79(1):68–70.
45. Goldstein JA, Balter S, Cowley M, Hodgson J, Klein LW, on behalf of the Interventional Committee of the Society of Cardiovascular Interventions. Occupational hazards of interventional cardiologists: Prevalence of orthopedic health problems in contemporary practice. *Physics.* 2012;39(7Part1):4537–4546. doi:10.1118/1.4730504
46. McCaffrey JP, Shen H, Downton B, Mainegra-Hing E. Radiation attenuation by lead and nonlead materials used in radiation shielding garments. *Med Physics.* 2007;34(2):530–537. doi:10.1118/1.2426404
47. Uthoff H, Peña C, West J, Contreras F, Benenati JF, Katzen BT. Evaluation of novel disposable, light-weight radiation protection devices in an interventional radiology setting: A randomized controlled trial. *Am J Roentgenol.* 2013;200(4):915–920. doi:10.2214/AJR.12.8830
48. Marichal DA, Anwar T, Kirsch D, et al. Comparison of a suspended radiation protection system versus standard lead apron for radiation exposure of a simulated interventionalist. *J Vasc Intervent Radiol.* 2011;22(4):437–442. doi:10.1016/j.jvir.2010.12.016

2

How to Use Intracardiac Echocardiography to Reduce Fluoroscopy

Cameron Willoughby, DO

Using intracardiac echocardiography (ICE) is essential to reduce or eliminate fluoroscopy during cardiac ablation procedures. ICE allows real-time visualization of catheters and cardiac structures, monitoring for procedural complications, and direct visualization of structures that are not identifiable with fluoroscopy or 3D anatomical mapping. ICE also allows monitoring of ablation progression by edema formation and tissue–catheter contact, though it cannot measure force of contact.[1] This chapter describes the techniques for obtaining views of all cardiac structures using phased-array ICE. Image resolution in terms of ultrasound frequency and other such modifications are specific to consoles and laboratories and thus are not discussed here.

Becoming comfortable with ICE typically has a short learning curve. Rapid and precise identification of cardiac structures seen with ICE is facilitated by having an accurate knowledge of cardiac anatomy and the 3D relationships of cardiac structures. It may be beneficial to have an accurate 3D heart model available for reference during procedures. If one is new to ICE or has limited experience, we recommend integrating ICE during simple ablation procedures at first: manipulating the catheter and identifying structures during downtime of procedures, such as following anticoagulation reversal, while allowing tissue edema to subside, or at the conclusion of the case.

The most basic view with ICE is the "home view," which can be found by advancing the ICE catheter in a neutral position into the mid right atrium (**Figure 2.1** and **Video 2.1**). Visible structures are right atrium (RA), cavotricuspid isthmus (CTI), tricuspid valve anterior and posterior leaflets, and right ventricle (RV) and right ventricular outflow tract (RVOT).[2]

In our lab, the ICE catheter is the first catheter advanced to the RA. An initial survey of the heart is performed to assess the cardiac anatomy, variants or possible obstacles, and baseline pericardial effusions.

Catheter Manipulation

The catheter may be moved with four basic maneuvers: advancing/withdrawing, anterior/posterior tilt, catheter rotation, right/left tilt. Slight manipulations of the catheter can significantly enhance the resolution of the structure in interest. In this text, unless otherwise noted, ICE catheter movement will be in reference to the home view. We assume a standard, out-of-the-box setup to the ICE console in terms of left-to-right scrolling and an up-down configuration, with up being the tip of the catheter at the top and center of the screen. We utilize a clock face to describe the structure location seen on the viewscreen of ICE, that is, 12 o'clock being the top and center of the screen, 6 o'clock being the bottom and center of the screen (**Figure 2.2**).[3] The descriptions that follow are agnostic to the specific ICE system manufacturer. Any specific and important differences will be pointed out. The most

Fluoroscopy Reduction Techniques for Catheter Ablation of Cardiac Arrhythmias. © 2019 Mansour Razminia, Paul C. Zei, eds. Cardiotext Publishing, ISBN: 978-1-942909-30-9.

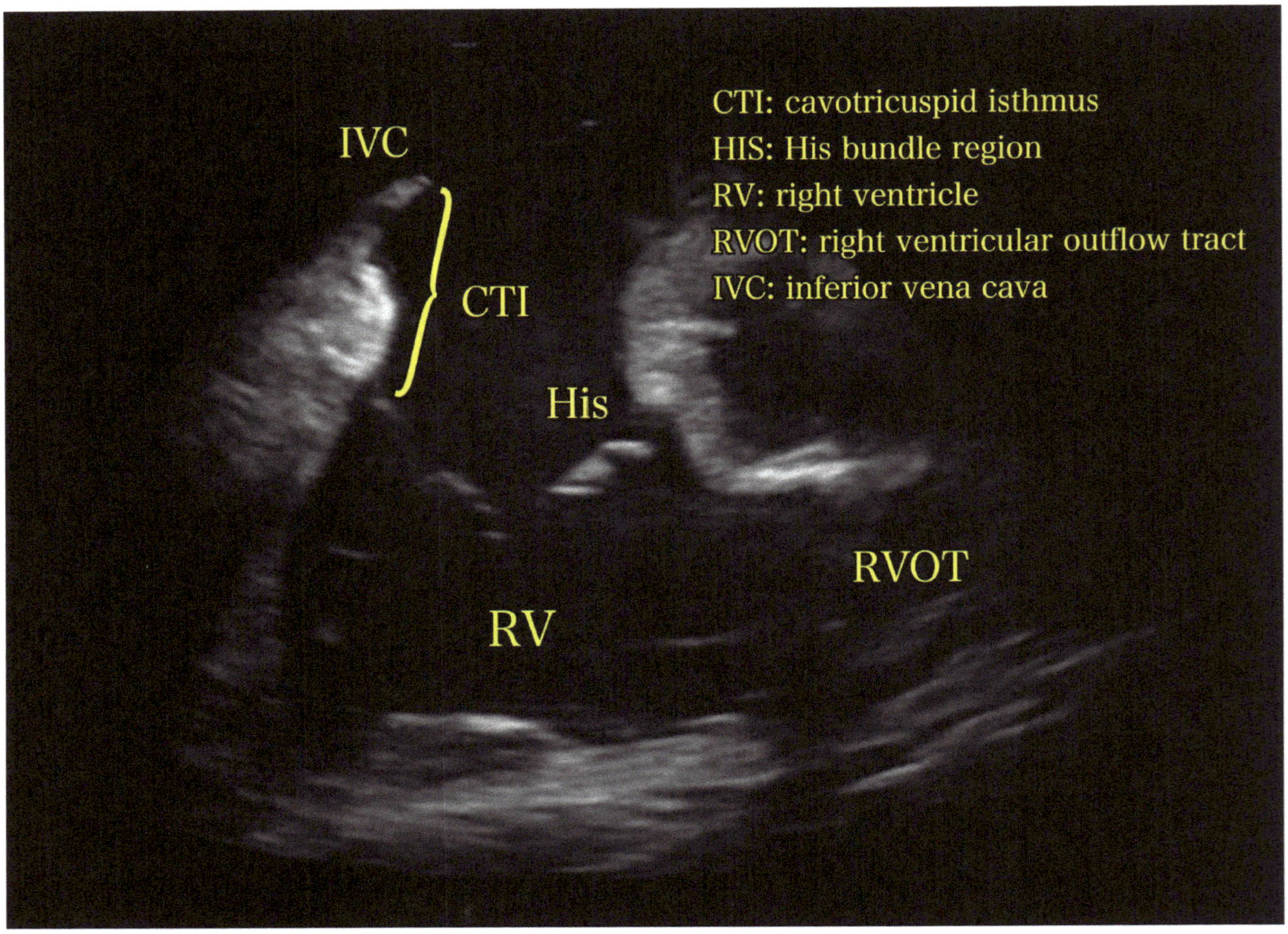

Figure 2.1 Home view. ICE catheter in the neutral position. RA is on the upper half of the screen. Tricuspid valve and RV on the lower half. The long-axis aortic valve (AV) at 1–2 o'clock and RVOT at 4–5 o'clock.

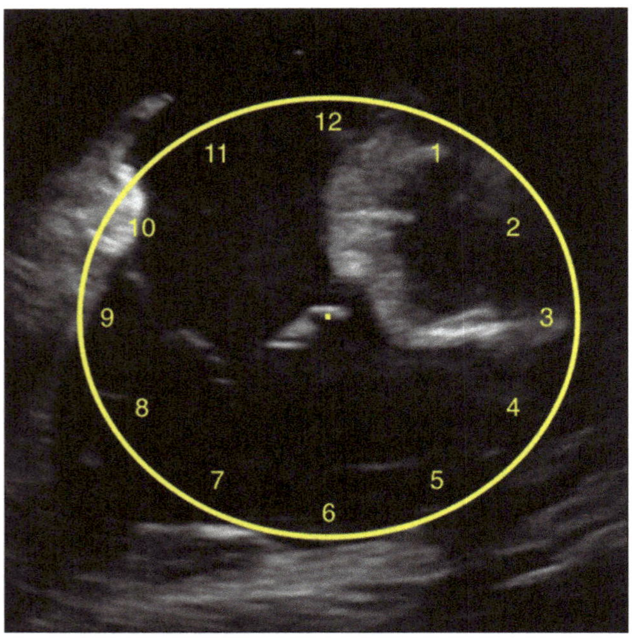

Figure 2.2 Clock face. A clock face is superimposed on the image of the home view. The CTI is located at 10–11 o'clock. The long-axis AV is at 1–2 o'clock, and the RVOT is at 4–5 o'clock.

commonly utilized ICE catheters include the ViewFlex (Abbott, Abbott Park, IL), CARTOSOUND (Biosense Webster, Irvine, CA), and Acuson (Siemens, Tarrytown, NY). Commonly perceived particulars for the ViewFlex catheter are a stiffer shaft, as well as the highest quality imaging. For the CARTOSOUND catheter, a soft catheter shaft is noted, and the ICE images can be integrated into the electroanatomic mapping system.

Advancing the ICE catheter brings structures from the right side of the viewscreen (3 o'clock) to the center of view. Withdrawing the catheter will bring structures from the left of the viewscreen (9 o'clock) to the center of view.

Applying anterior tilt to the catheter will bring the tip of the catheter towards the structure in center view, typically bringing that structure towards the 3 o'clock position. Applying posterior deflection will bring the tip of the catheter away from the structure in center view, typically bringing that structure towards the 9 o'clock position.

Clockwise (CW) rotation of the catheter itself sweeps posteriorly from an anterior starting position, crossing septal views, bringing posterior structures into center view, such as the coronary sinus os and left atrium (LA). Counterclockwise (CCW) rotation generally sweeps anteriorly from a posterior starting position, bringing anterior structures into center view, such as the aorta and right ventricular outflow tract. It is typically necessary to apply slight CW/CCW rotation to keep a region of interest in focus; this is particularly important when entering cardiac chambers.

Turning the right-left dial to the right will sweep the tip of the catheter and bend the tip of the catheter to the right relative to the neutral position of the catheter. Turning that dial left will bend and sweep the tip left relative to the neutral position. This is most useful for fine tuning the resolution of structures and in particular in assessing the interatrial septum (IAS) and left atrial structures through the IAS.

ICE is particularly useful for placing a catheter in the region of interest during ablations. One may follow a catheter (i.e., ablation catheter) to the location targeted with ICE guidance. First, locate the structure/target via ICE, then locate the ablation catheter (often with CW/CCW rotation). Relocate the structure/target and move the ablation catheter with the same manipulation used with the ICE catheter to bring the ablation catheter to the structure/target. Typically, CW/CCW is all that is needed, but steps may need to be repeated to get to the precise location.[2,3]

Advancing ICE Without Fluoroscopy

As a standard, we obtain venous access for the ICE catheter via the left common femoral vein. Due to tortuosity common to that vessel, a long sheath (35 cm) is commonly used for direct access to the inferior vena cava (IVC). This is particularly useful for the ViewFlex ICE catheter, which is stiffer than the Acuson or CARTOSOUND catheters. The ICE catheter may be freely advanced throughout the vessels and cardiac structures if the leading edge (right side of screen at roughly the 3 o'clock position) has an echo-free space (**Figure 2.3** A–B). Hepatic veins can be easily sub-selected, as evidenced by hepatic tissue dominating the viewscreen. Catheter withdrawal and redirection are typically all that is required to enter the RA. If difficulties arise with ICE advancement, advance another catheter from the same vessel accessed by the ICE catheter, such as the coronary sinus catheter, until it is known to be in the heart based on intracardiac electrograms. Reintroduce the ICE catheter, locate the catheter with CW/CCW rotation as needed, and follow that catheter to the heart (**Figure 2.4**). If a short sheath is used for ICE placement, vessel bifurcation may present a challenge. This may be overcome by applying anterior tilt to bring the ICE catheter tip to the junction of the vessels. Apply slight CW/CCW rotation as needed to maintain the junction in view, then advance the catheter once the aperture is at the 3 o'clock position (**Figure 2.5** A–C). The same principle may be applied to the IVC-RA junction (**Figure 2.6**).

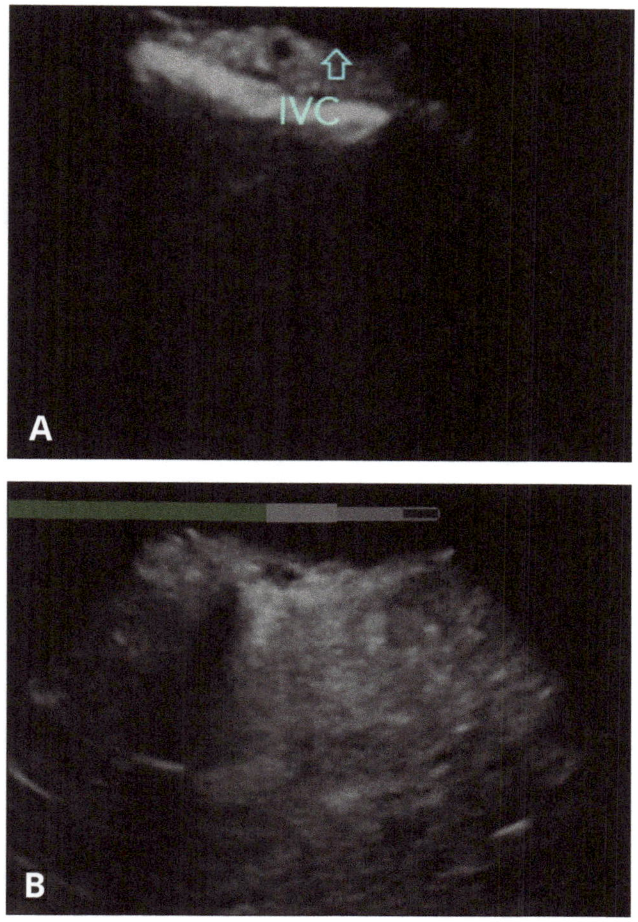

Figure 2.3 Advancing ICE. **A:** The IVC is the echo-free horizontal space indicated by the arrow. **B:** Illustration of the ICE catheter's path through the IVC.

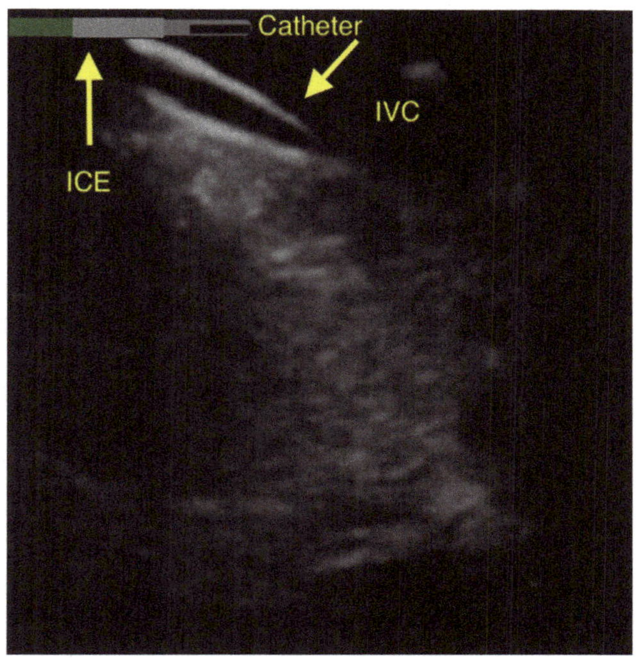

Figure 2.4 Using an EP catheter to guide ICE. An EP catheter that was advanced to the RA with guidance from the 3D map and intracardiac electrograms is seen in the IVC.

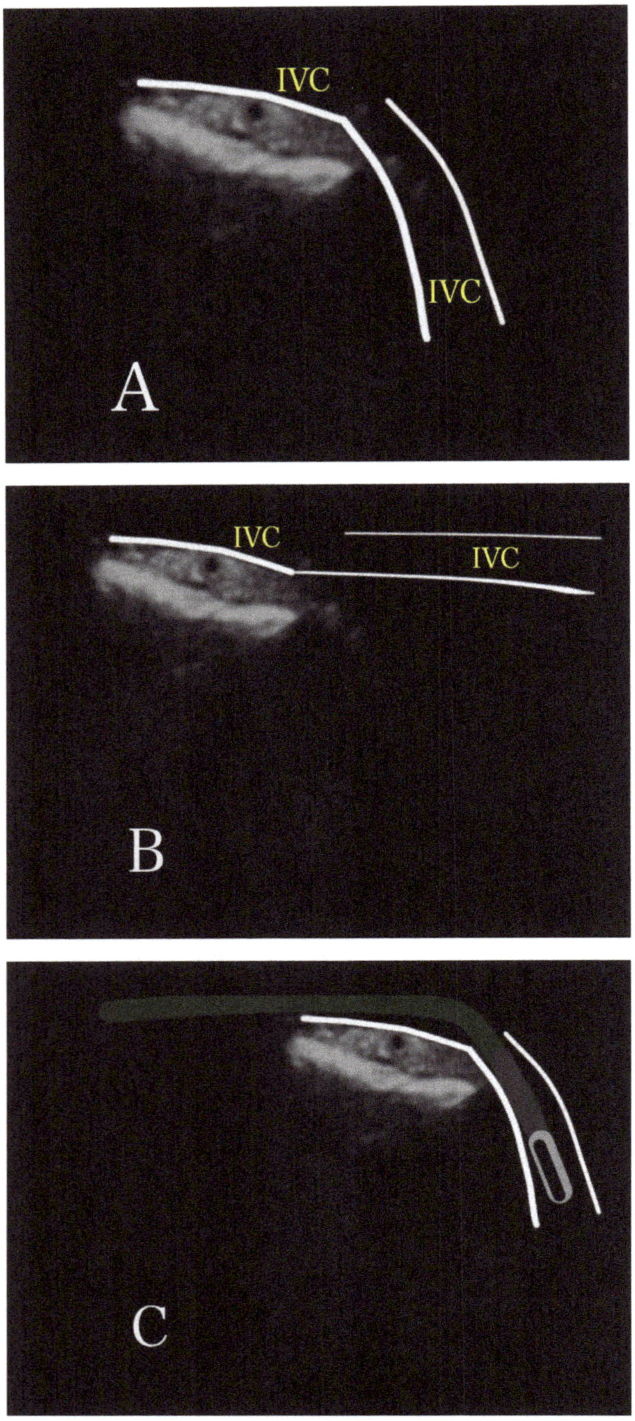

Figure 2.5 **A:** The IVC deviates at a sharp angle, into which the ICE catheter cannot freely enter. **B:** Applying anterior tilt tc the ICE catheter brings that deviated portion toward a path (3 o'clock position) to allow free advancement of the ICE catheter **C:** Illustration showing the path the ICE catheter takes. Once in this deviated component, the anterior tilt should be removed and returned to neutral.

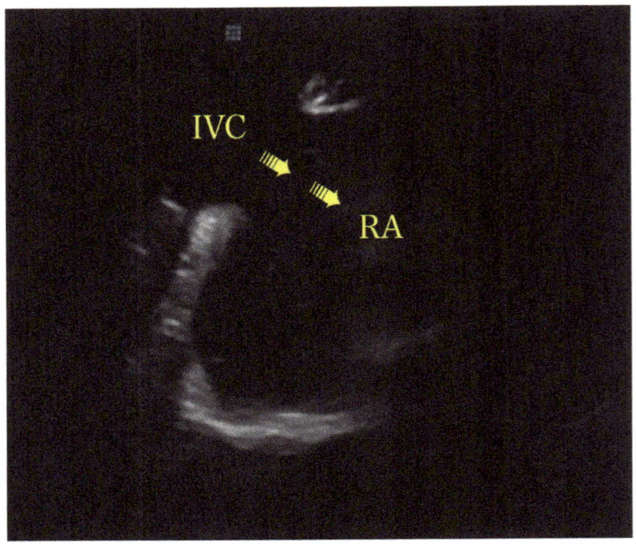

Figure 2.6 IVC-RA junction. A small aperture at the IVC-RA may make it challenging to advance the ICE catheter into the RA. Anterior will allow the tip of the ICE catheter to cross the junction.

Right Atrium

The CTI may be found in the home view. The image may be enhanced with slight anterior deflection and withdrawal of the catheter. Use CW (posterior/septal) and CCW (anterior/lateral) rotation to interrogate the CTI. Identify the best path to avoid obstacles, such as ridges, pouches, and crypts, and see the precise location of the CTI edges.

The coronary sinus os may be found by CW rotation from the home view. You will see the fossa ovalis and the inferior limbus in the 1–3 o'clock quadrant, and the coronary sinus os at the 6 o'clock position (**Figure 2.7**). With a large enough os, the coronary sinus may be cannulated with the ICE catheter from this view by applying anterior tilt and maintaining the os in view with slight CW or CCW rotation while gently advancing the catheter. This can be useful for enhanced visualization of the LA.

The region of the triangle of Koch may be seen, albeit in an unsatisfying way, by slight CCW rotation from home view bringing in the long-axis aortic valve. Having a His catheter placed will help define the region.

The right atrial appendage may be found with CCW rotation from the home view, with slight advancing of the ICE catheter in the 3–6 o'clock quadrant. Turning the right–left dial to the left may help refine the area of interest. This can be useful for focal atrial tachycardias and observing the manipulation of other catheters in a patient with an atrial pacing lead (**Figure 2.8**).

In the area of loss of pectinate muscles, the crista terminalis may be found with CCW rotation from the home view, beyond the right atrial appendage.

The superior vena cava (SVC) may be seen by CW rotation from the home view until the fossa ovalis is seen, and then adding posterior tilt and advancing the ICE catheter. The SVC will be seen in the 4–5 o'clock position (**Figure 2.9**).

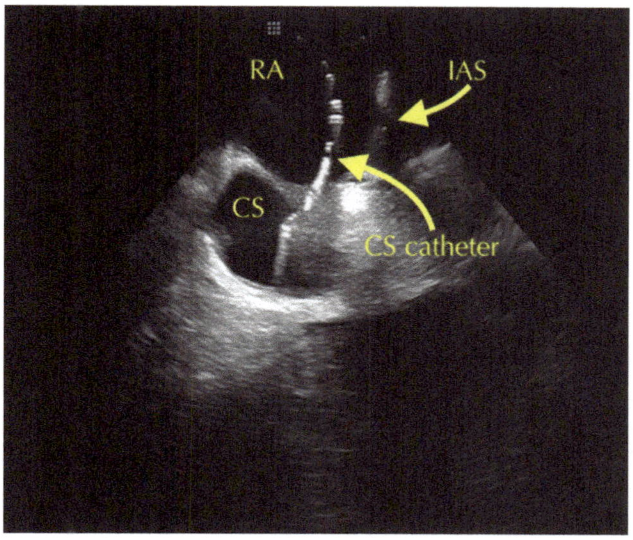

Figure 2.7 Coronary sinus. By CW rotation from the home view, the CS will be seen at the 6 o'clock position. CS catheter is seen cannulating the CS os.

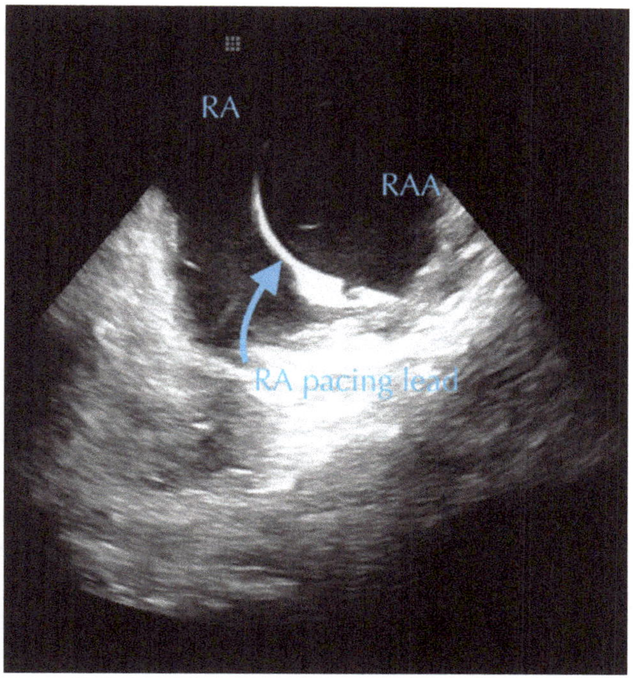

Figure 2.8 Right atrial pacing lead. A pacing lead is seen in the RAA, found by CCW rotation from the home view.

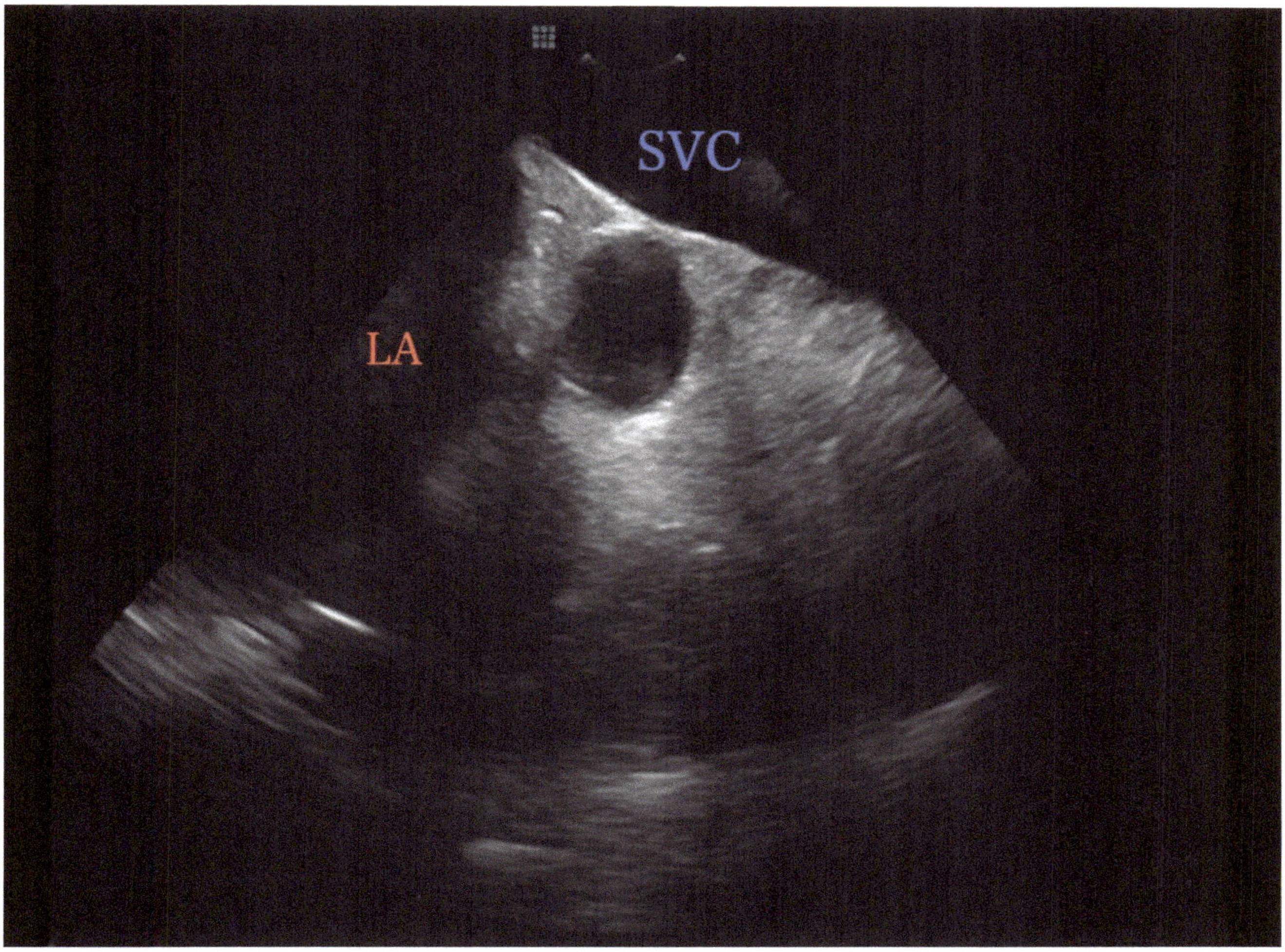

Figure 2.9 The superior vena cava may be seen by CW rotation from the home view until the fossa ovalis is seen, and then adding posterior tilt and advancing the ICE catheter.

Right Ventricle

The RV may be seen in the home view with anterior tilt and CW and CCW rotation applied as needed to bring the area of interest into view.

The region of the His bundle may be found by slight CCW rotation from the home view. A long-axis view of the aortic valve and proximal ascending aorta should be seen in the 2–3 o'clock position.

The right ventricle view may be obtained by cannulating the RV with the ICE catheter itself by applying anterior tilt from the home view with slight CW and CCW rotation as needed to continuously maintain the opening and closing of the tricuspid valve leaflets in view, and gently advancing the catheter. During this maneuver, the tricuspid valve apparatus will move from the 6 o'clock to the 3 o'clock position. Once across the tricuspid valve, return the ICE dials to the neutral position (**Figure 2.10** A–C and ▶ **Video 2.2**). The RVOT may be seen in this view at the 4–6 o'clock position with CW/CCW rotation and slight advancing and withdrawal of the catheter. If desired, the image may be flipped up-down through a setting change in the ICE console, such that the RVOT is seen at the 10–12 o'clock position (**Figure 2.11** A–B).

Interatrial Septum

The IAS can be seen by CW rotation from the home view with posterior tilt as needed, showing the septal view (**Figure 2.12** and ▶ **Video 2.3**). The IAS may also be seen from the right ventricle view (see right ventricle section). Once the RV is cannulated, apply CW rotation to sweep posteriorly through the RV, interventricular septum, left ventricle (LV), and mitral valve (MV), until the LA is seen. The IAS will be in the 8–11 o'clock position. Slight withdrawal is often needed to bring the IAS in view. This should be performed cautiously as the catheter may be easily expelled from the RV in this position. If present, pericardial effusions can be readily seen in this view[2,3] (**Figure 2.13**), as free-flowing fluid will tend to collect in the most dependent space, posterior to the LV base with a patient in the supine position.

After appropriate anticoagulation, the IAS may be crossed with the ICE catheter itself via a PFO/ASD or transseptal puncture. The defect may be directly visualized or a transseptal wire may be placed/retained through the defect. To cross the defect, apply anterior tilt to bring the catheter tip towards the defect/wire and advance the catheter, keeping the defect/wire in view with slight CW/CCW rotation as needed. The IAS and defect/wire will be brought to the 3 o'clock position. The catheter will be in the LA once there is no further visualization of the IAS, one will also see greater resolution of LA cardiac structures.

Left Atrium

The LA may be seen with the ICE catheter in the RA, LA, or RV. As ICE allows for direct, real-time visualization of the catheters and cardiac structures, one can readily determine if the catheter is within a pulmonary vein or antral. To view the LA with ICE in the RA, use the septal view. As the fossa ovalis is thin, bring the catheter tip to the fossa ovalis with slight anterior tilt. A thickened septum will generally lead to poor image resolution of the LA. This is particularly true in patients with a thickened limbus of the interatrial septum. To orient oneself, find the MV, with CCW rotation. Once the MV is in view, rotate the catheter CW to sweep posteriorly through the structures. The left atrial appendage (LAA) will be near the MV in the 4–5 o'clock position. Further CW rotation will sweep through to the left pulmonary veins (PV). The left superior PV will come into view first, typically in the 3–4 o'clock position. The left inferior PV will follow, typically in the 4–5 o'clock position. Further CW rotation will sweep though the posterior wall of the LA, where the esophagus may be seen coursing somewhat horizontally[2,4,5] (**Figure 2.14**). With further CW rotation, the right PVs will come into view. At this point the right-left dial should be turned to the left to better visualize the right PVs (**Figure 2.15**). The right inferior PV will be visualized first, then the right middle PV if present, followed by the right superior PV, sweeping the 7–5 o'clock position. The right superior PV may be easily recognized by being adjacent to the pulmonary artery (▶ **Video 2.4**).

With the ICE catheter in the LA, the anatomy is similarly viewed as above, though the resolution tends to be superior. The ability to utilize ICE to exclude thrombus in the LAA remains to be validated, but views of the LAA can be quite clear in these views.

The LA may be seen via the right ventricle view as well (see right ventricle section). Once the RV is cannulated, apply CW rotation to sweep posteriorly through the RV, interventricular septum, LV, and MV, until the LA is seen. Further CW rotation will sweep through the following structures at the 5 o'clock position: the LAA near the MV, the appendage ridge, the left superior PV, and to a lesser degree the left inferior PV (**Figure 2.16** and ▶ **Video 2.5**). Again, interrogation of the LAA for thrombus may be feasible, although there is still need for rigorous validation. Though difficult to view, the right PVs may be seen adjacent to the IAS at the 7–6 o'clock position with significant CCW rotation and withdrawal of the catheter.

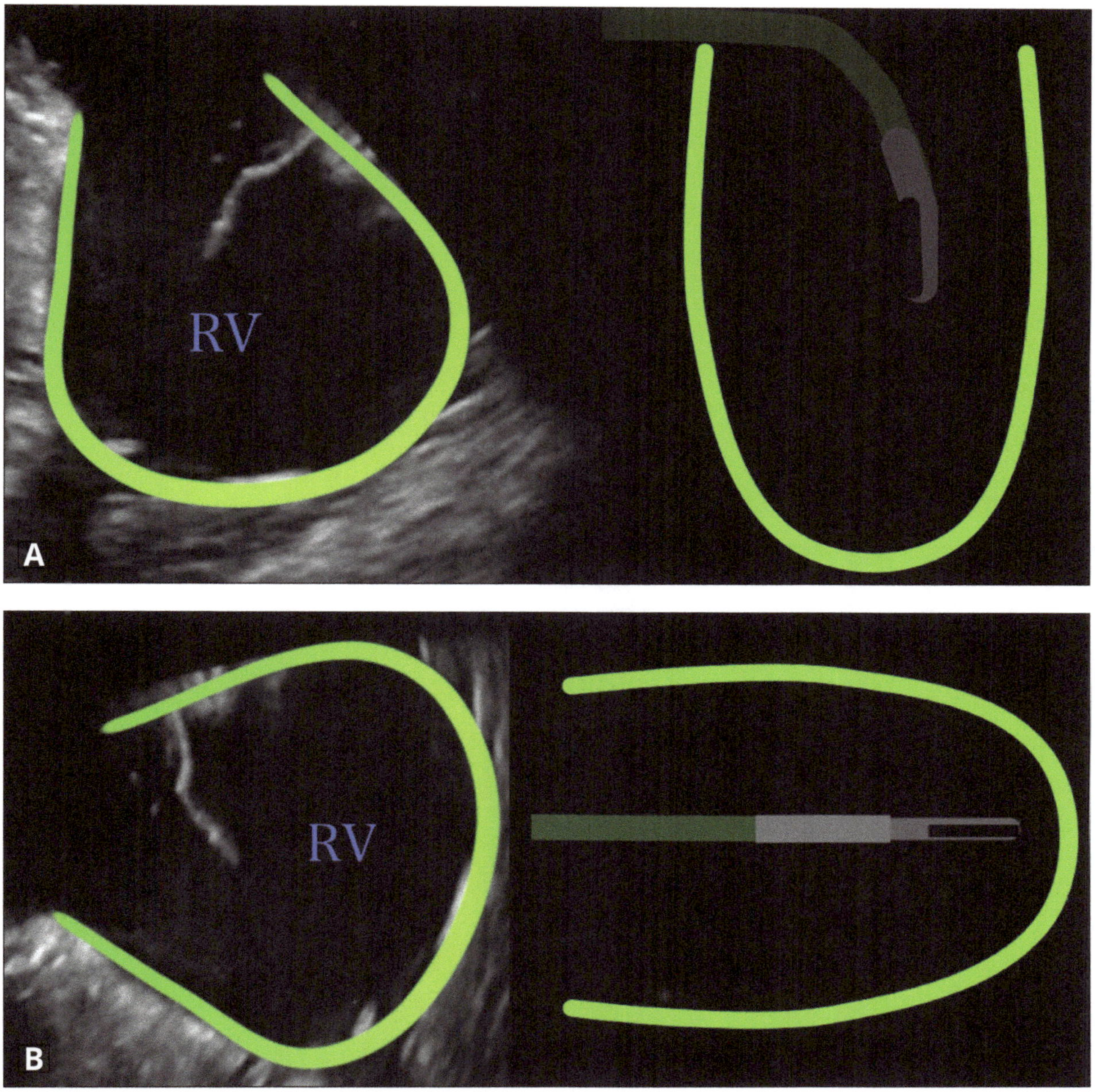

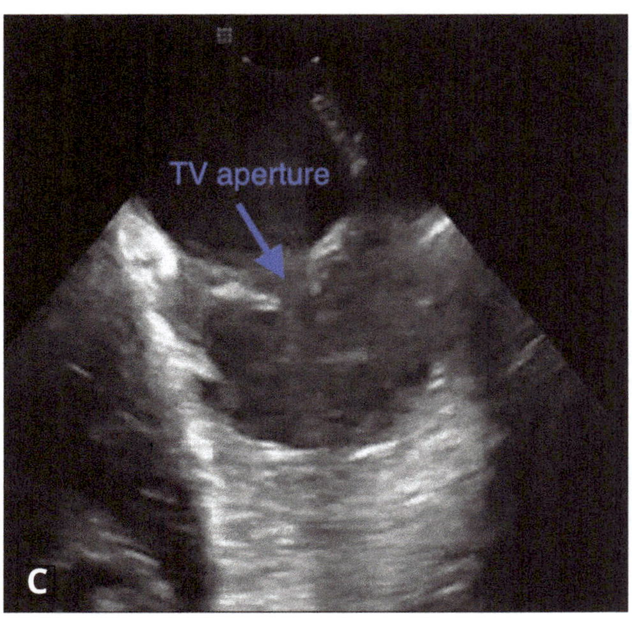

Figure 2.10 ICE in the right ventricle. **A:** RV seen from the home view. **B:** Cannulating the RV with the ICE catheter by applying anterior tilt from the home view will bring the RV to the 3 o'clock quadrant. **C:** When entering the RV, always maintain the valve aperture in center view.

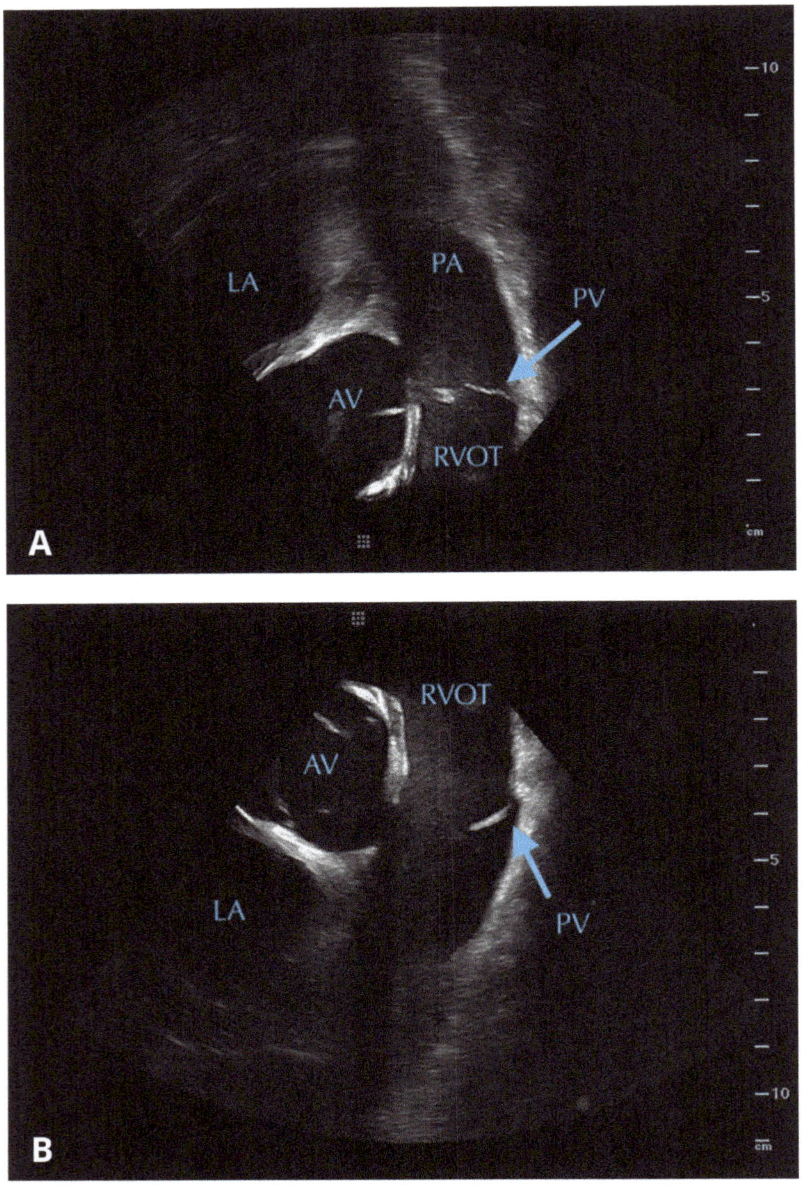

Figure 2.11 Right ventricular outflow tract. **A:** RVOT seen from the right ventricle. Also seen is AV and LA. **B:** The image may be flipped if that orientation is preferred.

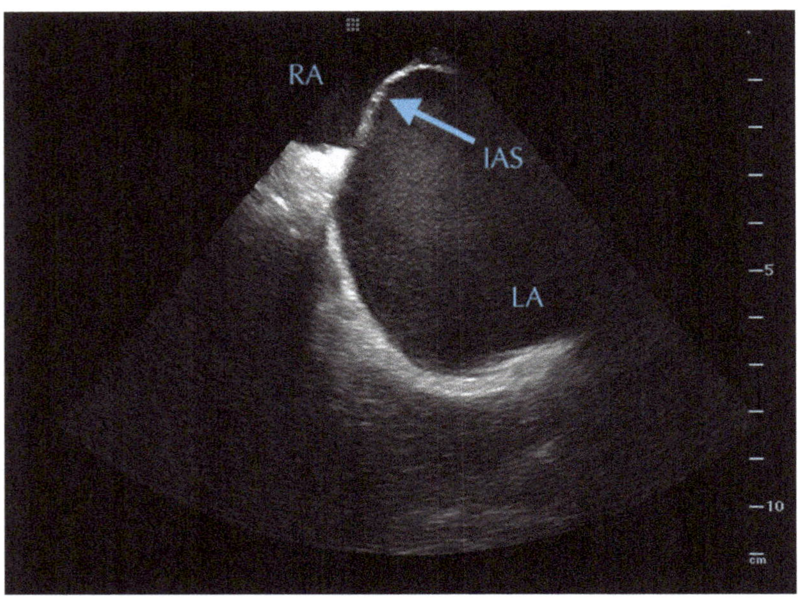

Figure 2.12 Interatrial septum. IAS seen by CW rotation from home view.

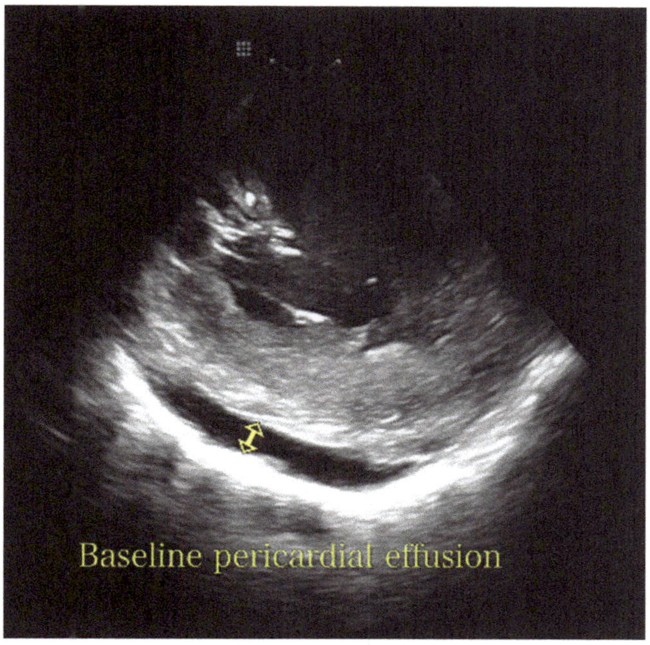

Figure 2.13 Pericardial effusion. A pericardial effusion is seen with the ICE in the RV. Baseline effusions are assessed at the beginning of each case by sweeping the ICE catheter anteriorly and posteriorly with the ICE in the RV.

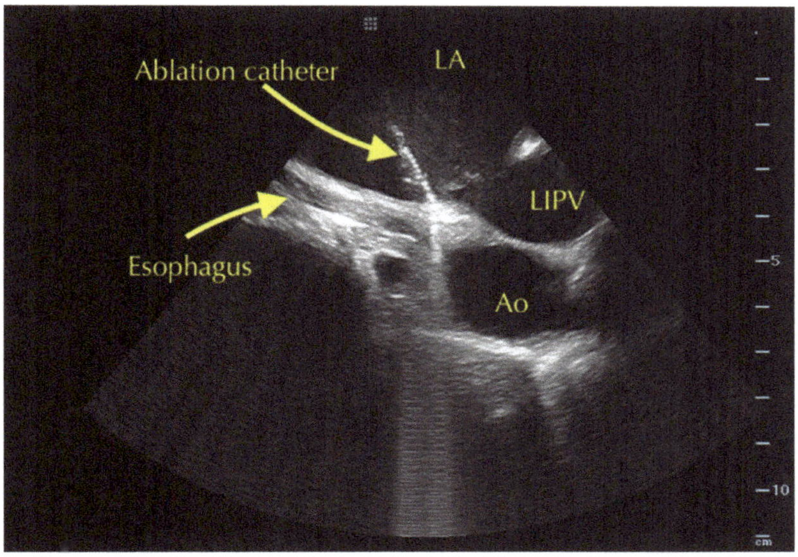

Figure 2.14 Left atrium seen with ICE in LA. Esophagus seen coursing horizontally.

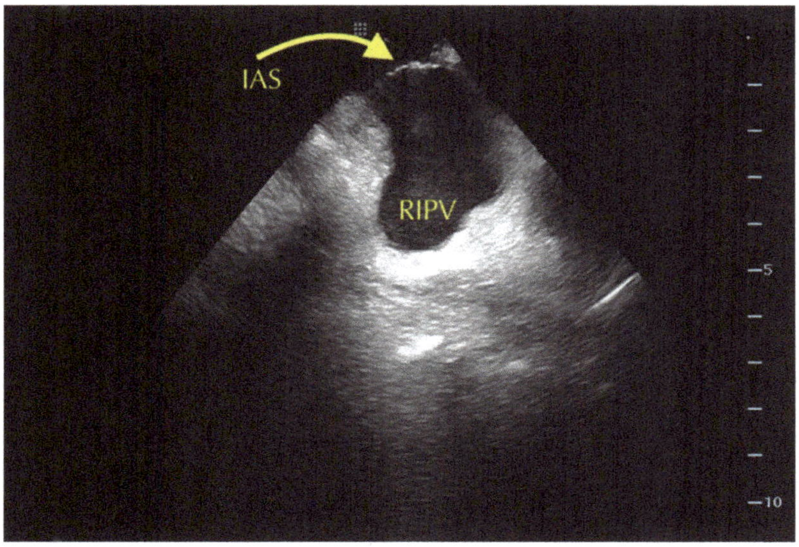

Figure 2.15 Right inferior pulmonary vein. Left tilt applied to ICE to better visualize RIPV through IAS.

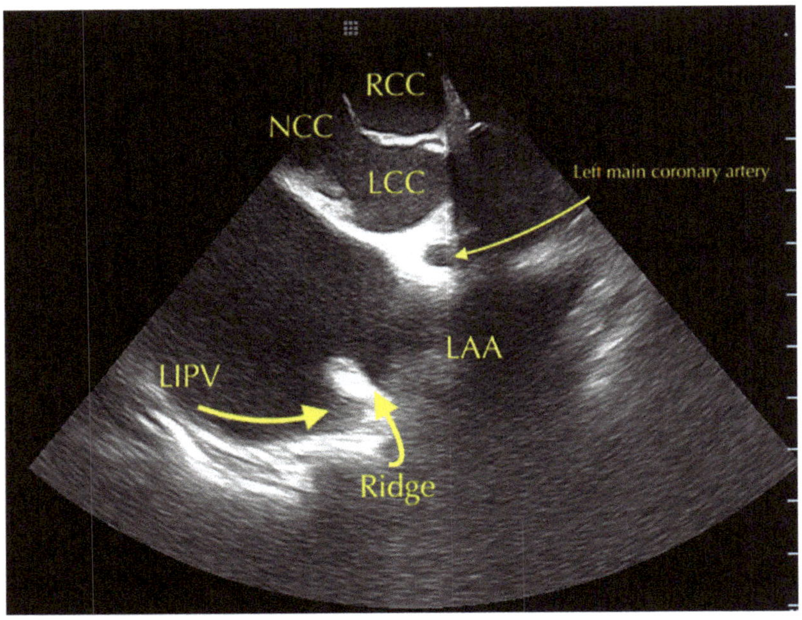

Figure 2.16 Left atrium from right ventricle view. AV at 11–12 o'clock. Right coronary cusp is at the top, non-coronary cusp along the IAS and left coronary cusp near the MV. Note the left main coronary artery in the left coronary cusp. The LAA is in the center of the screen, with ridge separating it and the LSPV.

Left Ventricle

The LV is best visualized through the right ventricle view (see right ventricle section). Once the RV is cannulated, apply CW rotation to sweep posteriorly through the RV and the interventricular septum to encounter the LV.

If desired, through a setting change with the console, the image may be flipped right to left such that the image will resemble a parasternal long-axis view seen with transthoracic echocardiography[2] (**Figure 2.17**).

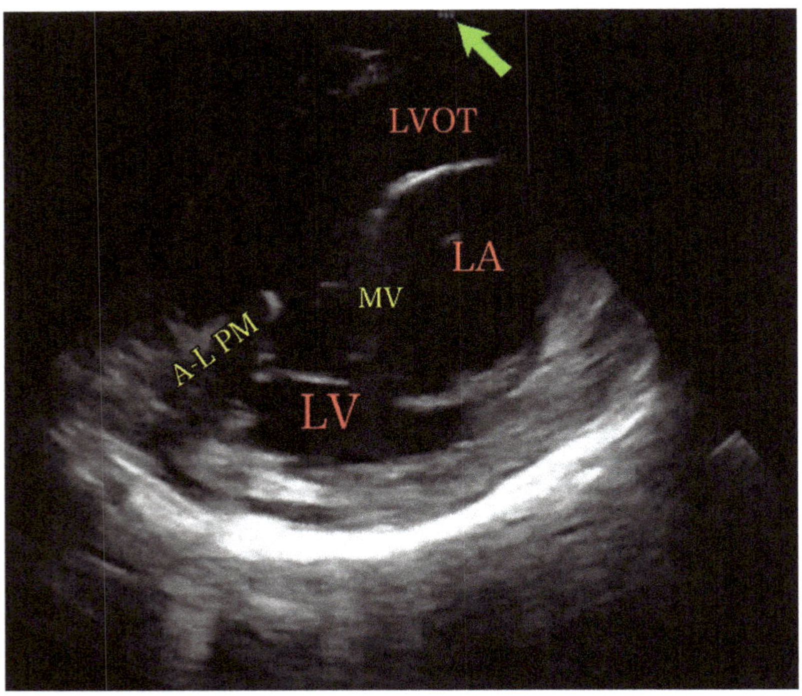

Figure 2.17 Left ventricle seen through right ventricle. LV is seen through RV; the image has been flipped left to right to appear similar to a parasternal long-axis view as seen on transthoracic echocardiography.

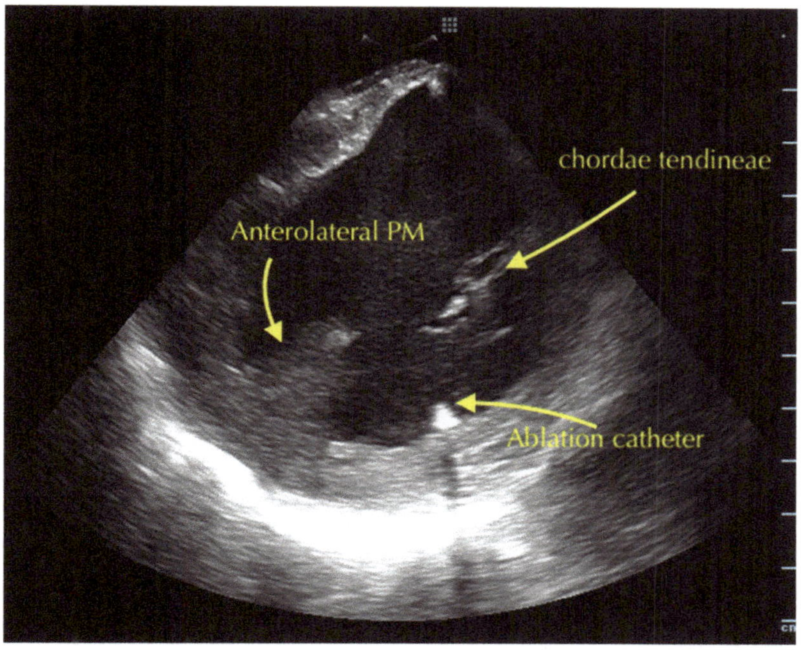

Figure 2.18 Anterolateral papillary muscle. The anterolateral papillary muscle seen with ICE catheter in RV.

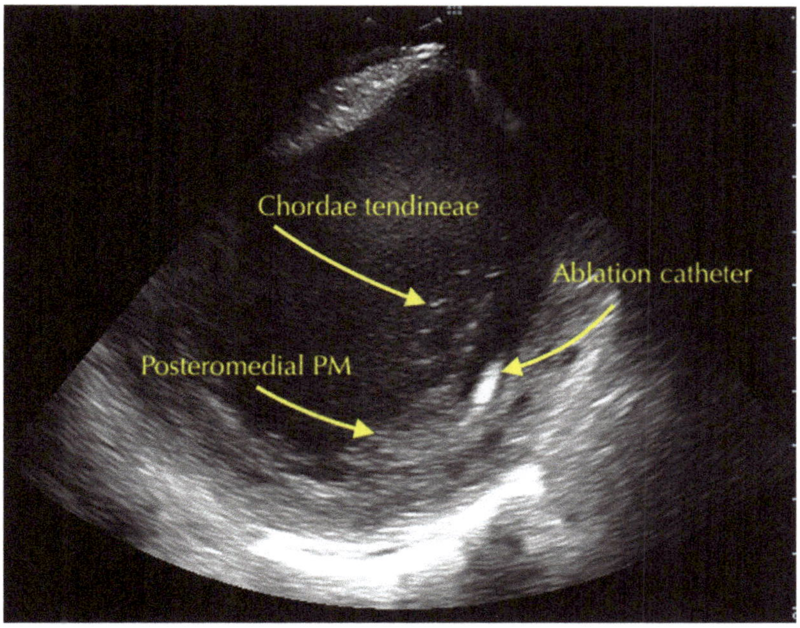

Figure 2.19 Posteromedial papillary muscle. The ICE catheter in RV. Ablation catheter is adjacent to the posteromedial papillary muscle.

Distinguishing the papillary muscles may be challenging. In general, the anterolateral papillary muscle will be seen with CW rotation and the LV will appear foreshortened. The posteromedial papillary muscle will be seen with CCW rotation and the LV will appear fuller (**Figure 2.18**, **Figure 2.19**, and **Video 2.6**).

The MV can be seen with the septal view and adding anterior tilt. CCW rotation shows the anterior aspect of the valve apparatus, and CW rotation shows the posterior components of the valve apparatus. With the right ventricle view, the MV can be scanned with CW/CCW rotation. The anterior component is near the LV outflow, and posterior component is near the LAA.

Catheters can be seen to enter the LV from the MV valve either from the right ventricle view or septal view. If a retrograde approach is taken, the catheter can be seen to prolapse across the aortic valve via the home view with slight CCW rotation to see the long axis of the aortic valve (AV).

Aortic Valve and Proximal Ascending Aorta

The AV can be seen in the long axis or short axis. The long-axis view may be seen with CCW rotation from the home view. Two coronary cusps should be seen in the 3–4 o'clock quadrant, with the proximal ascending aorta projecting to the right. The non-coronary cusp (NCC) will be the cusp on "top" (closest to the ICE catheter), and either the right or left coronary cusp at the bottom of the pair seen. In this view, determination between left and right coronary cusps may be challenging. Applying more CCW (anterior) rotation will bring the right coronary cusp (RCC) into view and applying CW (posterior) rotation will display the left coronary cusp (LCC)[2,6] (**Figure 2.20**).

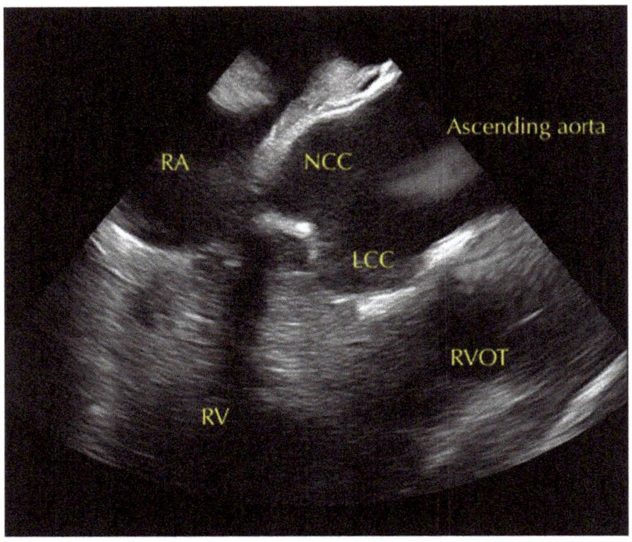

Figure 2.20 Long-axis view of aortic valve. AV is seen in the long axis, with NCC and LCC seen in this view.

The short-axis view of the aortic valve provides more precise identification of the coronary cusps. This view can be obtained from the right ventricle view (see right ventricle section). Once the RV is cannulated, apply CW rotation to sweep posteriorly through the RV, interventricular septum, LV, and MV, until the LA is seen; slight withdrawal of the catheter may be needed. The LCC should be seen in the 4–6 o'clock position, the RCC in the 12–3 o'clock position, and the NCC in the 7–11 o'clock position (**Figure 2.16** and **Video 2.5**). The right and left coronary artery ostia can be seen on ICE, aided by color flow Doppler.

Conclusion

ICE is an invaluable tool to perform fluoroless ablations. It provides real-time imaging of nearly all of the cardiac structures and allows for monitoring of catheter movement and catheter–tissue interface. This enables one to confidently and safely manipulate catheters during cardiac ablations. We are still finding new ways to utilize ICE during ablations and update our view library. Becoming familiar with ICE will enable the operator to discover practical and detailed views to facilitate ablations.

References

1. Bartel T, Müller S. Why is intracardiac echocardiography helpful? Benefits, costs, and how to learn. *Eur Heart J.* 2014 Jan 7;35(2):69–76.
2. Jongbloed MR, Schalij MJ. Clinical applications of intracardiac echocardiography in interventional procedures. *Heart.* 2005 Jul;91(7):981–990.
3. Hijazi ZM, Shivkumar K. Intracardiac echocardiography (ICE) during interventional and electrophysiological cardiac catheterization. *Circulation.* 2009; Feb 3:119(4):587–596.
4. Cummings JE, Schweikert RA, Saliba WI, et al. Assessment of temperature, proximity, and course of the esophagus during radiofrequency ablation within the left atrium. *Circulation.* 2005;112:459–464.
5. Ren JF, Marchlinski FE, Callans DJ. Real-time intracardiac echocardiographic imaging of the posterior left atrial wall contiguous to anterior wall of the esophagus. *J Am Coll Cardiol.* 2006;48:594. author reply, 594–595.
6. Armstrong WF, Ryan T. Feigenbaum's *Echocardiography,* 7th ed. Philadelphia, PA. Lippincott Williams & Wilkins. 2011.

Video Legends

Video 2.1 Home view. ICE catheter in the neutral position. RA is on the upper half of the screen. Tricuspid valve and RV on the lower half. The long-axis AV at 2 o'clock and RVOT at 4–5 o'clock. [00:06]

Video 2.2 Right ventricle view. The ICE catheter in the home view anterior tilt is applied with slight CW and CCW rotation to continuously maintain the opening and closing of the tricuspid valve leaflets in view. The catheter is advanced, once across, returned to neutral. The catheter is rotated CW to scan through the RV, interventricular septum, LV, and LA. [00:30]

Video 2.3 Septal view. CW rotation of ICE from home view until the IAS comes into view. [00:06]

Video 2.4 Left atrium from septal view. MV seen first at 6 o'clock. With CW rotation, the PV come into view as follows: left superior PV at 4 o'clock, followed by left inferior PV at 5 o'clock, followed by right inferior PV at 6 o'clock, and finally right superior PV at 5 o'clock. The esophagus is seen along the posterior wall between the left and right PV. Note left tilt was not needed to visualize the right PV in this case. [00:15]

Video 2.5 Left atrium from right ventricle view. CW rotation from the right ventricle view to scan through the left atrium. Left PV at 5 o'clock. AV at 11–12 o'clock. Right coronary cusp is at the top, non-coronary cusp along the IAS, and left coronary cusp near the MV. Note the left main coronary artery in the left coronary cusp. [00:15]

Video 2.6 Left ventricle from right ventricle view. Note the image has been flipped left to right. CW rotation from the right ventricle view, the posteromedial papillary muscle comes into view first with an ablation catheter adjacent to it. With further CW rotation the anterolateral papillary muscle then LV outflow tract comes into view. [00:10]

Video 2S Chapter summary and step-by-step procedures by Mansour Razminia. [19:00]

3

How to Use Electroanatomic Mapping to Reduce Fluoroscopy

Kristen Breedlove, MPAS, PA-C; John Clark, MD

Introduction

Medical radiation exposure has dramatically increased over the last 30 years. From the early 1980s until 2006, there was a more than 7-fold increase in exposure per U.S. citizen.[1] That increase has triggered a new public awareness and led to measures to both track and minimize exposure. Fortunately, in the electrophysiology (EP) lab there has been an equally dramatic decrease in radiation exposure over the last 10 years. Today, it is possible to achieve zero fluoroscopy in the majority of procedures. This is primarily due to technology advancements in three-dimensional (3D) mapping systems and intracardiac echocardiography (ICE). This chapter will review reasons to minimize fluoroscopy, discuss the currently available mapping tools for reducing or eliminating radiation, and point out some of the various methods employed to maximize their utility.

Reasons to Reduce Radiation

As previously stated, in the United States, over a roughly 25-year period, there was a dramatic increase in the amount of medical radiation exposure per capita.[1] In the early 1980s, medical radiation accounted for roughly 15% of our total exposure. By 2006, the amount had increased to nearly one-half (48%; **Figure 3.1**).

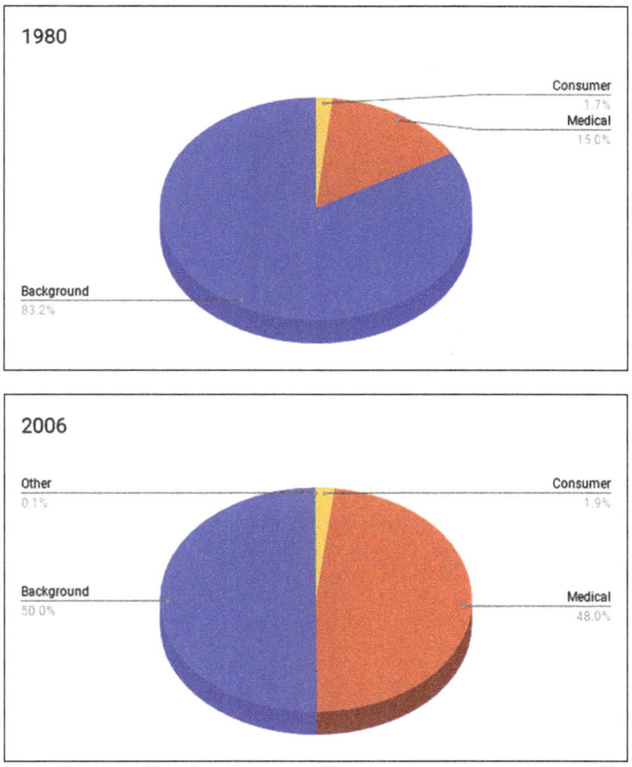

Figure 3.1 Change in medical radiation exposure between early 1980s and 2006.

Fluoroscopy Reduction Techniques for Catheter Ablation of Cardiac Arrhythmias. © 2019 Mansour Razminia, Paul C. Zei, eds. Cardiotext Publishing, ISBN: 978-1-942909-30-9.

While the risks of the current levels of exposure remain low, they are not negligible. Risks to the patient include deterministic (predominantly radiation dermatitis) and stochastic (malignancy and birth defects). Risks to the staff include deterministic (mostly cataracts) and stochastic (malignancy), as well as orthopedic problems related to wearing lead. All of these issues are worthy of continuing efforts to eliminate radiation in the electrophysiology lab.

History

In 1997, Gepstein et al. published "A Novel Method for Non-fluoroscopic Catheter-Based Electroanatomical Mapping of the Heart."[2] In it, they described a new system (CARTO, Biosense Webster) that uses magnetic technology to determine the location of a catheter tip in 3D space, and simultaneously records the local electrogram from the tip. When multiple points are sampled during a stable rhythm, the system is capable of creating a 3D geometry of the chamber sampled, overlaying it with a color representation of the electrical activation of the tissue. This was the first time that electrical information could be linked to the anatomic information. In their porcine study, they found the system to be highly accurate and reproducible. In 1999, Varanasi et al. published the first human experience with this new system.[3] They reported using the system to guide ablation in 3 patients: a focal atrial tachycardia, typical atrial flutter, and a right ventricular outflow tract (RVOT) tachycardia. With eventual regulatory approval world-wide, a new tool was now available to the catheter-based electrophysiologist.

In the early period soon after, as EP labs began to gain experience with the new technology, it was not immediately clear if the utility of the technology justified its expense. Indeed, one of the supportive manuscripts published in 2000 was titled, "Non-fluoroscopic Three-Dimensional Mapping for Arrhythmia Ablation: Tool or Toy?"[4] It was that group's conclusion that the technology was, in fact, a tool. They found that fluoroscopy time was significantly reduced without increasing procedure time. Shortly after this publication, Drago et al. published a series in which CARTO was used in children to minimize or eliminate fluoroscopy.[5] In 21 patients, they were able to successfully perform the ablation without fluoroscopy in 9 (42%). The magnitude of this accomplishment can hardly be overstated, given that they were using the first-generation CARTO system. That system could only visualize one catheter: the Navistar radiofrequency catheter. No other mapping catheters could be visualized in the system, and the only energy source was radiofrequency (RF). Geometry creation was a slow process, and the field of view of the system was limited to a small volume within the thorax. Given all of those handicaps, it is no surprise that it would take 5 years of further technological advancements, including an alternative electroanatomic mapping (EAM) system before further significant advances and widespread adoption.

Systems

The first system released for clinical use was CARTO (Biosense Webster). In its original version, this system utilized magnetic fields. The patient was positioned supine over a magnetic field generator containing 3 magnets of different field strengths. Navistar catheters contain metal coils in their tip. Electric current is generated by the coil when within the magnetic field. Based on the field strength detected, a computer could localize the tip in 3D space. It also had the ability to store points for reference.

Within a few years of the release of CARTO, there were 2 competitors: Localisa (Medtronic, Inc.) and EnSite (Abbott, Abbott Park, IL). Localisa could not display electrical information onto a 3D map, and so adoption was poor, and its availability clinically was of limited duration. EnSite could display both 3D anatomy and electrical activation, and became the primary alternative to CARTO. EnSite utilized different technology for its mapping functions. The system uses 6 surface patches on the torso to set up 3 orthogonal electrical fields. Any electrode within the body can detect those electrical signals, and a computer can use impedance information to triangulate the location of the electrode in space. The benefits of the EnSite system were that it could function with all available EP catheters, it enabled visualization of catheters using different energy sources (cryo or RF), it had a far field of view, and could draw highly detailed geometry rapidly. **Figures 3.2** and **3.3** show geometries obtainable with early versions of CARTO and EnSite. **Figure 3.4** shows the more complex geometries available with current equipment.

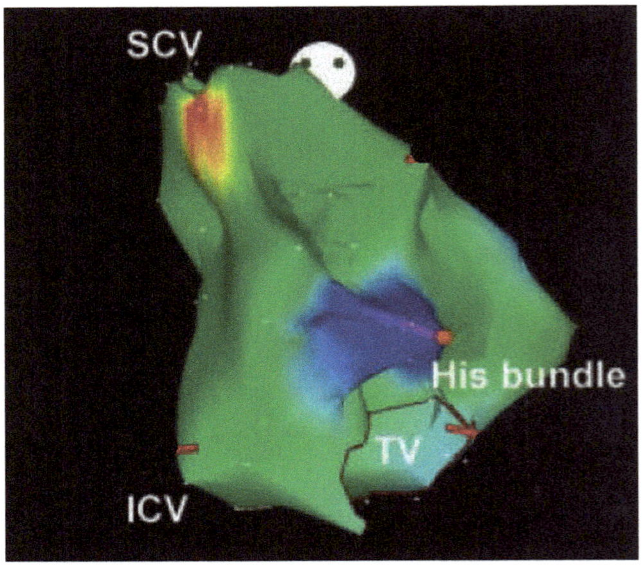

Figure 3.2 Typical geometry created with the early versions of CARTO.

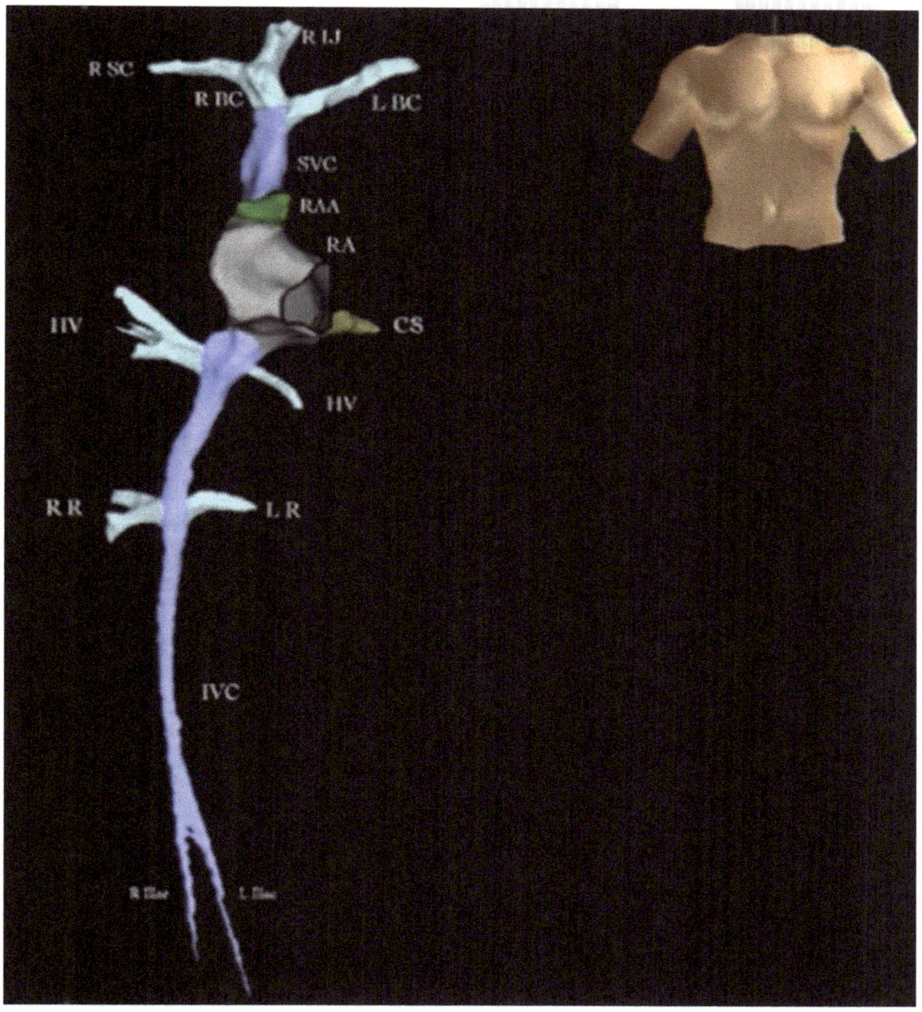

Figure 3.3 Typical geometry created with the early versions of EnSite.

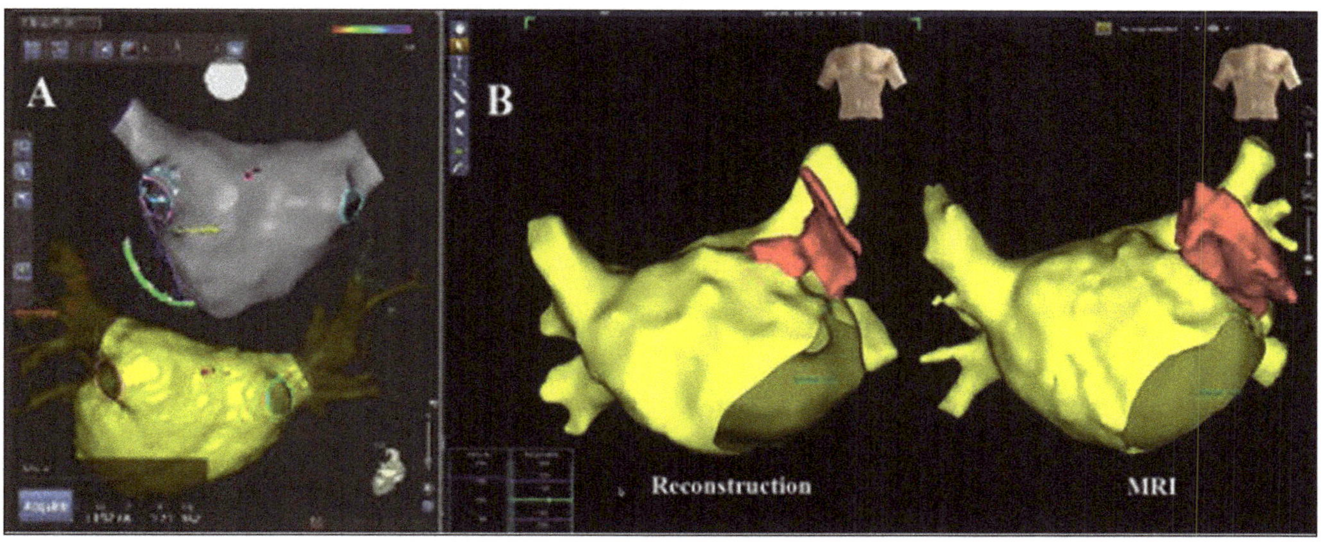

Figure 3.4 Detailed geometry obtainable with later versions of mapping systems. **A (gray image):** CARTO 3 electroanatomic reconstruction of the left atrium obtained with the mapping catheter (postero-anterior view); **(yellow image):** MRI of the left atrium. **B (reconstruction):** EnSite NavX electroanatomic reconstruction of the left atrium obtained with the mapping catheter (antero-posterior view); **B (MRI):** MRI of the left atrium. With both EAM systems, the reconstructed cardiac anatomy is very similar to that obtained with MRI.

In 2007, Tuzcu and Smith each independently published their experience with elimination of fluoroscopy using the EnSite system.[6,7] Multiple other centers subsequently reported similar results for differing substrates, such as atrioventricular nodal reentrant tachycardia (AVNRT),[8] right-sided pathways,[9] left-sided accessory pathways,[10] atrial fibrillation (AF),[11] and ventricular tachycardia (VT).[12] Both systems have improved and matured. With advent of CARTO 3, the possibility of routine zero fluoroscopy became available to CARTO users, largely matching the EnSite features of wider field of view, visualization of most other catheters including alternate ablation energy catheters, as well as several additional mapping features. Today, both systems provide high-quality maps with an array of additional mapping features to aid in the mapping and ablation process. Scaglione et al., in 2013, was the first to report a CARTO 3 series. Their study involved 21 children with AVNRT undergoing cryoablation. They had 100% acute success. In 19 of the cases no fluoroscopy was used. Two of the cases required brief fluoroscopy to guide a catheter from the femoral vein.[13] Macias compared CARTO 3 to their lab standard, EnSite, and found equal ability to successfully ablate typical cavotricuspid isthmus-dependent flutter without fluoroscopy.[14] Scaglione reported 44 children with accessory pathway mediated tachycardia, all successfully ablated without fluoroscopy. They chose a retrograde approach for left-sided substrates if the patient did not have a patent foramen ovale.[15] Kuhne reported using CARTO 3 plus CARTOMERGE MRI for AF ablation.[16] Today, it is possible to routinely perform zero-fluoroscopy ablation with either system. The first step needed to eliminate fluoroscopy is the decision to utilize EAM as much as possible, and use fluoroscopy only when necessary. There will be a learning curve during this adoption process, and certainly safety must be maintained. With that in mind, we can walk through a procedure.

Femoral venous access is obtained in the usual way (please refer to Chapter 5 for further details). Once access is established, a catheter can be advanced. A deflectable multipolar catheter is of some utility at this point if using the EnSite system. An ablation catheter is required with the current CARTO system at the time of this publication. While the catheter is within the sheath, it will appear distorted on the screen in EnSite, usually being upside down. As the electrodes exit the sheath, the distortion will resolve, and the catheter will assume a normal orientation. As the catheter is advanced, its motion and direction are accurately displayed on the screen. For CARTO, gentle resistance-free advancement will move the catheter within the mapping field, which typically is located above the mid-IVC. If the catheter inadvertently enters the opposing femoral vein, the course of the catheter makes that readily apparent. Similarly, as the catheter ascends the IVC it may course into a renal or hepatic vein. By following the catheter from the sheath to the heart, any different path which it may take is seen. There is no need to move the table in order to track the catheter, as the EAM software can change the focal point to anywhere needed.

Whether or not geometry is drawn from the femoral vein to the heart is a matter of operator choice. Without drawing geometry, it remains clear that the catheter is moving toward the patient's head. It will advance in a fairly straight, superior direction until it reaches the liver. At the liver, the catheter will take a noticeable turn toward the patient's left shoulder. This turn is the indication that the catheter is about to enter the right atrium. Advancing the catheter further will result in atrial electrograms being visible on the recording system, as the catheter reaches the atrium. Once the catheter is within the heart, the system is usually optimized and respiratory compensation is collected to stabilize the catheter position during respiration. Now a cardiac geometry can be created.

From this position it is easy to create geometries for the superior vena cava, inferior vena cava (IVC), right atrium, and tricuspid valve. In most instances, the coronary sinus can also be entered and displayed on the map. While drawing the tricuspid valve, a shadow or tag can be placed to mark the location of the His bundle. For the majority of supraventricular tachycardia ablations, this degree of geometry creation will suffice to complete the procedure. For all right-sided accessory pathways and AVNRT, no other geometry will be needed, although more detailed mapping of the triangle of Koch region will be useful. For left-sided accessory pathways, left atrial geometry can be drawn if desired, but the coronary sinus geometry can function quite well as an adequate landmark for ablation. For ectopic atrial tachycardias and intra-atrial reentrant tachycardia (IART), more right or left atrial geometry may be needed. For VT, a right or left ventricular geometry will be necessary. Creating the geometry rarely takes more than a few minutes. It might be expected that minimal fluoroscopy procedures will take longer than a traditional fluoroscopy-guided procedure due to the need to draw geometry, although this may be counterbalanced by quicker and more confident catheter movement and positioning; the overall procedure time differences remain unclear, but data thus far demonstrates comparable procedure times in skilled hands. While there is indeed a learning curve, the literature consistently fails to show longer procedure times.[4,7,17] There is no time consumed stepping on the fluoroscopy pedal and orienting the location of the catheters.

One of the handicaps of both EnSite and CARTO is the inability to visualize most sheaths, dilators, and guidewires. However, if a long sheath is needed for the procedure, it can be indirectly visualized. First the sheath is positioned in the IVC. A catheter is advanced through it into the right atrium. The sheath is then advanced over the catheter. When the sheath reaches the proximal electrode of the catheter, it will distort the appearance of the catheter on the screen for EnSite, and for CARTO, the proximal electrode of an ablation catheter will display as within the sheath. This allows identification of the end of the sheath relative to the electrodes. Another hurdle to be overcome is positioning circular catheters that require advancing through a long sheath. This is often the case with RVOT ablation. If a circular catheter needs to be positioned in the RVOT, a deflectable catheter can first be advanced through a long sheath and positioned within the pulmonary arterial tree. The long sheath is then advanced over the catheter. When the proximal electrode distorts/marks as in the sheath, the sheath will then be within the pulmonary artery also. The deflectable catheter is then removed and replaced with the circular catheter. As the distal electrode emerges from the sheath, it is recognized by the amount of distortion visible. The long sheath can then be pulled back to expose the remaining electrodes, allowing the catheter to assume its normal shape and appearance. The catheter and sheath can then be pulled back as a unit to be positioned in the RVOT. With these simple maneuvers, there are very few arrhythmias that cannot be approached with zero fluoroscopy. A new sheath available for the CARTO 3 system at the time of this publication, Vizigo (Biosense Webster), allows sheath visualization, including sheath curvature, on the CARTO mapping system. **Figure 3.5** shows a left atrial EAM created using CARTO 3, with a Vizigo sheath visualized in the chamber. Note the ablation catheter exiting the sheath. As experience grows with this sheath, its benefit in a fluoroscopy-free ablation approach remains to be determined. Transseptal puncture will require additional tools, namely ICE, and that will be discussed in a later chapter.

The primary motivation for most EP labs to pursue a zero-fluoroscopy approach is for the safety of the patients and the staff, relative to radiation exposure. However, there are other benefits to the approach that are not usually considered until the practice has become established within the lab. The first, and most welcome, benefit is the ability to eliminate the requirement for lead protective gear. Once the degree of comfort with the procedure is high enough, the staff can stop wearing lead aprons. When this point is reached, everyone in the lab will appreciate having gone through the learning curve to reach that milestone. The appreciation from the staff is almost palpable. Once staff has been liberated from lead, they will never go back to the traditional way of doing things.

Another benefit is procedures during pregnancy. While ablation on a pregnant female will be discussed in another chapter, there is also the issue of pregnant staff members. We have been fortunate in that, 4 times thus far, there has been a staff member who was pregnant but did not have to be reassigned to other duties. The ability to keep experienced staff working in the EP lab throughout pregnancy because they are not getting exposed to radiation is great for continuity of care and workflow.

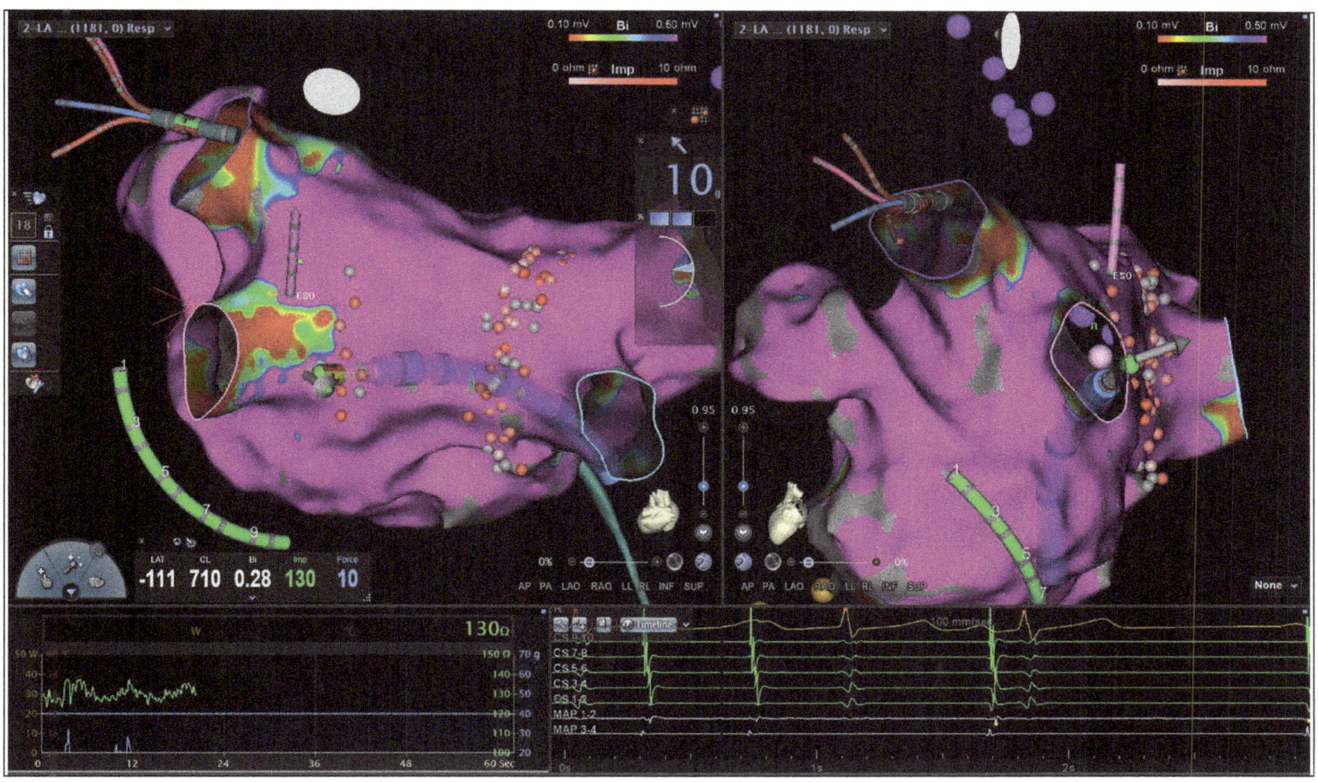

Figure 3.5 EAM created using CARTO 3 of the left atrium in 2 views, posteroanterior and right anterior oblique, demonstrating a steerable guide sheath (Vizigo, Biosense Webster) in the left atrium, with the ablation catheter exiting the sheath. Note that the direction and curve of the sheath is visible, based on markers placed along the distal curve of the sheath.

Finally, there is the benefit of being able to perform ablation procedures outside the EP lab. While we have performed ablations outside the lab in more than 100 cases,[18] there is no pressing need to do so. The reason to continuously sharpen EP labs skills for this situation is the rare patient who presents with tachycardia-induced cardiomyopathy and requires extracorporeal membrane oxygenation (ECMO). If an ablation is necessary with the patient in tachycardia, then the patient must be taken to the EP lab while on ECMO, which is fraught with risk. If the lab is highly experienced in zero-fluoroscopy ablation, then a safer option is to transport the EP lab to the patient. However, it should be kept in mind that ablation in a procedure setting that does not have a fluoroscopy system in the room as a backup remains outside the bounds of accepted clinical practice, even if an experienced operator has not required fluoroscopy for a long time.

Conclusion

Three-dimensional electroanatomic mapping has revolutionized the field of electrophysiology. To date, more than 200 manuscripts have been published which support the safety and utility of these tools for treating virtually any arrhythmia. Some of the more significant publications are noted in the reference list.[17,19–26] As the tools continue to evolve and improve, all labs will eventually transition to a fluoroscopy-free approach. In subsequent chapters of this book, you will learn valuable insights to shorten the learning curve of that transition.

References

1. Schauer DA, Linton OW. National Council on Radiation Protection and Measurements Report shows substantial medical exposure increase. *Radiology*. 2009;253(2):293–296. doi:10.1148/radiol.2532090494
2. Gepstein L, Hayam G, Ben-Haim SA. A novel method for non-fluoroscopic catheter-based electroanatomical mapping of the heart. In vitro and in vivo accuracy results. *Circulation*. 1997;95(6):1611–1622.
3. Varanasi S, Dhala A, Blanck Z, Deshpande S, Akhtar M, Sra J. Electroanatomic mapping for radiofrequency ablation of cardiac arrhythmias. *J Cardiovasc Electrophysiol*. 1999;10(4):538–544.
4. Khongphatthanayothin A, Kosar E, Nademanee K. Nonfluoroscopic three-dimensional mapping for arrhythmia ablation: Tool or toy? *J Cardiovasc Electrophysiol*. 2000; 11(3):239–243.
5. Drago F, Silvetti MS, Pino AD, Grutter G, Bevilacqua M, Leibovich S. Exclusion of fluoroscopy during ablation treatment of right accessory pathway in children. *J Cardiovasc Electrophysiol*. 2002;13(8):778–782.doi:10.1046/j.1540-8167.2002.00778.x
6. Tuzcu V. A non-fluoroscopic approach for electrophysiology and catheter ablation procedures using a three-dimensional navigation system. *Pacing Clin Electrophysiol*. 2007;30(4):519–525. doi:10.1111/j.1540-8159.2007.00702.x
7. Smith G, Clark JM. Elimination of fluoroscopy use in a pediatric electrophysiology laboratory utilizing three-dimensional mapping. *Pacing Clin Electrophysiol*. 2007; 30(4):510–518.doi:10.1111/j.1540-8159.2007.00701.x
8. Gist K, Tigges C, Smith G, Clark J. Learning curve for zero-fluoroscopy catheter ablation of AVNRT: Early versus late experience. *Pacing Clin Electrophysiol*. 2011;34(3):264–268. doi:10.1111/j.1540-8159.2010.02952.x
9. Ma Y, Qiu J, Yang Y, Tang A. Catheter ablation of right-sided accessory pathways in adults using the three-dimensional mapping system: A randomized comparison to the conventional approach. *PLoS One*. 2015;10(6):e0128760. doi:10.1371/journal.pone.0128760
10. Clark J, Bockoven JR, Lane J, Patel CR, Smith G. Use of three-dimensional catheter guidance and trans-esophageal echocardiography to eliminate fluoroscopy in catheter ablation of left-sided accessory pathways. *Pacing Clin Electrophysiol*. 2008;31(3):283–289. doi:10.1111/j.1540-8159.2008.00987.x
11. Reddy VY, Morales G, Ahmed H, et al. Catheter ablation of atrial fibrillation without the use of fluoroscopy. *Heart Rhythm*. 2010;7(11):1644–1653. doi:10.1016/j.hrthm.2010.07.011
12. Razminia M, Willoughby MC, Demo H, et al. Fluoroless catheter ablation of cardiac arrhythmias: A 5-year experience. *Pacing Clin Electrophysiol*. 2017;40(4):425–433. doi:10.1111/pace.13038
13. Scaglione M, Ebrille E, Caponi D, et al. Single center experience of fluoroless AVNRT ablation guided by electroanatomic reconstruction in children and adolescents: Fluoroless AVNRT cryoablation in children. *Pacing Clin Electrophysiol*. 2013;36(12):1460–1467. doi:10.1111/pace.12183
14. Macías R, Uribe I, Tercedor L, Jiménez-Jáimez J, Barrio T, Álvarez M. A zero-fluoroscopy approach to cavotricuspid isthmus catheter ablation: Comparative analysis of two electroanatomical mapping systems: zero-fluoroscopy catheter ablation. *Pacing Clin Electrophysiol*. 2014;37(8): 1029–1037.doi:10.1111/pace.12376
15. Scaglione M, Ebrille E, Caponi D, et al. Zero-fluoroscopy ablation of accessory pathways in children and adolescents: CARTO3 electroanatomic mapping combined with RF and cryoenergy: Fluoroless WPW ablation in children and adolescents. *Pacing Clin Electrophysiol*. 2015;38(6):675–681. doi:10.1111/pace.12619
16. Kühne M, Knecht S, Mühl A, et al. Fluoroscopy-free pulmonary vein isolation in patients with atrial fibrillation and a patent foramen ovale using solely an electroanatomic mapping system. *PLoS One*. 2016;11(1):e0148059.doi:10.1371/journal.pone.0148059
17. Sporton SC, Earley MJ, Nathan AW, Schilling RJ. Electroanatomic versus fluoroscopic mapping for catheter ablation procedures: A prospective randomized study. *J Cardiovasc Electrophysiol*. 2004;15(3):310–315. doi:10.1111/j.1540-8167.2004.03356.x
18. Bigelow AM, Smith PC, Timberlake DT, et al. Procedural outcomes of fluoroless catheter ablation outside the traditional catheterization lab. *Europace*. 2017;19:1378–1384. doi:10.1093/europace/euw207

19. Marini M, Del Greco M, Ravanelli D, et al. The benefit of a general, systematic use of mapping systems during electrophysiological procedures in children and teenagers: The experience of an adult EP laboratory. *Pediatric Cardiol.* 2016;37(4):802–809. doi:10.1007/s00246-016-1354-2
20. Tuzcu V. Significant reduction of fluoroscopy in pediatric catheter ablation procedures: Long-term experience from a single center. *Pacing Clin Electrophysiol.* 2012;35(9):1067–1073. doi:10.1111/j.1540-8159.2012.03472.x
21. Scaglione M, Ebrille E, Clemente FD, Gaita F, Bradfield JS. Catheter ablation of atrial fibrillation without radiation exposure using a 3D mapping system. *J Atr Fibrillation.* 2015;7(5). doi:10.4022/jafib.1167
22. Ozturk E, Ergul Y, Tanidir IC, Akdeniz C, Tola HT, Tuzcu V. Electroanatomic mapping guided cryoablation of Mahaim pathways in children with limited fluoroscopy exposure. *Pacing Clin Electrophysiol.* 2015;38(3):362–367. doi:10.1111/pace.12559
23. Nguyen MB, Ceresnak SR, Janson CM, et al. A multicenter review of ablation in the aortic cusps in young people. *Pacing Clin Electrophysiol.* 2017;40(7):798–802. doi:10.1111/pace.13126
24. Caponi D, Corleto A, Scaglione M, et al. Ablation of atrial fibrillation: Does the addition of three-dimensional magnetic resonance imaging of the left atrium to electroanatomic mapping improve the clinical outcome? A randomized comparison of CARTOMERGE vs. CARTO-XP three-dimensional mapping ablation in patients with paroxysmal and persistent atrial fibrillation. *Europace.* 2010;12(8):1098–1104. doi:10.1093/europace/euq107
25. Koca S. Electroanatomic mapping guided pediatric catheter ablation with limited/zero fluoroscopy. *Anatolian J Cardiol.* 2018. doi:10.14744/AnatolJCardiol.2018.72687
26. Nedios S, Sommer P, Bollmann A, Hindricks G. Advanced mapping systems to guide atrial fibrillation ablation: Electrical information that matters. *J Atr Fibrillation.* 2016;8(6). doi:10.4022/jafib.1337

4

How to Use Technologies such as MediGuide and CARTOUNIVU to Reduce Fluoroscopy During Catheter Ablation

Martin Borlich, MD; Philipp Sommer, MD

Introduction

Catheter ablation of cardiac arrhythmias has quickly become established as standard therapy, is indispensable for rhythm control, and rightly ensures a steady increase in electrophysiological (EP) examinations worldwide. Fluoroscopy is still often required in modern ablation strategies despite continuous further development of 3D mapping systems and image integration technology. The least possible use of fluoroscopy time and dose is essential to avoid stochastic or deterministic radiation risks to both our patients and the entire EP laboratory staff and should be a marker of good procedure quality. Here we aim to highlight the potential and importance of modern image integration tools like MediGuide and CARTOUNIVU for reduction of fluoroscopy and to illustrate the integration into a modern workflow for the interventional therapy of cardiac arrhythmias.

MediGuide

MediGuide (Abbott, Abbott Park, IL) is a non-fluoroscopic catheter visualization system (NFCV) enabling real-time catheter navigation superimposed to prerecorded x-ray sequences. The technology was first described in 2008 as technical report,[1] followed by published first-in-man experience in 2009.[2] The system is composed of a transmitter unit generating a 3D electromagnetic field. This unit is attached to the fluoroscopy detector of an x-ray imaging system aligning automatically the fluoroscopy field with the 3D magnetic sensor field. A miniaturized single-coil sensor (<1 mm^3) is attached to the tip of a MediGuide-capable catheter and thus can be tracked in real time without fluoroscopy in the electromagnetic sensor field. Two algorithms are used to compensate for primary and secondary organ movement: A magnetic field reference sensor is attached to the patient, serving as reference sensor for calculation of catheter location and compensation for movement artifacts through respiration and patient activity. ECG signals are used to compensate the artifacts caused by cardiac motion. MediGuide is auto-registered due to system integration on hardware level. A maximum of 9 catheters can be displayed simultaneously by the system.

For initialization, recording of 2 short fluoroscopy loops (usually in right and left anterior oblique views) is required.[3,4] Subsequently, a MediGuide-capable diagnostic catheter (e.g., Lifewire diagnostic catheter, MediGuide Enabled, Abbott) can be placed in the coronary sinus. Depending on the planned type of ablation, anatomical structures such as the superior vena cava (SVC), inferior vena cava (IVC), and fossa ovalis are then marked via the MediGuide System as a first step for pulmonary vein isolation. If no intracardiac echocardiography (ICE) is used, the subsequent transseptal puncture and contrast agent imaging of the pulmonary veins are the final steps in the entire procedure that require the use of fluoroscopy. In the

Fluoroscopy Reduction Techniques for Catheter Ablation of Cardiac Arrhythmias. © 2019 Mansour Razminia, Paul C. Zei, eds. Cardiotext Publishing, ISBN: 978-1-942909-30-9.

subsequent steps, lead aprons and other personal protective equipment against x-rays can be removed. If desired, cardiac CT or MRI data sets may be loaded into the NFCV platform. Using the landmarks of anatomical structures, the 3D CT or MRI data set is registered. For pulmonary vein isolation, usually landmarks of PV ostia are used (**Figure 4.1**). A 3D mapping system is then used in conjunction with the MediGuide System for geometry creation (**Figure 4.2**). After electroanatomical reconstruction, the map can be fused with the CT or MRI data set.

The benefits of using MediGuide System for ablation of atrial fibrillation (AF) are well described. Rolf et al. demonstrated in 2012 that using diagnostic MediGuide-compatible catheters can reduce fluoroscopy time and dose by approximately 50% in patients undergoing ablation of AF.[5] Sensor-equipped ablation catheters for MediGuide were available since May 2012. Rolf et al. published their first clinical experience with the all-MediGuide-catheter approach for ablation of AF in 2013. The technology was easy to integrate in the standard workflow of AF ablation and fluoroscopy duration could be reduced to 4.6 minutes in average. No major complications occurred.[6] Recently published data demonstrated the consistent and safe performance of an AF ablation procedure with the non-fluoroscopic catheter visualization technology in conjunction with a 3D electroanatomical mapping system in a cohort of 1000 patients. A short learning curve is described (25–50 procedures), low complication rate (2%), a median procedure duration of 120 minutes, median fluoroscopy time of 0.9 minutes and median fluoroscopy dose of 345 cGy · cm^2. The most common intervention in interventional electrophysiology can therefore be performed with a fluoroscopy time of less than 1 minute and a correspondingly low dose-area product.[4] For the last 250 procedures, only 0.5 minutes of fluoroscopy were required with a cumulative dose of 152 cGy · cm^2. There is a limited number of devices for this system; however, a TactiCath contact force ablation catheter, sensor enabled (Abbott, Abbott Park, IL) is obtainable to exploit the advantages of contact force technology by using EnSite Precision 3D mapping system. An additional multipolar, high-density mapping catheter (Advisor HD Grid Mapping Catheter, Sensor Enabled, Abbott) recently became available and revolutionizes the mapping process.

Apart from the use of NFCV for AF ablations, there is also available data demonstrating the benefit of MG system for ablation of other cardiac arrhythmias. The application of MediGuide for ablation of typical atrial flutter was published in 2012 by Sommer et al., showing low fluoroscopy time of approximately 2.5 minutes for the entire cavotricuspid isthmus (CTI) ablation.[7] In a prospective study, Schöne et al. was able to demonstrate the significant reduction of radiation dose and fluoroscopy time by using the MG system compared to a group treated with use of conventional fluoroscopy.[8] The successful use of the technology for implantation of left ventricular leads in cardiac resynchronization therapy has been described,[9,10] as well as the use of MediGuide for other cardiac arrhythmias.[3] ▶ **Video 4.1** illustrates the beneficial utilization of these technologies for the treatment of atypical atrial flutter (aAFL). Data for the use of MediGuide in treatment of ventricular arrhythmias are rare. Besides that, MediGuide can be used to investigate local wall motion patterns by its ability to store and analyze point trajectories in 3D space very accurately.[11,12]

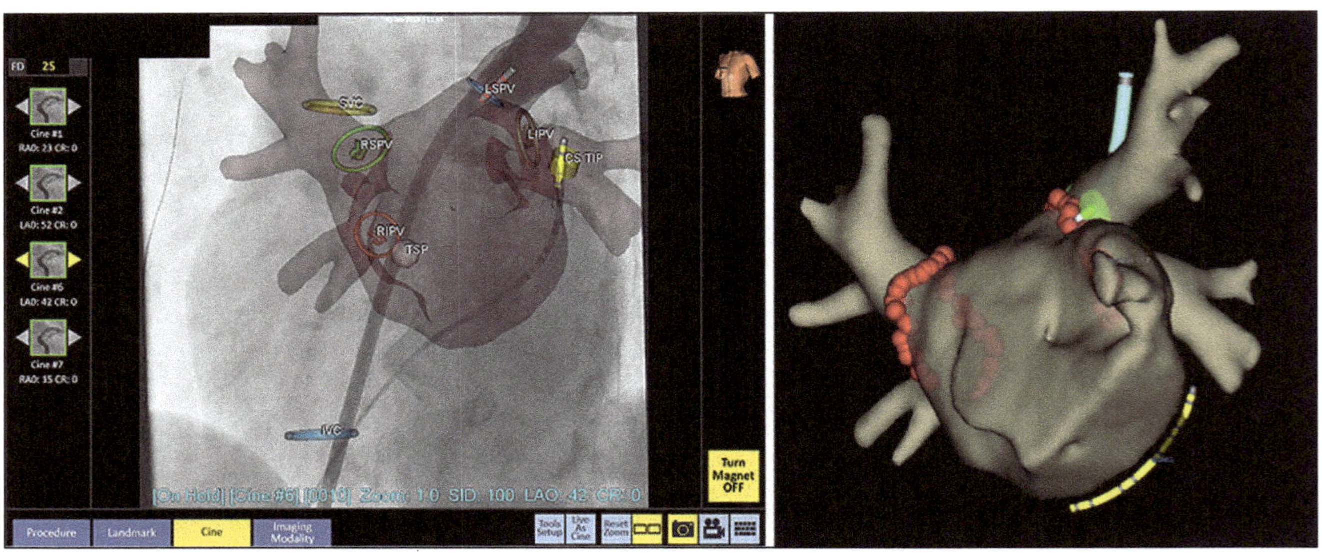

Figure 4.1 Screenshot of the MediGuide System and the corresponding 3D reconstruction of the left atrium using EnSite Precision cardiac mapping system. Image of a short fluoroscopy loop is displayed on the left side in LAO view (42 degrees). Ostia of the 4 pulmonary veins are marked together with the transseptal puncture side, the tip of the ablation and CS catheter, and the inferior and the superior vena cava. In the corresponding map on the right side the marked ablation points are displayed together with the esophageal probe, the CS, and ablation catheter.

Apart from limited number of available catheters, the limited compatibility to one x-ray company, and high costs for system acquisition, MediGuide represents an outstanding component of a modern catheter system helping to limit the procedural and cumulative dose and reduce lifelong radiation risk for the electrophysiologic laboratory staff and our patients.

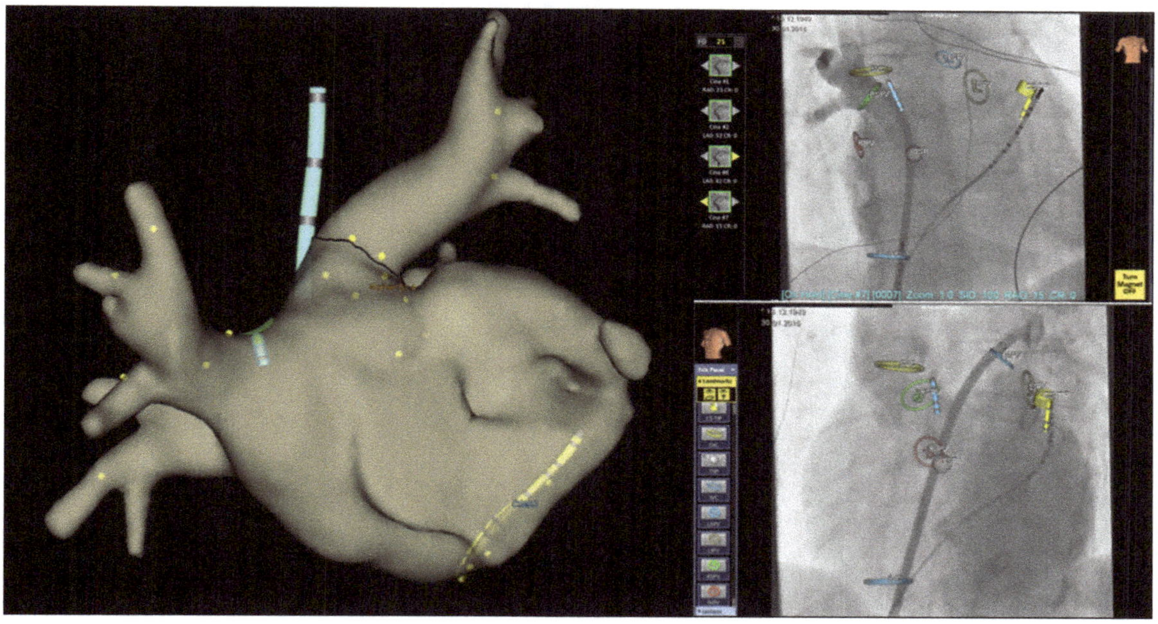

Figure 4.2 Illustration of an anatomic reconstruction of the left atrium created with EnSite Precision cardiac mapping system being displayed in RAO view (15-degree angle). The corresponding view of MediGuide System in RAO (**upper picture**) and additional LAO view (**lower picture**) can be seen on the right side.

CARTOUNIVU

The CARTOUNIVU Module (Biosense Webster, Diamond Bar, CA) is an advanced image integration tool for the CARTO 3 electroanatomical mapping system (Biosense Webster). It combines the information provided by the fluoroscopy system with the 3D map created by the CARTO 3 system. It is compatible with most different fluoroscopy models of different manufacturers. The initial installation of the CARTOUNIVU Module software package is specific to the x-ray system used in the respective catheter laboratory. There is no need for separate disposable ablation material when CARTOUNIVU is to be used.

To utilize the module after installation, open patient setup and select your fluoroscopy system. A symbol will show the successful connection. After initialization, the registration window appears. The fluoroscopy detector must be therefore in AP orientation, ideally in 0 degrees with no tilt, cradle, or rotation in the patient table. The patient table must be moved, guided by the tracking tool, so that the fluoroscopy detector is located above the registration disc being attached to the existing location pad. Align the red rectangle superimposed to the green rectangle and record an image or cine loop. The table must not be moved during the registration process. CARTOUNIVU automatically detects the radio-opaque markers over the registration plates. The system recognizes the disc and marks it green (**Figure 4.3**). The recorded x-ray image with the registration disc will be saved. This allows the system to calculate the exact location between the location pad and the C-arm of the fluoroscopy system. The now registered relationship between the 2 systems is valid for recording all other images and cine loops of each procedure. Each fluoroscopy image or cine loop taken with the fluoroscopy system is automatically transferred via the hospital network to the CARTOUNIVU Module and will accurately be stored at its acquisition projection. When the map is rotated to a projection with a stored fluoroscopic image, real-time catheter locations are shown together with the registered fluoroscopy image. With the CARTOUNIVU toolbar, the map can be rotated to the last saved x-ray image/cine or to the x-ray image/cine in the neighboring angle, or it can be used to rescale recorded x-ray images/loops. Defining favored perspectives as "view X" makes it possible to quickly set up a frequently requested perspective, such as LAO or RAO.

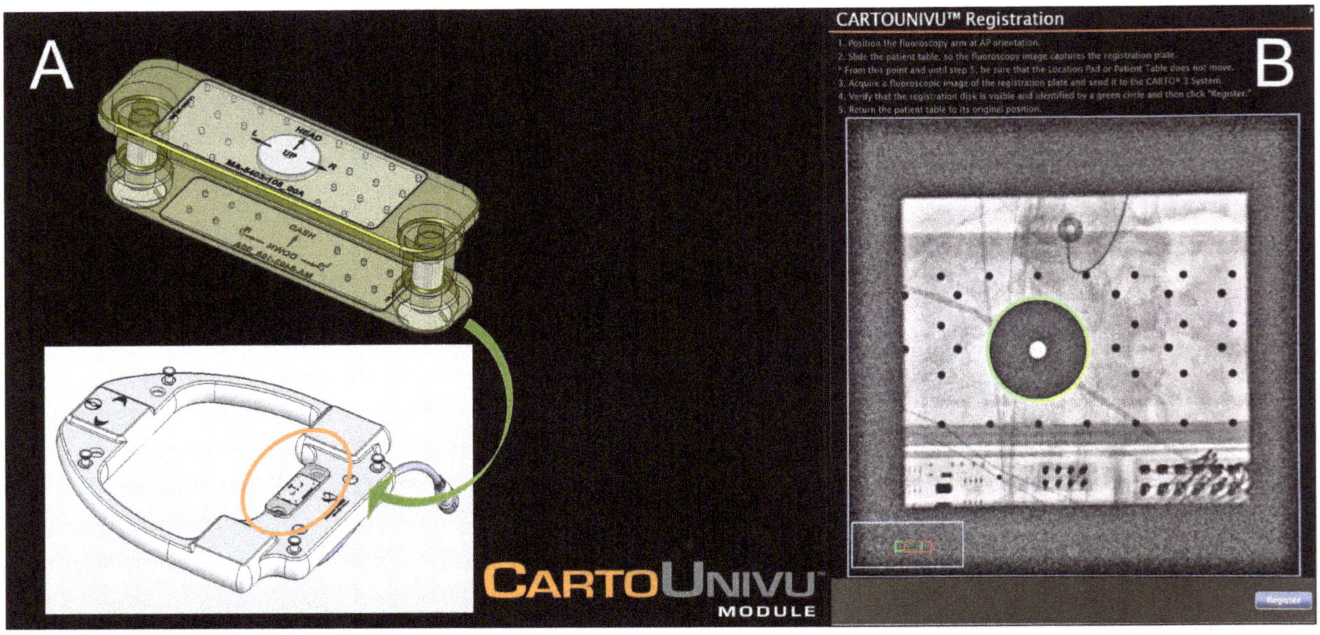

Figure 4.3 **A:** Illustration of the registration plate attached to the location pad of CARTO 3 system. (Reproduced with permission from © Johnson & Johnson.) **B:** Registration window of CARTOUNIVU with successful detection of registration disc.

In order to further improve the anatomical accuracy of the map, image integration of CT or MRI data sets as well as images obtained with intracardiac ultrasound should be considered.[13] Another possibility involves the use of 3D rotational angiography images. This method allows reconstruction of tomographic slices of a volume of interest with the advantage of real-time creation during the current procedure, avoiding mismatch due to changes in heart rhythm or volume status.[14] CARTOUNIVU supports rotational angiography. The respective fluoroscopy system must therefore be able to do this. Images of a 180-degree rotational scan can be sent to the CARTOUNIVU Module. By mirroring the images, a 360-degree view can be made possible. A perceptive use of the appropriate image-integration tools available today allows near-zero radiation workflows.

In 2015, Cano et al. published the first experience in the use of CARTOUNIVU. They investigated the influence of the module in reducing fluoroscopy levels in patients undergoing complex arrhythmia ablation procedures. Twenty-eight patients with left atrial arrhythmia and 13 patients with ventricular tachycardia were treated using the CARTOUNIVU Module and were compared with a retrospective cohort of patients (16 patients with left atrial arrhythmia and 8 patients with ventricular tachycardia [VT]) treated without using this image integration tool. Using CARTOUNIVU resulted in significantly reduced total fluoroscopy time and mean radiation dose (lowered by about 60%) without influencing procedure duration.[15]

This seems to apply to a wide spectrum of cardiac arrhythmias (**Figure 4.4**), except in the treatment of accessory pathways and premature ventricular complexes (PVCs).[16] In the same year, Reents et al. from Munich also demonstrated a reduction in fluoroscopy time and dose in patients receiving VT ablation and use of CARTOUNIVU compared to conventional fluoroscopy supplemented by electroanatomical mapping with CARTO 3 system.[17] A minimally fluoroscopic approach (<1 mSv) is possible in ischemic VT ablation in approximately 50% of patients, especially among those who only need endocardial access.[18] Akbulak et al. from Hamburg evaluated whether the use of the image integration module could help to reduce fluoroscopy time and burden and has influence on procedure duration in patients undergoing PVI due to paroxysmal AF. In a prospective 1:1-randomized trial that enrolled 60 patients, the use of CARTOUNIVU was investigated as an interventional therapy for paroxysmal AF, and also showed a significant reduction in fluoroscopy time and dose without any influence on the duration of the procedure.[19] Similar results were reported by Huo et al. for the ablation of AF.[20]

The CARTOUNIVU system is easy to integrate into an ablation workflow, is a great help in reducing radiation exposure, and has no negative impact on the procedure duration and complication rate.

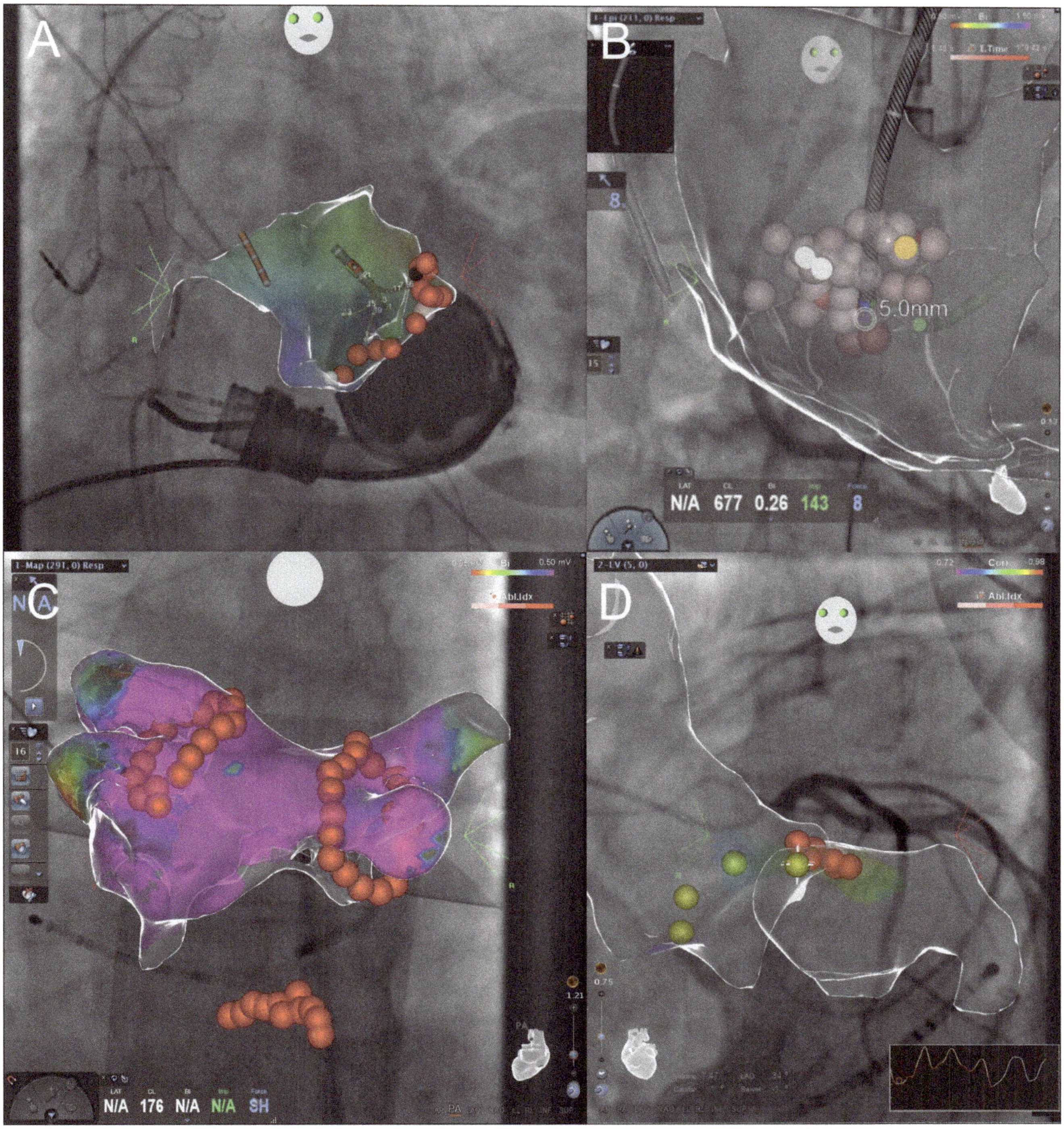

Figure 4.4 Illustration of using CARTOUNIVU technology. **A:** LAT-map and ablation of VT in a patient with left ventricular assist device (LVAD). **B:** Ablation of PVC with epicardial origin. The angiography of the right coronary artery was integrated via CARTOUNIVU and helped to maintain a sufficient distance during ablation. **C:** 3D reconstruction and bipolar voltage map of the left atrium and subsequent pulmonary vein isolation and cavotricuspid isthmus ablation in a patient with paroxysmal atrial fibrillation and typical atrial flutter. **D:** Ablation of PVC from the LCC with using CARTOUNIVU to visualize the distance to left coronary arteries.

General Recommendations

The presented image-integration tools contribute significantly to the reduction of fluoroscopy, but general rules of radiation protection should always be kept in mind. The effective reduction of radiation dose with low or extremely low frame-rate fluoroscopy without relevant impairment of therapeutic efficacy is well documented.[21,22]

Collimating to the minimum required visual fluoroscopy field as well as using low magnification and low tube voltages also leads to reduction of radiation exposure.[23] In addition, the possibility of intracardiac echocardiography reduces need for fluoroscopy, may improve outcomes, leads to shortening of procedure time, and offers early detection of complications such as pericardial effusion or thrombus formation.[24] This system is not widely used in Europe. The functionality and quality of the self-protective equipment should be observed at regular intervals.

Conclusions

Modern ablation strategies include low fluoroscopy time and radiation exposure as an important quality feature. The Non-Fluoroscopic Catheter Visualization (NFCV) Systems (MediGuide and the CARTOUNIVU Module) contribute significantly to this safety aspect and are easy to integrate into our ablation workflow without compromising patients' safety or procedure duration. Numerous studies have demonstrated the benefit of both systems in reducing need of fluoroscopy in catheter ablation of cardiac arrhythmias.

Acknowledgments

We thank Sebastian Riedel from Biosense Webster for carefully reading the chapter and providing technical advice.

References

1. Flugelman MY, Shiran A, Nusimovici-Avadis D, et al. Medical positioning system: A technical report. *EuroIntervention*. 2008;4(1):158–160.
2. Jeron A, Fredersdorf S, Debl K, et al. First-in-man (FIM) experience with the magnetic medical positioning system (MPS) for intracoronary navigation. *EuroIntervention*. 2009;5(5):552–557.
3. Sommer P, Richter S, Hindricks G, Rolf S. Non-fluoroscopic catheter visualization using MediGuide™ technology: Experience from the first 600 procedures. *J Interv Card Electrophysiol.* 2014;40(3):209–214.
4. Sommer P, Bertagnolli L, Kircher S, et al. Safety profile of near-zero fluoroscopy atrial fibrillation ablation with non-fluoroscopic catheter visualization: Experience from 1000 consecutive procedures. *Europace.* 2018.
5. Rolf S, Sommer P, Gaspar T, et al. Ablation of atrial fibrillation using novel 4-dimensional catheter tracking within autoregistered left atrial angiograms. *Circ Arrhythm Electrophysiol.* 2012;5(4):684–690.
6. Rolf S, John S, Gaspar T, et al. Catheter ablation of atrial fibrillation supported by novel non-fluoroscopic 4D navigation technology. *Heart Rhythm.* 2013;10(9):1293–1300.
7. Sommer P, Wojdyla-Hordynska A, Rolf S, et al. Initial experience in ablation of typical atrial flutter using a novel three-dimensional catheter tracking system. *Europace.* 2013;15(4):578–581.
8. Schoene K, Rolf S, Schloma D, et al. Ablation of typical atrial flutter using a non-fluoroscopic catheter tracking system vs. conventional fluoroscopy—results from a prospective randomized study. *Europace.* 2015;17(7):1117–1121.
9. Richter S, Döring M, Gaspar T, et al. Cardiac resynchronization therapy device implantation using a new sensor-based navigation system: Results from the first human use study. *Circ Arrhythm Electrophysiol.* 2013;6(5):917–923.
10. Döring M, Sommer P, Rolf S, et al. Sensor-based electromagnetic navigation to facilitate implantation of left ventricular leads in cardiac resynchronization therapy. *J Cardiovasc Electrophysiol.* 2015;26(2):167–175.
11. Piorkowski C, Breithardt OA, Razavi H, et al. Mapping-guided characterization of mechanical and electrical activation patterns in patients with normal systolic function using a sensor-based tracking technology. *Europace.* 2017;19(10):1700-1709.
12. Piorkowski C, Arya A, Markovitz CD, et al. Characterizing left ventricular mechanical and electrical activation in patients with normal and impaired systolic function using a non-fluoroscopic cardiovascular navigation system. *J Interv Card Electrophysiol.* 2018;51(3):205–214.
13. Borlich M, Iden L, Kuhnhardt K, Paetsch I, Hindricks G, Sommer P. 3D Mapping for PVI- geometry, image integration and incorporation of contact force into work flow. *J Atr Fibrillation.* 2018;10(6):1795.
14. De Potter T, Bardhaj G, Viggiano A, Morrice K, Geelen P. Three-dimensional rotational angiography as a periprocedural imaging tool in atrial fibrillation ablation. *Arrhythm Electrophysiol Rev.* 2014;3(3):173–176.
15. Cano Ó, Alonso P, Osca J, et al. Initial experience with a new image integration module designed for reducing radiation exposure during electrophysiological ablation procedures. *J Cardiovasc Electrophysiol.* 2015;26(6):662–670.
16. Christoph M, Wunderlich C, Moebius S, et al. Fluoroscopy integrated 3D mapping significantly reduces radiation exposure during ablation for a wide spectrum of cardiac arrhythmias. *Europace.* 2015;17(6):928–937.
17. Reents T, Buiatti A, Ammar S, et al. Catheter ablation of ventricular arrhythmias using a fluoroscopy image integration module. *Pacing Clin Electrophysiol.* 2015;38(6):700–705.
18. Cano Ó, Andrés A, Osca J, et al. Safety and feasibility of a minimally fluoroscopic approach for ventricular tachycardia ablation in patients with structural heart disease: Influence of the ventricular tachycardia substrate. *Circ Arrhythm Electrophysiol.* 2016;9(2):e003706.
19. Akbulak R, Schäffer B, Jularic M, et al. Reduction of radiation exposure in atrial fibrillation ablation using a new image integration module: A prospective randomized trial in patients undergoing pulmonary vein isolation. *J Cardiovasc Electrophysiol.* 2015;26(7):747–753.

20. Huo Y, Christoph M, Forkmann M, et al. Reduction of radiation exposure during atrial fibrillation ablation using a novel fluoroscopy image integrated 3-dimensional electroanatomic mapping system: A prospective, randomized, single-blind, and controlled study. *Heart Rhythm.* 2015; 12(9):1945–1955.
21. Lee JH, Kim J, Kim M, et al. Extremely low-frame-rate digital fluoroscopy in catheter ablation of atrial fibrillation: A comparison of 2 versus 4 frame rate. *Medicine (Baltimore).* 2017;96(24):e7200.
22. Crowhurst J, Haqqani H, Wright D, et al. Ultra-low radiation dose during electrophysiology procedures using optimized new generation fluoroscopy technology. *Pacing Clin Electrophysiol.* 2017;40(8):947–954.
23. Walters TE, Kistler PM, Morton JB, Sparks PB, Halloran K, Kalman JM. Impact of collimation on radiation exposure during interventional electrophysiology. *Europace.* 2012;14(11):1670–1673.
24. Enriquez A, Saenz LC, Rosso R, et al. Use of intracardiac echocardiography in interventional cardiology: Working with the anatomy rather than fighting it. *Circulation.* 2018; 137(21):2278–2294.

Video Legend

Video 4.1 Ablation of atypical atrial flutter using Precision as the 3D mapping system and MediGuide for non-fluoroscopic catheter visualization. Mapping with a circular mapping catheter reveals counterclockwise perimitral flutter in LAT and sparkle map (TCL 211 ms). Ablation of anterior isthmus line prolongs TCL to 237 ms. New map shows localized septal reentry with a PPI = TCL at the septal annulus. Ablation here terminates the tachycardia. LAT map during SR proves the complete block of the septal line with a delay over the line of >150 ms. Final fluoroscopy time of the procedure is 0.3 min; radiation dose is 191 μGy · m^2. [3:11]

5

How to Obtain Central Vascular Access Using Real-Time Ultrasound

Carola Gianni, MD; Carlos Monreal, CVT; Zachary J. Rosenblatt, CVT; Jason T. Engel, CVT; Clayton Robison, CVT; Rodney P. Horton, MD; Andrea Natale, MD; Amin Al-Ahmad, MD

Introduction

Traditionally, vascular access is performed relying on landmarks based on the knowledge of the so-called "normal" anatomy. Yet, anatomic variations are common and cannot be identified using a landmark technique, leading to complications or unsuccessful cannulation. By allowing direct visualization of vascular targets, ultrasound (US) reduces the need for multiple attempts and inadvertent puncture of surrounding structures. US-guided central vascular access is standard of care and, as such, should be performed in every electrophysiology lab.[1,2] Of note, there are two strategies when using US for vascular access: *static* or *dynamic/real-time*. With static US-guided vascular access, US is used only to visualize the anatomy and identify the entry point on the skin over the vessel before obtaining access. However, to gain the most advantage, US has to be used dynamically throughout the procedure, with direct visualization of the needle finding its way into the vessel and to confirm correct placement of the wire before advancing the sheath.[3] Real-time US-guided access requires combining knowledge about anatomy with specific technical skills (i.e., probe manipulation, transforming 2D images into a 3D impression of the anatomy, hand-eye coordination), but when performed properly, it is both rewarding and de facto eliminates complications. This chapter will focus on the use of real-time US to facilitate access, a technique that can be employed safely by any trained operator involved in electrophysiology procedures.

Equipment

The following equipment (**Figure 5.1**) is needed:

- US machine with 2D and Doppler imaging
- linear, high-frequency (5 to 12 MHz) US probe
  - it provides appropriate resolution and penetration for central vascular access
- US conducting gel (can be nonsterile), applied to the head of the probe
- sterile sleeve
  - it covers the probe and its cord to maintain sterility
  - it is important to smooth the sleeve over the probe to remove any air bubbles and fasten it into place with one or two sterile elastic bands
- sterile saline (or equivalent sterile fluids)
  - it is used as a conductive medium over the skin instead of sterile gel (which is expensive and messy)

Fluoroscopy Reduction Techniques for Catheter Ablation of Cardiac Arrhythmias. © 2019 Mansour Razminia, Paul C. Zei, eds. Cardiotext Publishing, ISBN: 978-1-942909-30-9.

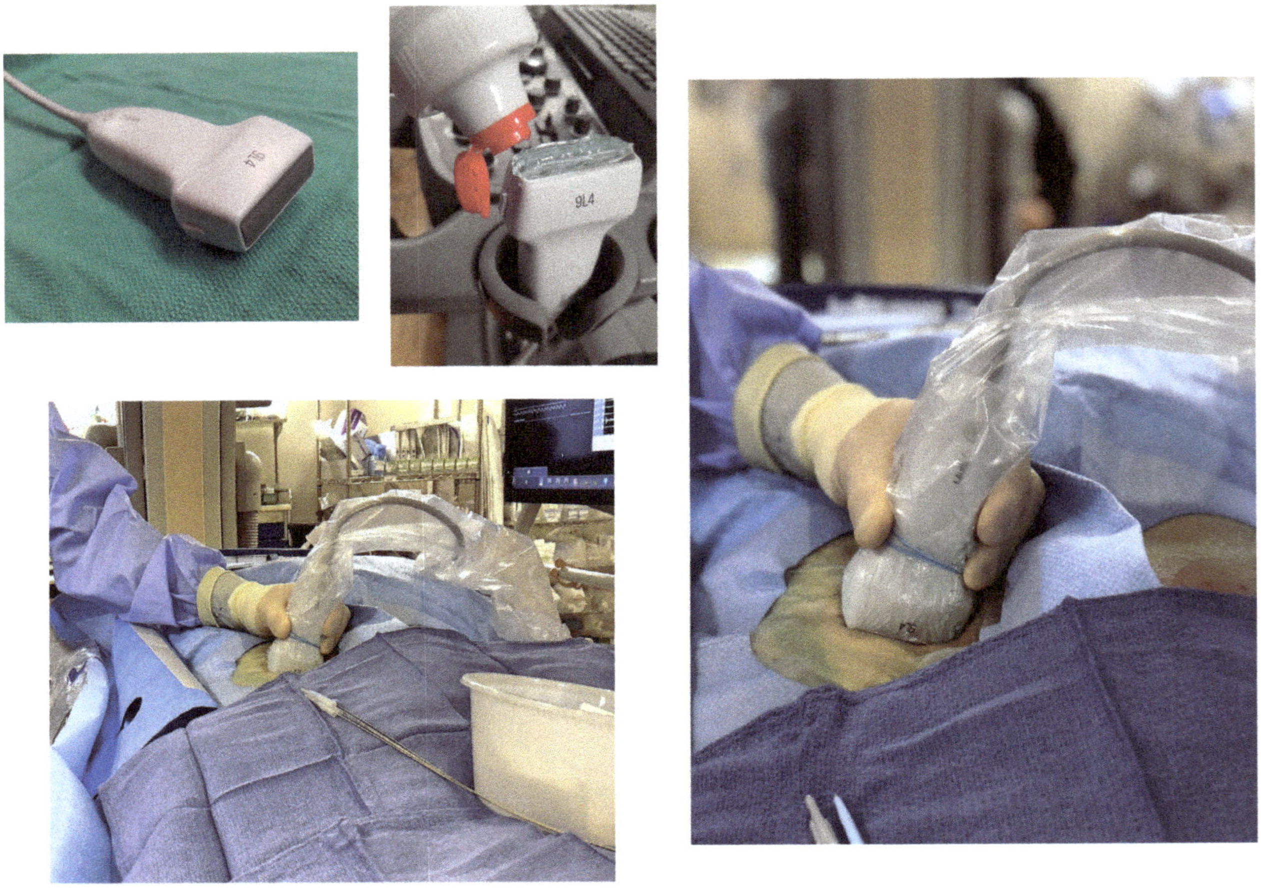

Figure 5.1 Equipment for ultrasound-guided central vascular access.

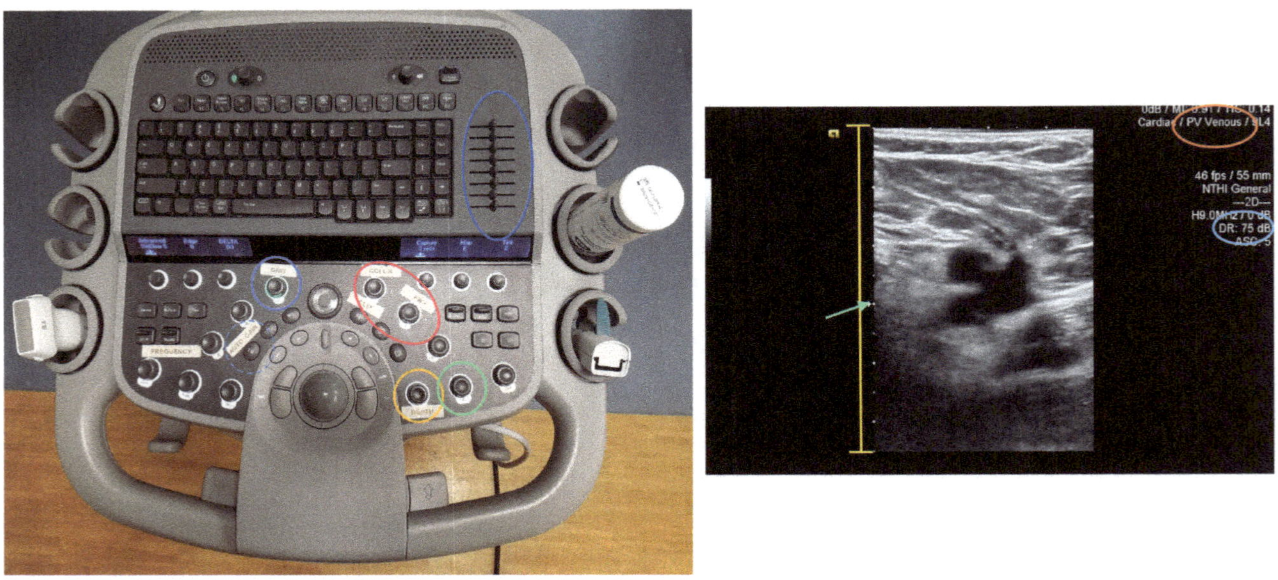

Figure 5.2 Relevant ultrasound machine settings.
Orange circle: preset; **yellow circle:** depth; **blue oval:** gain (light, overall gain; dark, time gain compensation); **green circle:** focus; **pink:** Doppler.

Ultrasound Machine Setup

There are a few image settings in every US machine that are important to optimize the image (**Figure 5.2**), and everyone involved in US-guided access should be familiar with:

- presets
  - most US machines have a "central vascular access" (or similar nomenclature) preset, which should be selected before starting the procedure
  - they usually need to be further optimized by adjusting the depth, gain, and—optionally—focus, according to the operator preference and patient's own anatomy
- depth
  - it is indicated by the *cm* markings on the side of the image (set at 0.5- to 1-cm increments)
  - it is useful to begin with a high depth to get a big picture and then gradually decrease the depth when the target vessel is found
  - depth should be set to keep the target vessel at about mid to three-quarters of the screen
    - this allows the operator to visualize important deep structures (i.e., another vessel or lung), which should be avoided by not advancing the needle past the target
  - in practice
    - a fixed depth of 5.5 to 6 cm is adequate for most femoral access sites and can be used for jugular and subclavian access, with no need to change the depth
    - for subclavian access, adjusting the depth to properly visualize the ribs/pleural lining is key to avoid complications
- gain, i.e., the brightness of the image
  - it can be changed either overall with a dedicated control knob (marked as *gain*) or with separate sliders that fine-tune the gain at different depths (near vs. far field gain; *time gain compensation*)
  - adjusting the gain helps to distinguish structures on the screen; the amount of gain depends on personal preference, but it should be adjusted so that vascular structures appear dark
  - most US machines have an *auto-gain* knob, which sets the gain to what the machine considers optimal (results may vary)
- focus (optional), i.e., the level of depth with the best image quality
  - it is usually marked as a small arrow/triangle on the side of the image and, by default, positioned at a mid-to-high depth
  - for central vascular access, it is not necessary to adjust the focus, unless good visualization of small structures is warranted (i.e., to locate small collaterals)
- Doppler
  - it helps to distinguish vascular structures and assess for patency (see below)

Probe Manipulation

To perform effective US imaging, one should be familiar with probe manipulation (**Figure 5.3**). The following are important to understand:

- orientation
  - before starting, care should be taken to identify the side of the probe with the *indicator mark* (usually, a small physical notch), which corresponds to the on-screen indicator
    - if the notch is not found, or the orientation is not clear, a finger can be rubbed on one side of the probe head: the corresponding movement localized on one side of the screen will confirm the orientation
  - the left side of the screen should display the right side of the patient; (i.e., if the on-screen indicator is positioned on the left side of the screen—standard for vascular access imaging—the probe marker should point to the patient's right)
- pressure
  - the right amount of pressure can improve the image quality, affecting the tissue echogenicity
    - too little pressure gives insufficient contact with the skin and a dark image result
    - too much pressure can distort or obliterate structures (most importantly, central veins and their collaterals)
- sliding
  - it can be done in a lateral-medial or cranial-caudal direction
  - it is used to find the target vessel and position it optimally on the screen for needle advancement

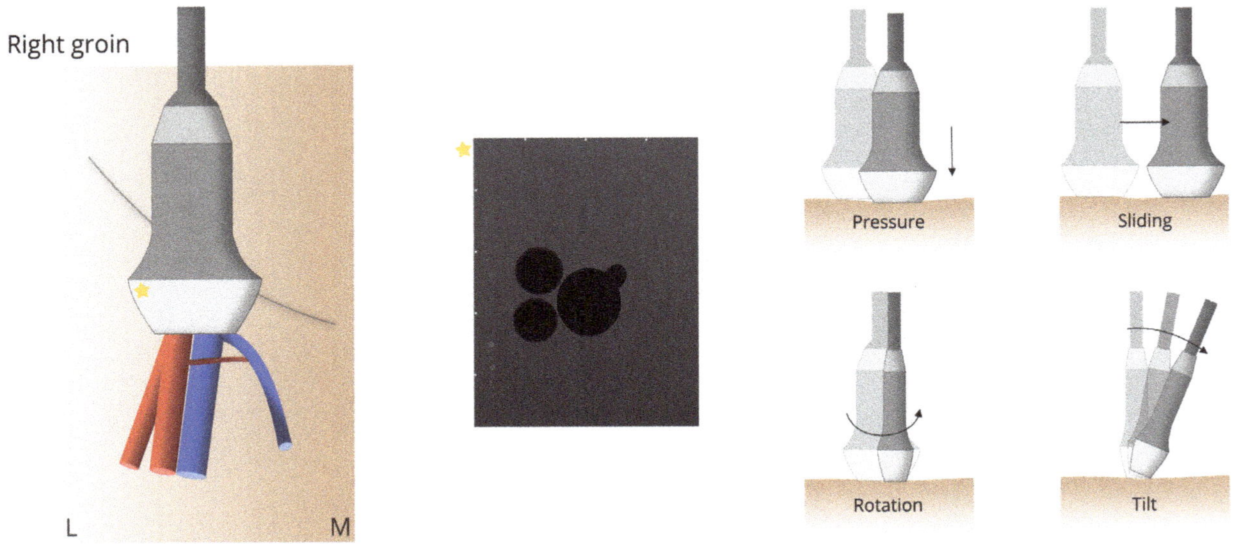

Figure 5.3 Probe orientation and manipulation.
L: lateral; M: medial.

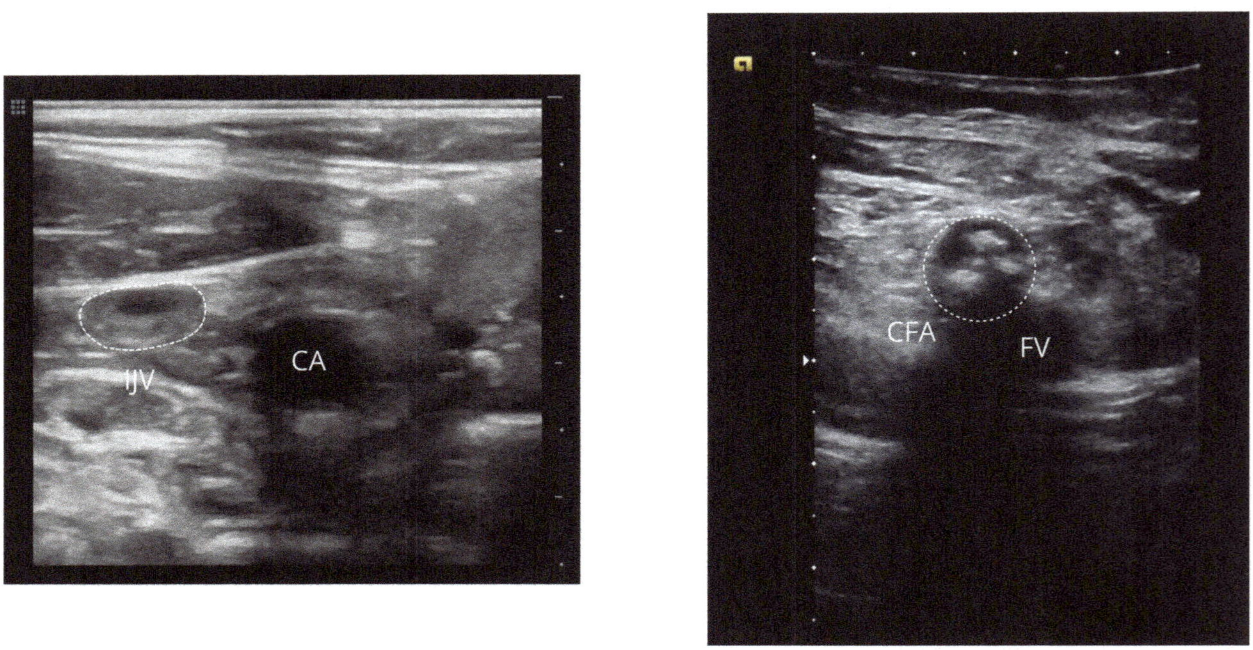

Figure 5.4 Partial thrombosis of the internal jugular vein (**left**), severe atherosclerosis of the common femoral artery (**right**).
CA: carotid artery; CFA: common femoral artery; FV: femoral vein; IJV: internal jugular vein.

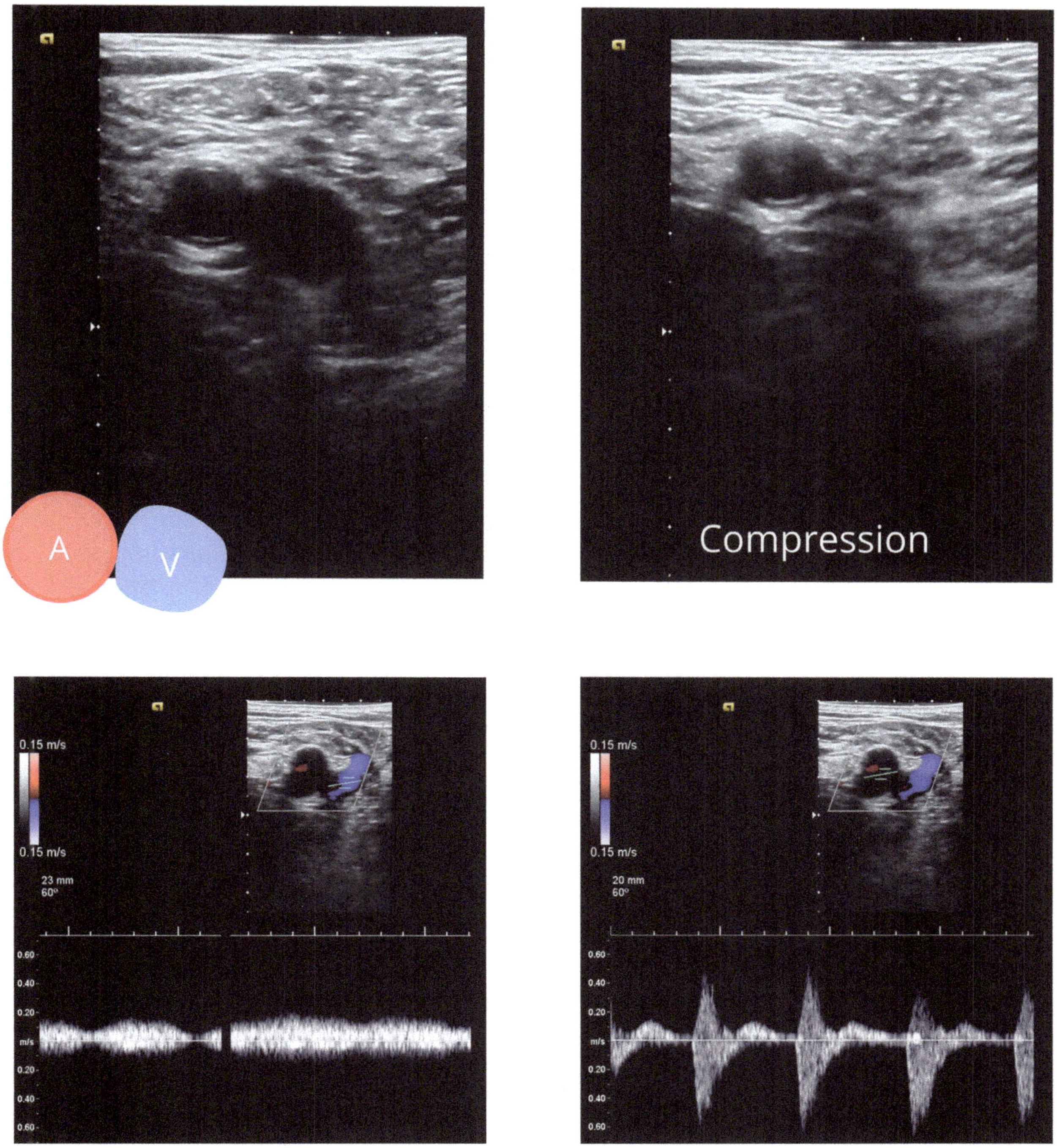

Figure 5.5 Artery vs. vein.

        - it is also important for scouting the vessel proximally and distally to the target site, in order to identify important surrounding structures
- rotation
    - it is used to obtain different axial views of the structure of interest
        - in the case of vessels, these are the so-called short- and long-axis view (see below)
        - for a long-axis view, it is good practice to rotate the probe so that the indicator mark points to the patient's head (the left side of the screen will display cranial structures)
- tilt
    - it is performed by changing the angle that the probe makes with the skin
    - for access, it is used to follow the needle when obtaining access with a short-axis view technique (see below)

Before Starting

A quick scan of the access site should be performed to identify the target vessel and surrounding anatomical structures. It is important to:

- confirm the patency of the target vessel (**Figure 5.4**)
    - exclude thrombosis (isoechoic/grey mass) or significant atherosclerosis (hyperechoic/white mass)
- assess its dimensions
    - relative to the diameter of the sheath(s) meant to be used
- assess its depth from the skin
    - this is critical to have an idea of the depth that the needle must pass to reach the vessel lumen
- visualize important surrounding structures (see relative sections)

Artery vs. Vein

Whether it is venous or arterial access, it is important to be able to distinguish between the two structures (**Figure 5.5**). As tubular fluid-filled vessels, arteries and veins have a similar appearance on a grayscale US image, i.e., they look like anechoic (black) circles surrounded by soft tissue. There are a few ways to distinguish an artery from a vein:

- arteries have thicker hyperechoic walls (the media)
- veins collapse with a relatively little pressure
    - however, both can collapse with enough pressure, i.e., > systolic blood pressure
    - full-lumen venous thrombosis will make the vein noncompressible
- arteries are pulsatile
    - pulsatility is accentuated with partial arterial compression
    - veins can be pulsatile in cases of high enough right atrial and/or central venous pressure
- Doppler imaging (color and pulsed-wave)
    - to identify the presence of blood flow (patency of the vessel)
    - to differentiate arterial (pulsatile, high velocity) and venous (continuous, low velocity) flow

Occasionally, the target vessel cannot be visualized. For the vein, this is usually due to hypovolemia: reducing the probe pressure or increasing the venous pressure (i.e., Valsalva, fluid administration) helps. In rare instances, the vessel might be absent, due to agenesis or chronic total occlusion (clot is similar in echogenicity to that of the surrounding tissues), and a different access point should be sought.

Short-Axis vs. Long-Axis Approach

When getting access, the US image plane can be oriented relative to the vessel in two ways (**Figure 5.6**):

- short-axis view
    - the US plane is perpendicular to the course of the vessel and needle
    - on the screen, vessels appear as anechoic circles while the needle is visualized as a hyperechoic point
    - it provides information about structures adjacent to the target vessel
    - it allows to direct the needle precisely over the center of the vessel
    - the needle artifact is only a cross section of the needle; therefore, it could be the tip but also any part of the shaft
        - care must be taken to fan the US plane by tilting/sliding the probe as the needle advances to always track the tip (see below)
- long-axis view
    - the US plane is parallel to the course of the vessel and needle

- the image shows the course of the vessel across the screen and the entire needle shaft and tip needle as it is advanced
- it does not allow to see simultaneously adjacent structures (typically, the artery) that might be important to avoid, nor to precisely aim toward the center of the vessel
- it is difficult to keep the US plane in line with the needle and the midline axis vessel: even a 1-mm slip of the US plane off to the side will result in a useless image

No technique is better than the other, and it is a matter of preference to decide which strategy to use. A short-axis approach is easier, but it is frequently performed incorrectly, keeping the probe still without following the needle, a de facto static US-guided approach. For this reason, the long-axis approach may be more appropriate to use when knowing the tip location is crucial (i.e., subclavian vein, to avoid inadvertent lung puncture). However, with experience and care, the short-axis approach is adequate to follow the needle tip location (see below). Alternatively, one may start with a short-axis view to ensure that the needle is centered over the middle of the vessel and then rotate the probe to a long-axis plane view as the needle is advanced.

Technique, General Aspects

These are the steps to follow to get access under US guidance:

- orientation of the target vessel
  - when using a short-axis approach, the target vessel is aligned to the center of the screen; this way, it lies underneath the center of the US probe
  - in the long-axis approach, care should be taken to visualize the vessel along the whole length of the screen
- if necessary, local anesthetic can be infiltrated above the vessel under US guidance
  - it is important to inject a small amount before getting access, because the image can become significantly clouded, preventing visualization
  - after confirming the correct position of the wire, before advancing the sheath, it is possible to add more anesthetic
- orientation of the needle
  - in the short axis-approach, the needle should enter the skin directly underneath the middle of the probe, with a 60- to 80-degree angle (depending on the depth of the vessel)
  - in the long-axis approach, the needle enters the skin directly underneath the probe, with a shallower angle (45 to 60 degrees) to facilitate visualization
- the focus of the operator should be on the screen and not the hands, looking for the hyperechogenic needle entering the skin and advancing through the subcutaneous tissue
  - the needle can be difficult to visualize; a surrogate visual cue is movement of the surrounding tissue, which is accentuated by slightly wiggling the needle
  - **it is important to follow the needle tip throughout**
    - this is easy with a long-axis approach, although keeping the US plane in line might be challenging
    - with a short-axis approach (**Figure 5.7**), it is easy to misinterpret the shaft of the needle as the tip
      - to maintain imaging of the tip, it is crucial to keep tilting or sliding the probe so that it is always slightly ahead of the needle
        - the needle artifact disappears as the US plane lies distal from the tip of the needle (vanishing target sign)
        - this is easier to do with a steeper angle of the needle relative to the skin surface (less distance to cover, less frequent probe movement)
      - tenting of the front wall may be seen as the tip of the needle is entering the vessel, but this is less evident with sharper needles and does not replace careful imaging of the tip
  - aspirate at all times, even when withdrawing the needle
    - when a flash of blood is aspirated, stop and locate the needle tip
      - if the needle is in the target vessel, proceed as described below
      - if the needle is in an adjacent vessel, withdraw the needle right below the skin and reorient its trajectory to avoid them
- a tactile "pop" of the needle may be experienced as the needle passes through the front wall of the vessel; at the same time a free-flowing flash of blood should be aspirated in the syringe

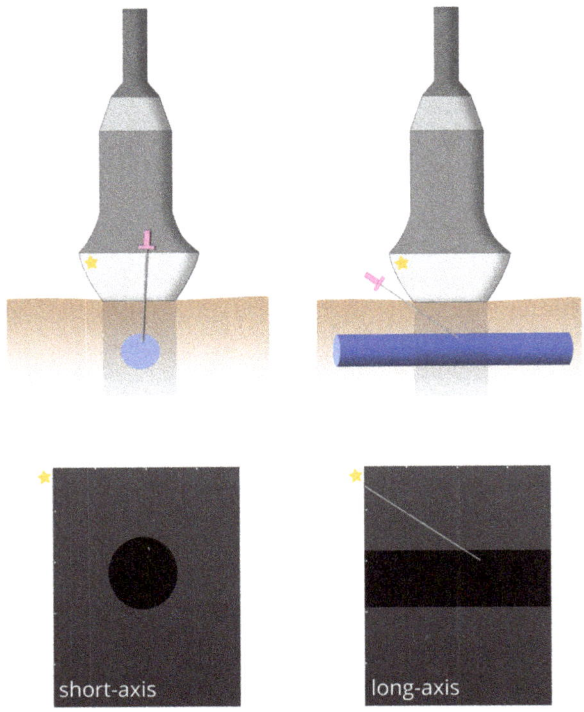

Figure 5.6 Short-axis vs. long-axis approach.

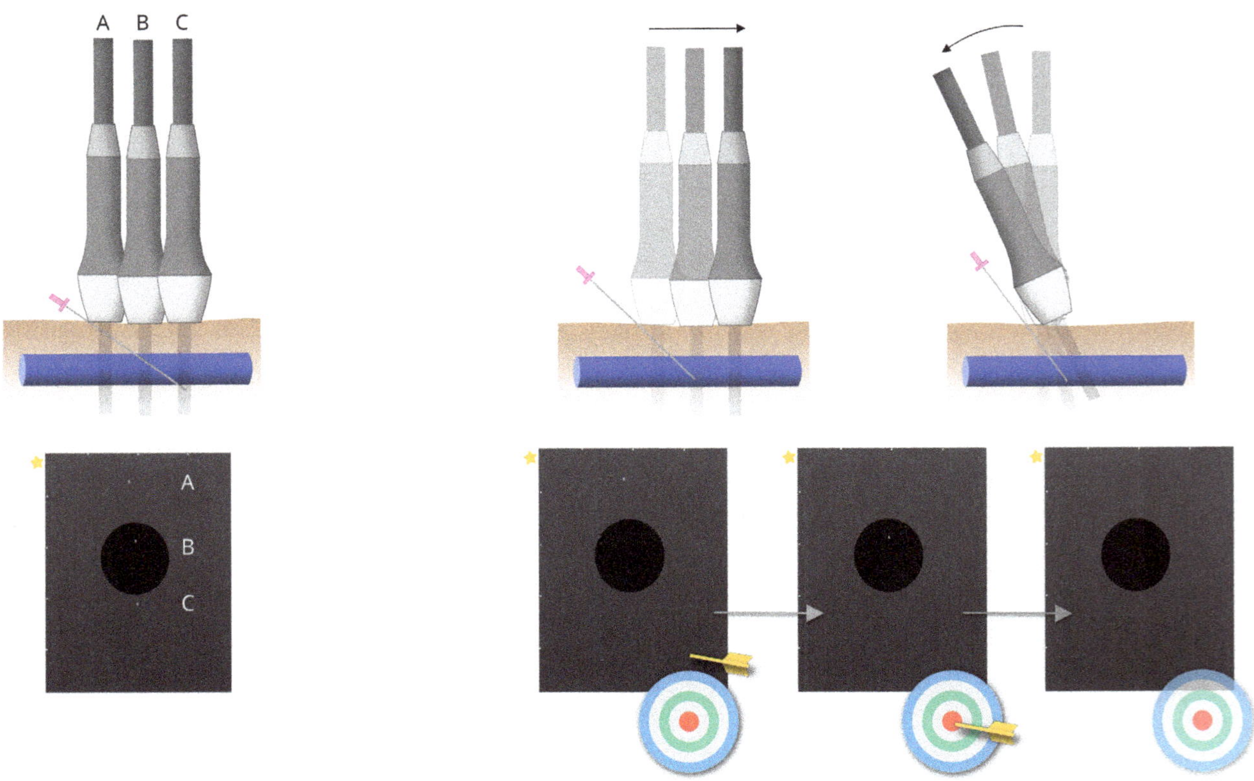

Figure 5.7 Keeping track of the needle tip in a short-axis approach.

- if there is no blood return, the needle is not within the lumen of the vessel
  - this is usually due to overshooting the needle and going through the posterior wall of the vessel ("back-walling"); gentle retraction of the needle is all that is needed
  - with arterial access, this is also observed when the tip is in a subintimal position; never advance the wire, as it might result in dissection
- if the flow is slow, this is usually secondary to the needle being close to the vessel wall
  - if the puncture is at the edge of the vessel, the best course of action is retracting the needle and starting over, aiming at the middle of the vessel anterior wall
  - if the needle is too close to the anterior or posterior wall of the vessel, this might result in losing access before advancing the wire, even with subtle movements of the needle
    - under US-guidance, the needle should be slightly advanced or retracted (according to the position of the needle tip) until free flow is achieved
- with good flow, the wire should advance freely; if any resistance is felt, it is better to stop and reassess the needle tip position to avoid advancing the wire outside of the target vessel leading to complications (i.e., surrounding soft tissue > hematoma, lung > pneumothorax, or subintima > dissection)

- with the needle tip confirmed to be in the middle lumen of the vessel, the US probe can be set aside, and the wire advanced without US guidance
  - to facilitate advancement of the wire, the angle of the needle can be decreased slightly while blood is continuously aspirated to confirm that an intraluminal location of the needle tip is maintained
  - with profound vessels (deeper than 6 cm), which are visualized only while compressing the soft tissue with the US probe, it is important to keep the probe in place when advancing the wire
    - removing the probe will result in expansion of the soft tissue, with subsequent retraction of the needle and loss of access
    - a single operator can hold both the probe and needle with one hand, while using the other to advance the wire
    - if someone else is scrubbed in, they can remove the syringe and advance the wire while the first operator keeps the probe and needle in place
- before advancing the sheath, it is important to visualize the wire with US (**Figure 5.8**)
  - long-axis view
    - both the artery and the vein should be visualized by sliding in a lateral-medial direction
    - it is important to confirm that the wire
      - is properly placed in the lumen of the target vessel (risk of hematoma/dissection, **Figure 5.9**)
      - is not going through surrounding vessels (risk of AV fistula/hematoma)
    - occasionally, to exclude back-walling of the wire, it might be necessary to pull it back and visualize the J-tip freely floating in the lumen
  - short-axis view
    - it is useful to confirm that the wire is entering the vessel at or close to the middle of the anterior wall
      - this is especially important when planning to use vascular closure devices
    - for internal jugular vein access, it allows confirmation of proper placement in the superior vena cava as opposed to the subclavian vein (see below)

Technique, Specific Tips

Femoral Vein

- important surrounding structures (**Figure 5.10**)
  - femoral artery and its collaterals
    - below the bifurcation, the femoral vein typically runs below the superficial femoral artery, whereas above, the common femoral artery lies next to the femoral vein
    - the most important collaterals are
      - external pudendal artery, a branch of the femoral artery (usually, superficial) which runs on top the femoral vein close to the saphenofemoral junction
      - medial circumflex femoral artery, a branch of the common femoral artery with runs below the femoral vein

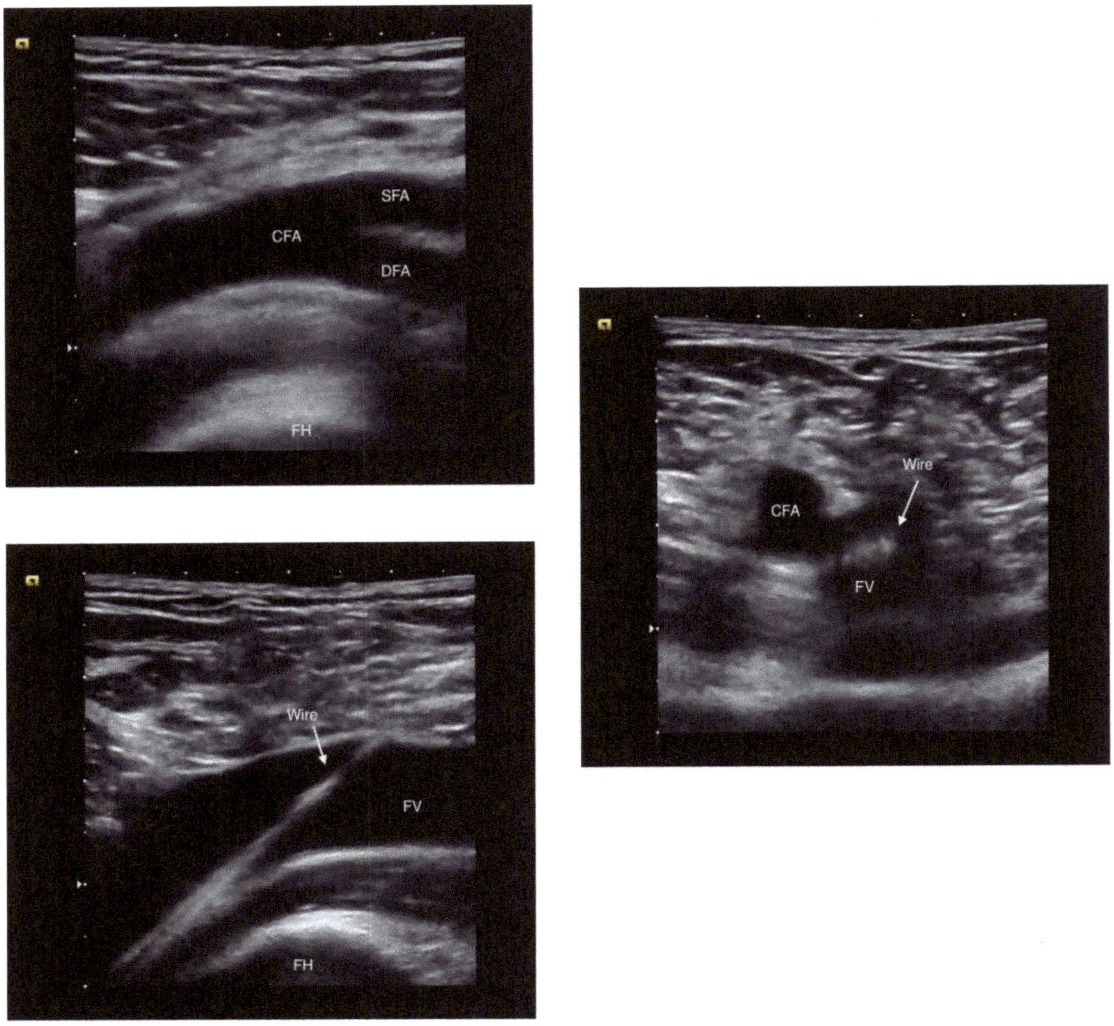

Figure 5.8 Wire visualization.
CFA: common femoral artery; DFA: deep femoral artery; FH: femoral head; FV: femoral vein; SFA: superficial femoral artery.

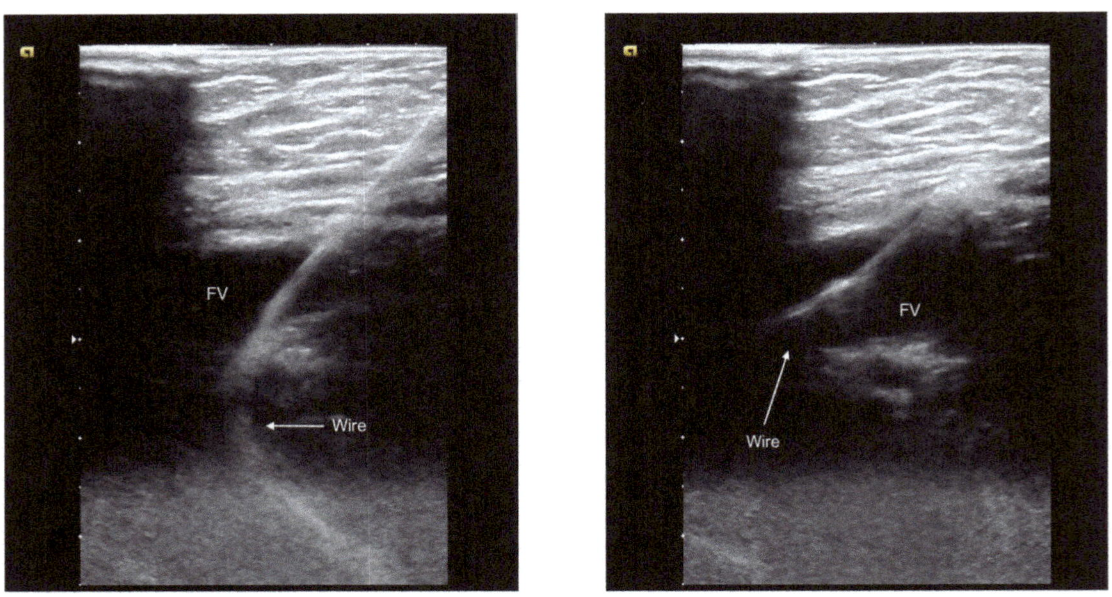

Figure 5.9 Wire back-walling the vein (**left**), subsequently repositioned (**right**).
FV: femoral vein.

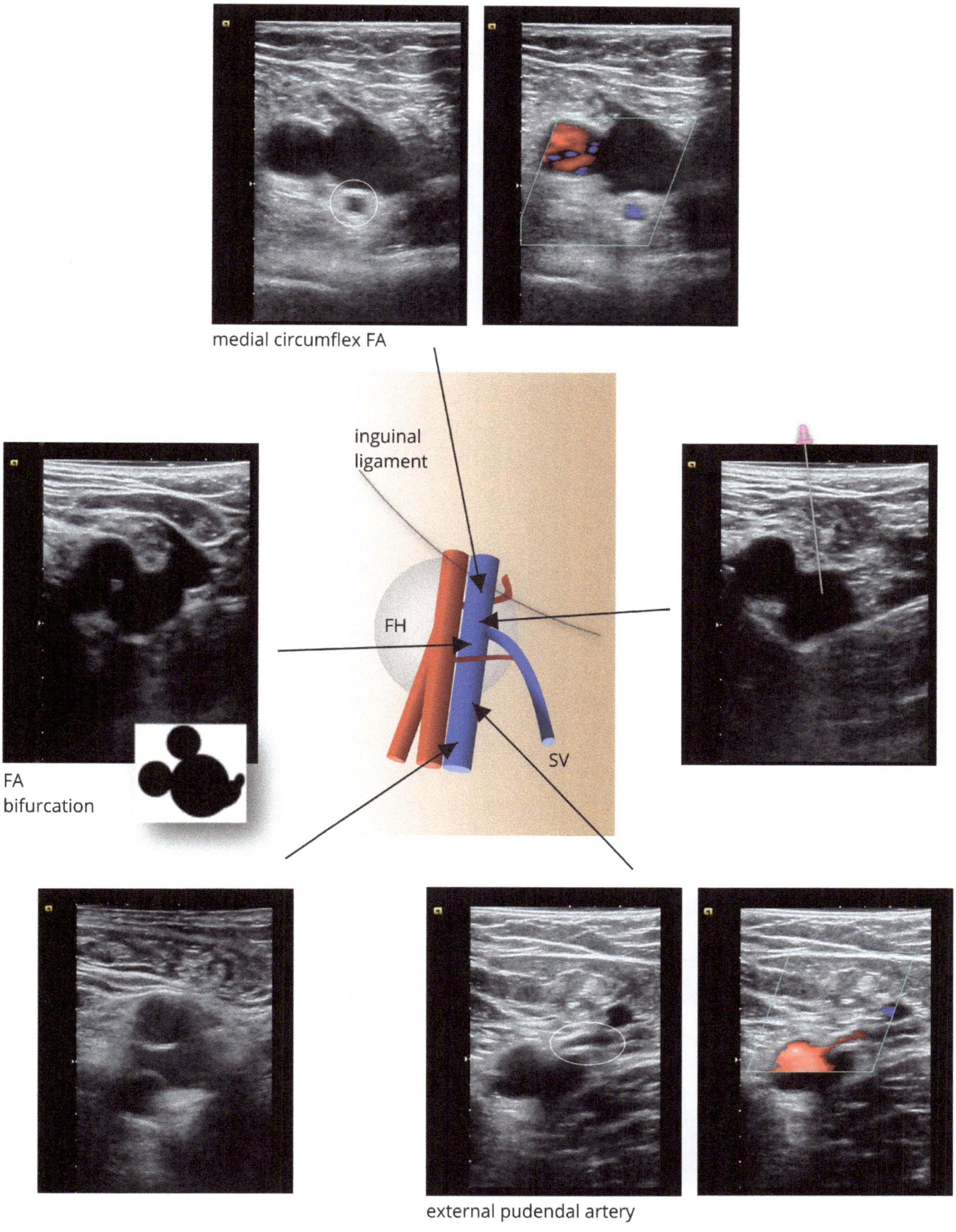

Figure 5.10 Femoral vein access.
FA: femoral artery; FH: femoral head; SV: saphenous vein.

- saphenous vein and its collaterals
  - these are easily visualized on US running on top of the femoral vein
  - they should be avoided by carefully following the needle tip throughout; going through a collateral might result in its laceration and subsequent hematoma
- peritoneal cavity
  - it is important to locate the inguinal ligament with bony landmarks as usual (i.e., anterior superior iliac spine and pubic tubercle)
  - access should never be obtained at or above the level where the vein dives down the abdominal cavity

- access should be obtained right above the femoral artery bifurcation (Mickey Mouse sign) at the level of the saphenofemoral junction (Figure 5.10)
  - this prevents going through most of the venous and arterial collaterals, even if the tip of the needle is not followed throughout
  - sometimes the femoral artery bifurcation is high, so it is always important to know where the inguinal ligament/femoral head lie to avoid an intraperitoneal puncture; in these cases, it is important to carefully scan the target access site looking for collaterals
- before inserting the sheath, it is good practice to confirm that the entry point of the wire is not too high or too low, relative to the femoral head (Figure 5.9), to prevent hematomas (both retroperitoneal and groin) due to inadequate compression at the time of sheath removal

Femoral Artery

- important surrounding structures
  - femoral vein and its collateral
    - easy to visualize and avoid with US
  - femoral nerve
    - it lies lateral to the femoral artery
    - obtaining access over the middle of the vessel prevents nerve injury
  - peritoneal cavity (see above)
- access should be obtained in the common femoral artery, above the femoral artery bifurcation (Mickey Mouse sign), in the middle of the anterior wall of the vessel, at the level of the femoral head (**Figure 5.11**)
  - for arterial access, the femoral head should be visualized (best seen in a long-axis view) before choosing the target site, which should always lie on top of the bone for effective compression after sheath removal
  - if the femoral artery bifurcation is high (see above), the superficial femoral artery at the level of the femoral head is the preferred target
- one should always confirm that the needle tip lies in the center of the vessel, with good blood flow, being careful not to move the needle any time before advancing the wire
  - partial needle insertion is possible, and advancing the wire when resistance is felt can lead to arterial dissection
- more importantly than with femoral vein access, before inserting the sheath it is essential to confirm that the entry point is over the femoral head to prevent hematomas (both retroperitoneal and groin) and pseudoaneurysms due to inadequate compression
- US is also useful when using vascular closure devices
  - to obtain access in an optimal location
    - middle of the anterior wall of the artery
    - above the bifurcation (if possible, and necessary)
  - to confirm proper deployment
    - most closure devices have distinctive features that can be sought; for example (**Figure 5.12**)
      - mixed hyper-hypoechoic (white-dark grey, black) areas are typically seen over the arterial wall access site for devices using collagen plugs
      - hyperechoic (white) lines can be seen at the level of the arterial wall access site, representing the intraarterial anchors/clips
    - suture-based devices can't be seen directly, but US can be used to confirm proper hemostasis
  - to confirm hemostasis

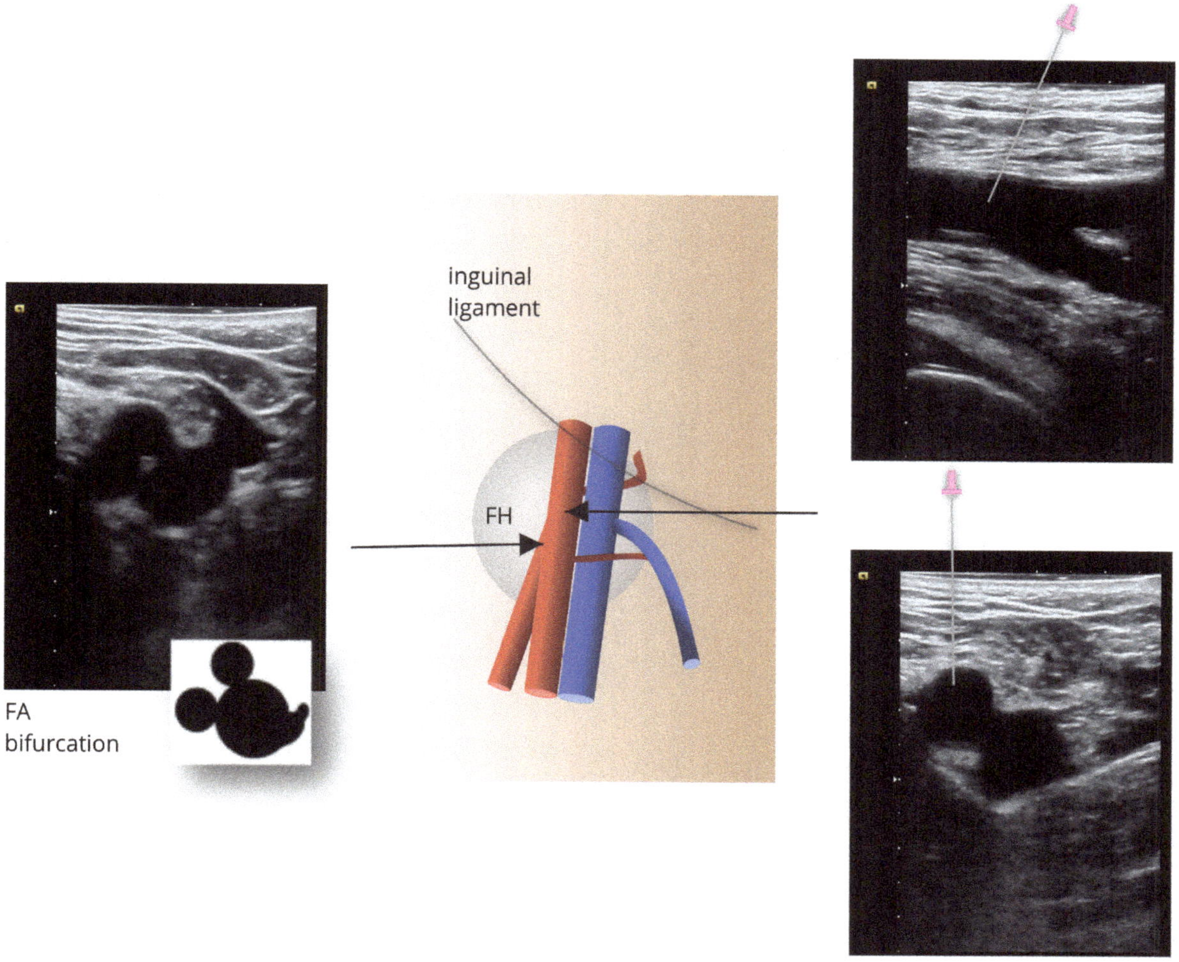

Figure 5.11 Femoral artery access.
FA: femoral artery; FH: femoral head; SV: saphenous vein.

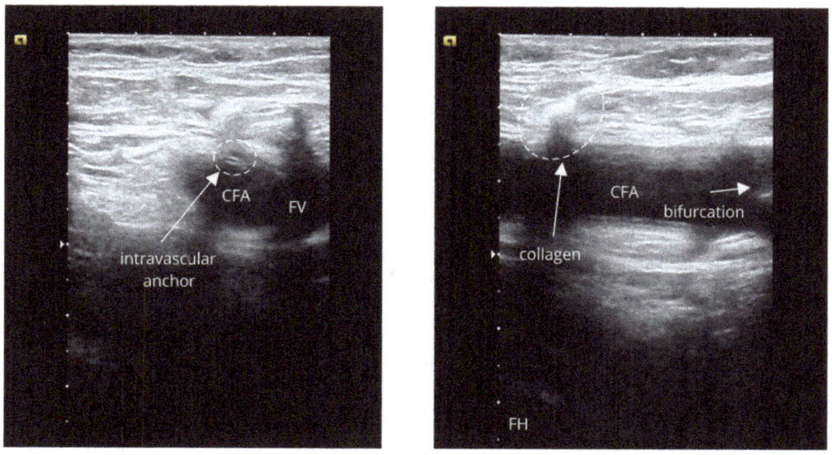

Figure 5.12 Vascular closure devices.
CFA: common femoral artery; FH: femoral head; FV: femoral vein.

Internal Jugular Vein

- important surrounding structures (**Figure 5.13**)
  - carotid artery
    - it usually lies medial to the internal jugular vein
    - sometimes, the carotid artery and internal jugular vein overlap
      - a full scan of the neck is useful to find a location without or with minimal overlap
      - rotation of the head is not necessary, and sometimes detrimental as it increases overlap
      - if overlap is still present, the best approach is choosing an angle of entrance so that, if the needle back-walls the vein, it won't enter the carotid artery
  - inferior thyroid artery
    - a collateral of the subclavian artery that lies below the internal jugular vein in the lower neck area
    - it is easily visualized with US and can be spared by either changing the angle of the needle or avoiding back-walling
  - external jugular vein
    - it usually runs lateral to the internal jugular vein
    - it is easy to compress with the probe, therefore can be missed on US
      - visual inspection of the neck before access should be performed to avoid going through (leading to hematoma)
  - subclavian artery
    - sometimes can run in the lower aspect of the neck, above the clavicle
    - it is easily visualized and avoided with US
  - nerves
    - they are usually lateral or deep and can be avoided by keeping the needle in line with the vein and avoid back-walling
  - lung
    - if one can see the pleural lining with US, the access site is too low; even if the lung is not punctured, compression will be difficult, leading to hematomas
    - even in higher neck areas, a steep angle of the needle is important to avoid inadvertent lung puncture
- if the vein is small or easily collapsible, a Valsalva maneuver effectively increases the internal jugular vein size (**Figure 5.14**)
- the best site for access is where the vein is more likely to be superficial and lateral to the carotid artery; this is usually in the mid to lower third of the neck
  - the angle of the needle should be as steep as possible (close to 90 degrees)
    - before advancing the wire, the angle can be reduced, making sure to retain access (either visualizing the needle tip or confirming good blood flow until removing the syringe)
  - care should be taken not to back-wall the needle, to avoid surrounding arteries and the lung
    - the vein is usually superficial
      - the needle should be advanced slowly and with small increments, always visualizing its tip on the US plane
      - never advance the needle beyond the anticipated depth of the vein (usually 1 to 2 cm), as assessed during the pre-access scan
    - the skin of the neck and internal jugular vein itself are fairly elastic: a sharp (arterial access needle) or smaller-gauge needle should be used to minimize tenting and subsequent back-walling
- before inserting the sheath, it is good practice to confirm that the wire goes down the superior vena cava vs. subclavian vein (**Figure 5.15**)
  - this is done by tilting the probe at the level of the clavicle until the superior vena cava is visualized with the wire running in it
- if any doubt of inadvertent lung puncture exists, lung sliding can be easily assessed using US to prove absence of pneumothorax
  - lung US is beyond the scope of this chapter, but as an easy and useful skill to master, it is highly recommended.

Subclavian/Axillary Vein

- the target is the extra-thoracic portion of the subclavian vein, also known as axillary vein
- important surrounding structures (**Figure 5.16**)
  - subclavian/axillary artery
    - it lies superior and below the vein and can be easily visualized/avoided with US

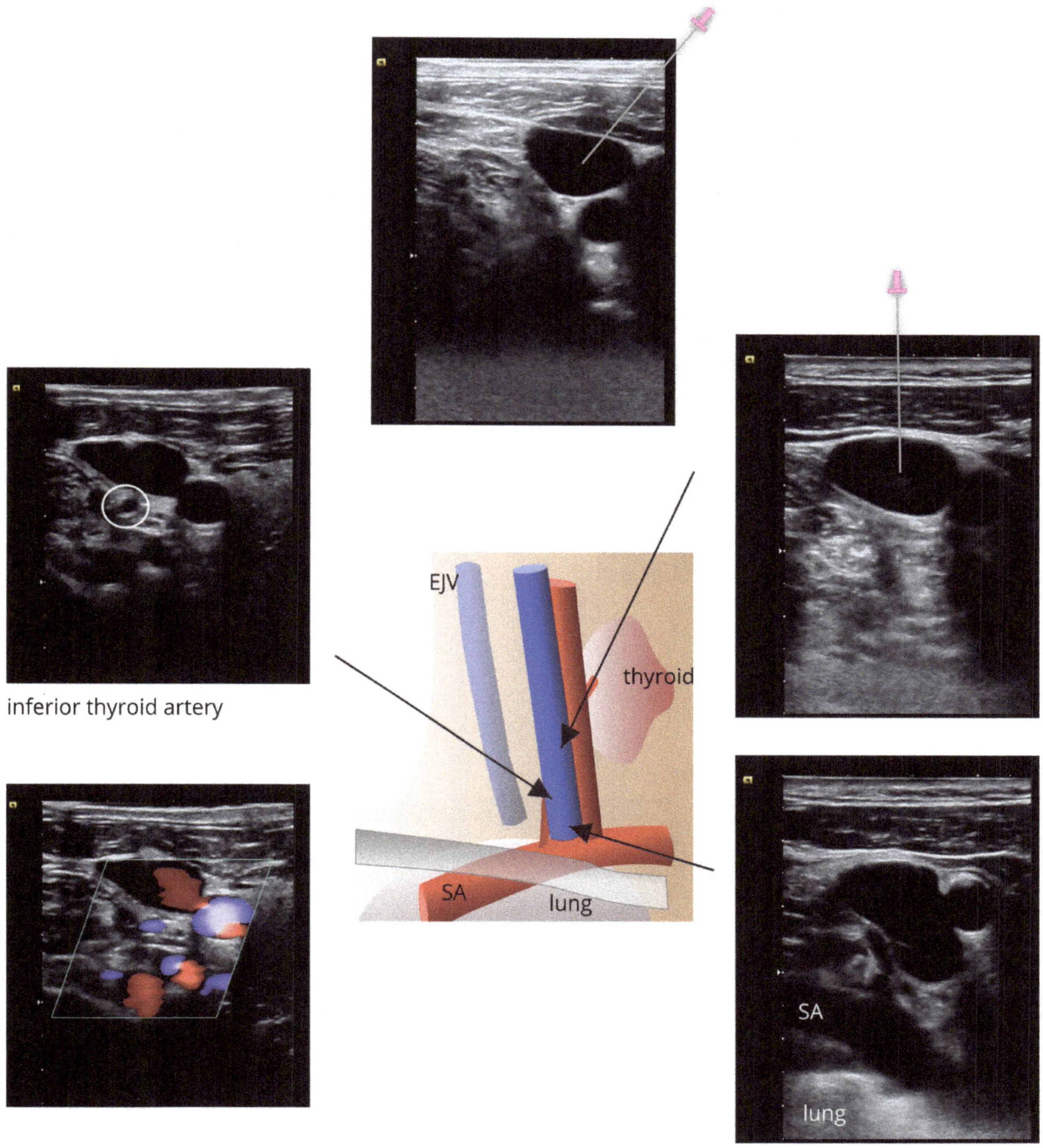

Figure 5.13 Internal jugular vein access.
EJV: external jugular vein; SA: subclavian artery.

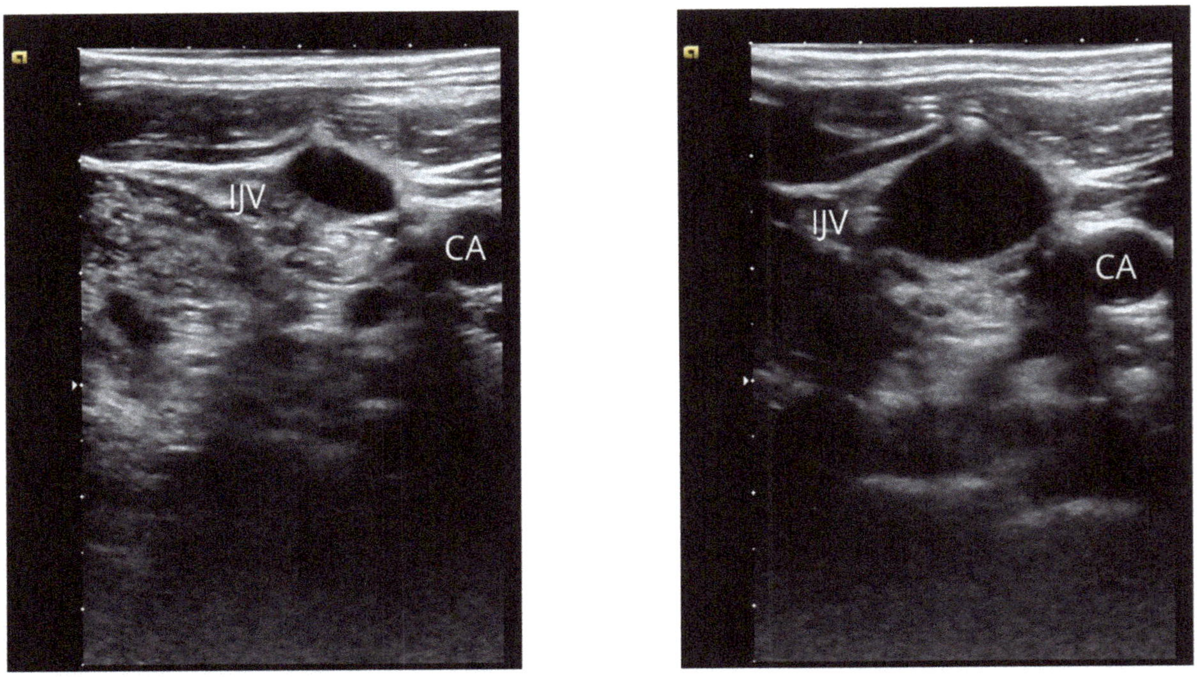

Figure 5.14 Valsalva maneuver.
IJV: internal jugular vein; CA: carotid artery.

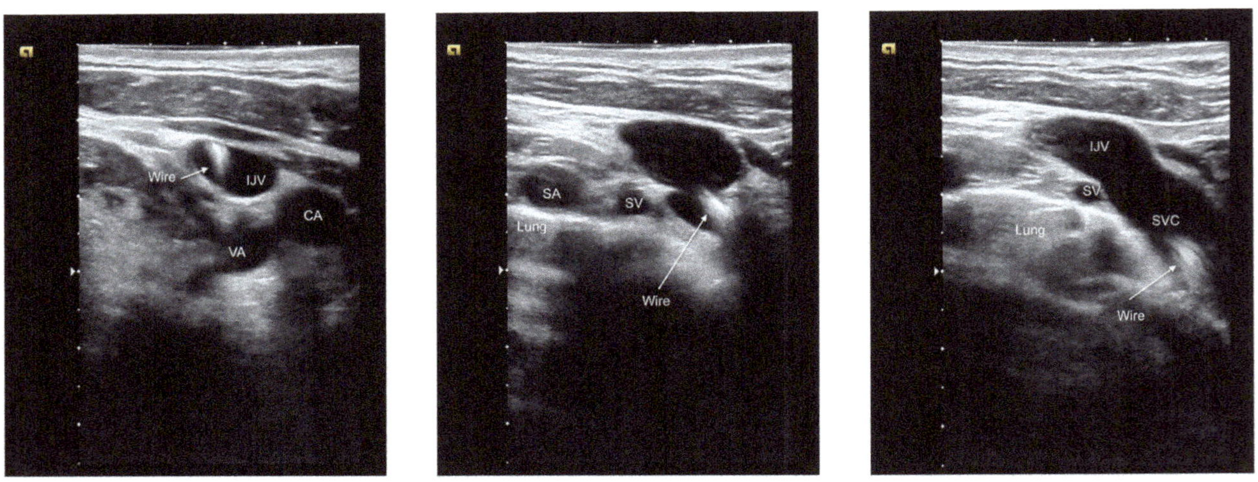

Figure 5.15 Wire in the superior vena cava.
CA: carotid artery; IJV: internal jugular vein; SA: subclavian arte-y; SV: subclavian vein; SVC: superior vena cava; VA: vertebral artery.

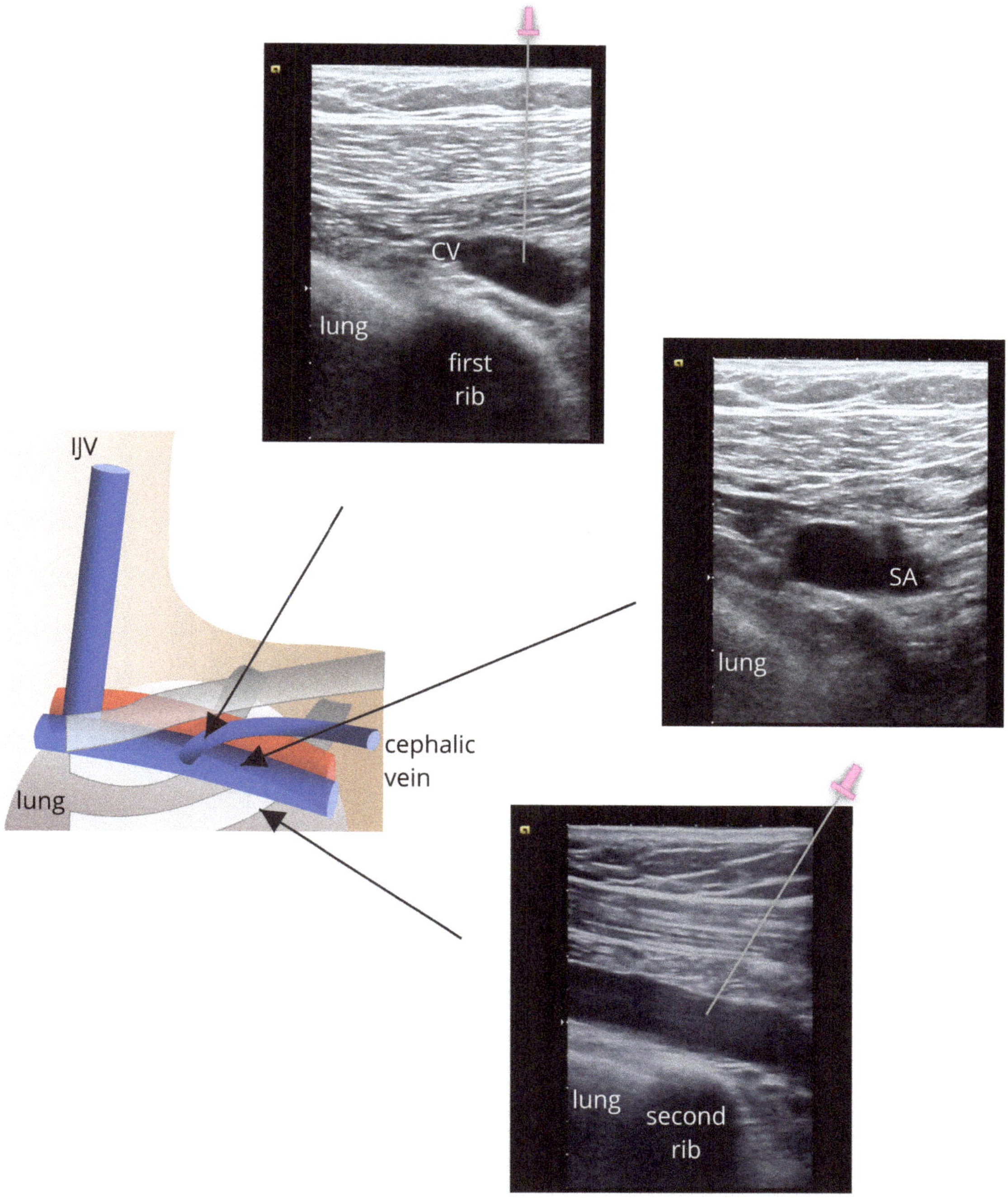

Figure 5.16 Subclavian/axillary vein access.
CV: cephalic vein; IJV: internal jugular vein; SA: subclavian artery.

- nerves
- the brachial plexus lies posterior to the subclavian and axillary artery; therefore, it is easily avoided by aiming at the vein

- lung
  - it lies below the vein and can be imaged with US by looking at the hyperechoic (white) line that slides along with every breath (sliding of the visceral pleura/lung relative to the parietal pleura), right under/between the ribs
  - to prevent pneumothorax, it is important to always precisely visualize the tip of the needle and never back-wall the subclavian vein
- ribs
  - they run between the subclavian vein and the pleura
  - they can act as a second line of defense against pneumothorax: if the needle is aimed toward them, even if it overshoots the vein, it will hit the rib
- cephalic vein
  - it usually joins the axillary vein at the level of the first rib, forming the subclavian vein
  - it should be avoided to prevent its laceration with subsequent hematoma
- shrugging the shoulder may help to open up the US window by pulling the clavicle upwards

- if the vein is small or easily collapsible, increasing venous return by ipsilateral arm squeeze or rapid fluid infusion is helpful
- the best site for access is where the vein does not lie directly over the lung or artery
  - ideally where it overlies the first or second rib (Figure 5.16); alternatively, where enough soft tissue is in between
  - it is crucial to always keep track of the needle tip
    - a long-axis approach is preferable as it allows to visualize the whole needle, along with the vein, the ribs, and underlying lung
    - especially for deep veins, a long-axis approach is challenging, as it is easy to lose vision of the vein or needle with even slight movements of the probe
      - a mixed short-axis/long-axis approach might be used; it is helpful to correct the needle trajectory and realign it with the vessel/US-plane
    - a short-axis only approach is adequate if the operator has enough experience with properly following the needle tip
- before advancing the sheath, it is useful to confirm that the wire goes down toward the superior vena cava vs. the ipsilateral jugular vein
  - this is facilitated by pointing the J-tip down, toward the heart
- this technique is useful also for device implant
  - whether to obtain access before or after creating the pocket depends on the operator preference
    - proper visualization within the pocket is challenging with a full-size linear probe: a smaller probe might be used, or access obtained outside/before the pocket

Complications

If US is used properly, it virtually eliminates complications related to central vascular access.[3] However, they are still possible, and, while a thorough discussion goes beyond the scope of this chapter, in order to prevent/recognize the most common complications it is important to know their causes and their appearance on US (**Figure 5.17**).

- hematoma
  - collection of blood in the soft tissue due to local hemorrhage
  - it looks like a mixed hyper-hypoechoic "cloudy" mass close to the target vessel, with ill-defined borders and no flow on Doppler examination
    - it might hinder visualization of deeper structures, preventing access if not already obtained
  - it is commonly caused by
    - multiple punctures or back-walling
      - follow the needle tip
      - aspirate at all times
    - poor hemostasis due to inadequate compression/failure of vascular closure devices
      - obtain access over bony structures
      - confirm proper closure device deployment/hemostasis
    - laceration of the target or adjacent vessels
      - follow the needle tip
      - obtain access in the center of the anterior wall of the vessel

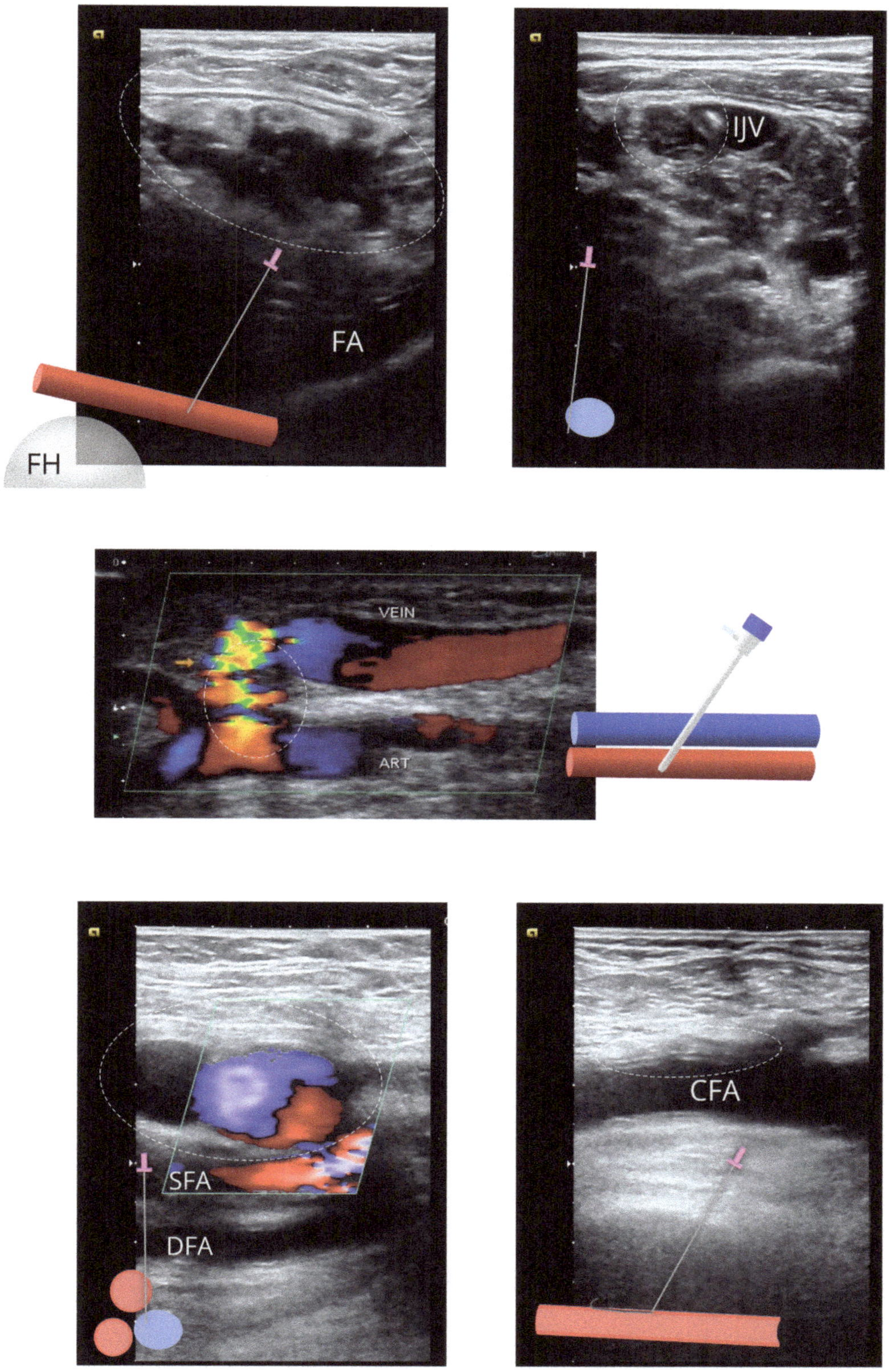

Figure 5.17 Examples of vascular complications and presumed mechanisms. From top to bottom, right to left: groin hematoma, neck hematoma, arteriovenous fistula*, pseudoaneurysm, arterial dissection.
CFA: common femoral artery; DFA: deep femoral artery; FH: femoral head; IJV: internal jugular vein; SFA: superficial femoral artery. (adapted from Dehghani et al. *Journal of Medical Case Reports*. 2013,7:2.)

        - never change the trajectory of the needle when close to vascular structures
        - do not advance the wire if any resistance is felt
    - retroperitoneal hematoma occurs with uncontrolled bleeding above the inguinal ligament (non-compressible area)
        - it cannot be directly visualized by US (CT scan being the diagnostic tool of choice)
        - but always suspect retroperitoneal hematoma in case of a high puncture
- pseudoaneurysm
    - collection of blood between the inner and the outer layers of an artery (usually between the intima/media and adventitia)
    - it looks like a discrete saccular mass close to the target vessel
        - it is usually anechoic, but can present with variable degrees of echogenicity according to the presence of thrombus
        - Doppler will reveal swirling blood flow (yin-yang sign) unless completely thrombosed
    - it is commonly caused by
        - arterial puncture/laceration along with poor hemostasis due to inadequate compression/failure of vascular closure devices
            - follow the needle tip
            - aspirate at all times
            - never change the trajectory of the needle when close to vascular structures
            - obtain access above bony structures
            - confirm proper closure device deployment/hemostasis
- arteriovenous fistula
    - a vascular communication between an artery and an adjacent vein
    - it can only be recognized by using Doppler in the suspect area, which will show arterialized blood flow in the vein along with turbulent/high-velocity flow at the level of the communication
    - it is usually caused by
        - back-walling of the target vessel into an adjacent vessel or through and through puncture of an adjacent vessel before reaching the target vessel
            - follow the needle tip
            - aspirate at all times
            - confirm the course of the wire before advancing the sheath
- arterial dissection
    - presence of variable length false lumen in the subintimal space
    - the dissected intimal layer with the underlying false lumen can be seen on US; the false lumen might by anechoic with flow on Doppler (parallel to true lumen blood flow), or iso-hyperechoic and without Doppler if filled by a thrombus
    - it is typically caused by
        - advancing the wire when the needle is partially inserted
            - confirm the needle tip location before advancing the wire
            - never advance the wire if any resistance is felt

References

1. Troianos CA, Hartman GS, Glas KE, et al. Guidelines for performing ultrasound guided vascular cannulation: Recommendations of the American Society of Echocardiography and the Society of Cardiovascular Anesthesiologists. *Anesth Analg.* 2012;114(1):46–72. doi:10.1213/ANE.0b013e3182407cd8
2. AIUM practice guideline for the use of ultrasound to guide vascular access procedures. *J Ultrasound Med.* 2013;32(1):191–215. doi:10.7863/jum.2013.32.1.191
3. Dietrich CF, Horn R, Morf S, et al. Ultrasound-guided central vascular interventions, comments on the European Federation of Societies for Ultrasound in Medicine and Biology guidelines on interventional ultrasound. *J Thorac Dis.* 2016;8(9):E851–E868. doi:10.21037/jtd.2016.08.49

6

How to Perform Transseptal Puncture Without Fluoroscopy

José Mauricio Sánchez, MD

History

Transseptal puncture is performed today with regularity in the modern world of clinical cardiac electrophysiology (EP) and structural heart interventions. However, it is important to recognize that this was not always the case. In fact, the idea is over 70 years old. Cournand et al. demonstrated the ability to measure left atrial (LA) pressure through an atrial septal defect in their 1947 report.[1] The necessity and desire for alternative methods and techniques to measure LA pressure drove the development of transseptal LA catheterization. Ross, Braunwald, and Morrow later demonstrated left heart catheterization through the transseptal route first in canine model and later in human subjects for pressure measurement.[2,3] Due to technical challenges and the risks of transseptal puncture, alternative methods for measurement of LA pressure such as pulmonary capillary wedge pressure were developed and remain more frequently utilized for this purpose. Retrograde catheterization with access to the left ventricle and mitral valve annulus resulted in decline in transseptal punctures. The advent of new techniques, including LA ablation of arrhythmias such as atrial fibrillation,[4] as well as structural procedures such as mitral valvuloplasty,[5] renewed interest in the transseptal approach. Over the last 20 years, the advent of advanced imaging systems including transesophageal echocardiography (TEE) and intracardiac echocardiography (ICE) have revolutionized the technique from a predominantly fluoroscopically guided procedure to one that can be performed safely without the use of fluoroscopy at all.[6]

While TEE can be utilized, the need for a second operator as well as the comparable or superior ICE images make ICE the standard of care in most modern EP labs. ICE has been demonstrated to be useful with transseptal puncture in the literature.[7] The practical use of ICE in transseptal puncture is nothing short of revolutionary with modern technology and the continued improvement in miniaturization of catheters. The amount of detail and resolution seen today is incredible. Additionally, phased-array ICE has also proved valuable in monitoring of interventional EP procedures which require transseptal LA access.[8]

A Revolution in Ablation Without Fluoroscopy

Imaging has improved to the point that operators have begun using multiple modalities of imaging, including 3D mapping systems and ICE, to perform ablations without the use of fluoroscopy.[9-11] While many operators can understand performing right-sided procedures without fluoroscopy, there remains some hesitancy with regard to transseptal procedures. Given that atrial fibrillation remains the most frequently ablated arrhythmia in adults, becoming comfortable and better appreciating the technique for

Fluoroscopy Reduction Techniques for Catheter Ablation of Cardiac Arrhythmias. © 2019 Mansour Razminia, Paul C. Zei, eds.
Cardiotext Publishing, ISBN: 978-1-942909-30-9.

transseptal puncture in the absence of fluoroscopy remains critical. Ablation of atrial fibrillation without fluoroscopy or with non-fluoroscopic imaging has been reported and is employed by an increasing number of operators and centers.[12-15] It is a technique that can be performed safely for both LA procedures as well as for procedures that cross the atrium in order to access the left ventricle.

Technique

As with any new technique, understanding a step-by-step approach is invaluable to success and safety of the procedure. Fluoroscopy-free transseptal puncture requires a thoughtful approach. The approach can be broken down into 3 critical steps:

1. Catheter placement
2. Wire placement and exchange of sheaths
3. Needle placement and puncture

While mapping systems will be needed for step 1, the key to steps 2 and 3 is excellent visualization and a disciplined approach to performing each step and maneuver only if the appropriate visualization is obtained on ICE.

Catheter Placement

While not essential to transseptal puncture itself, it is best to maintain a workflow as similar to the usual practice as possible. Catheter placement allows initial development of a geometry or 3D model, allowing for greater certainty of location of anatomy. Catheter placement can be performed with a variety of mapping systems including the EnSite system (Abbott, Abbott Park, IL) or CARTO 3 system (Biosense Webster, Irvine, CA). The EnSite system allows for direct visualization of any catheter as they are advanced through the venous system into the right atrium (RA). The current CARTO 3 system can visualize the majority of diagnostic catheters, but mapping to create the electroanatomic map requires placement of a proprietary ablation catheter. In addition, specific features such as creating ablation or other tags requires a mapping catheter such as the PentaRay or Lasso (Biosense Webster), an enabled navigational decapolar deflectable catheter, or a proprietary ablation catheter. The key to catheter placement includes visualization when possible, as well as tactile response. Gentle advancement is necessary with the ability to stop when any resistance is noted or buckling of the catheter is visualized. Construction of a RA map can then assist in position of a coronary sinus (CS) catheter and any additional catheters desired for the specific case and operator. Placement of an ICE catheter into the RA is the usual next step. An AcuNav 8-Fr ICE catheter (Siemens) may be introduced through an 8.5-Fr sheath in the left femoral vein. Advancement is performed while maintaining an echo-free space at the tip of the transducer. Some deflection may be needed at the junction of the left iliac vein into the inferior vena cava (IVC) to maintain the echo-free space at the transducer tip. Since catheters have already been placed, these catheters can be seen on ICE and following them can guide the operator through the pelvis and up through the abdomen into the IVC. Advancement into the RA allows visualization of the heart. While catheter placement prior to wire placement and exchange is not mandatory, the ability to place a catheter into the LA after transseptal puncture and already having a 3D understanding of the location in relation to the RA is very valuable. This practice also most closely follows most operators' current approach with fluoroscopy, making the transition more familiar.

Wire Placement and Sheath Exchange

Once electrophysiology catheters and an ICE catheter have been placed in desired position of the operator, initiation of wire exchange may begin. The author's preference is to gain access using modified Seldinger technique and utilize a short 8-Fr sheath in the right femoral vein, then exchange for a long sheath over a long 0.032-inch wire. In positioning the wire, one must find the position of the phased-array ICE catheter in the RA that provides the best field of view. ICE catheter placement is key in order to visualize exchange wire placement into the superior vena cava (SVC). Adjustments will likely be needed due to the variable nature of the heart's positioning in the chest wall. Once the ICE catheter is in the RA, counter clockwise rotation in order to see the RA, RV, aorta, and part of the SVC provides the most desirable view for wire positioning.

Placement of 0.032-inch exchange wire or wires into the SVC is then performed with direct visualization of the wires into the SVC (**Figure 6.1**). An ICE view that provides visualization of the greatest length of wire in the SVC is ideal, providing adequate visualization of the wire exchange process. Gentle advancement is always required with careful attention to any buckling of the wire or any resistance. Short 8-Fr sheaths can then be exchanged for 8-Fr long sheaths over 0.032-inch guidewires. The operator should choose a long sheath with which he or she is comfortable; the author prefers the Preface sheath (Biosense Webster), but there are a variety of sheaths that can be used, including steerable sheaths, with the same technique. Steerable or larger sheaths should utilize a stiff exchange wire. Careful attention is required to ensure that no excess wire buckled into the right atrial appendage (RAA) (**Figure 6.2**). The long sheath is then advanced slowly with tip point toward the intra-atrial septum. Advancement is performed with sheath being advanced into SVC under direct ICE visualization. Additionally, movement of the wire back and forth while advancing the sheath allows for detection of any resistance, which may denote possible buckling of the wire or bending of the wire. Any tension should result in immediate stop of movement and reassessment of the situation. Advancement over the wire should occur without any resistance and ability to shift the wire freely. The sheath can frequently be seen coming over the wire and advancing from the superior RA into the SVC (**Figure 6.3**). It should be understood that for much of the advancement, the sheath-over-wire advancement is not directly visualized. Therefore, care should be taken to ensure there is little to no resistance to advancement of the sheath to avoid buckling and "derailing."

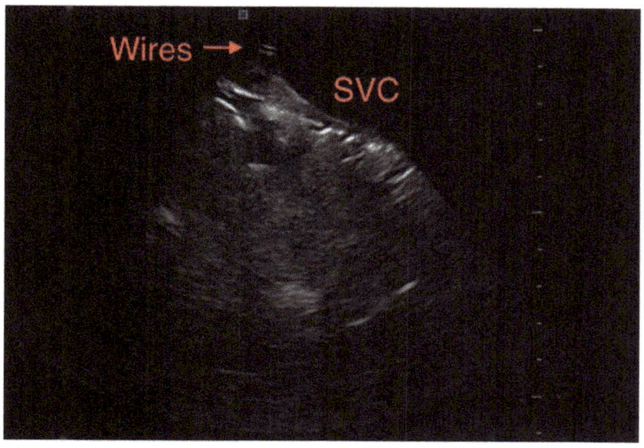

Figure 6.1 ICE visualization of exchange wire in SVC.

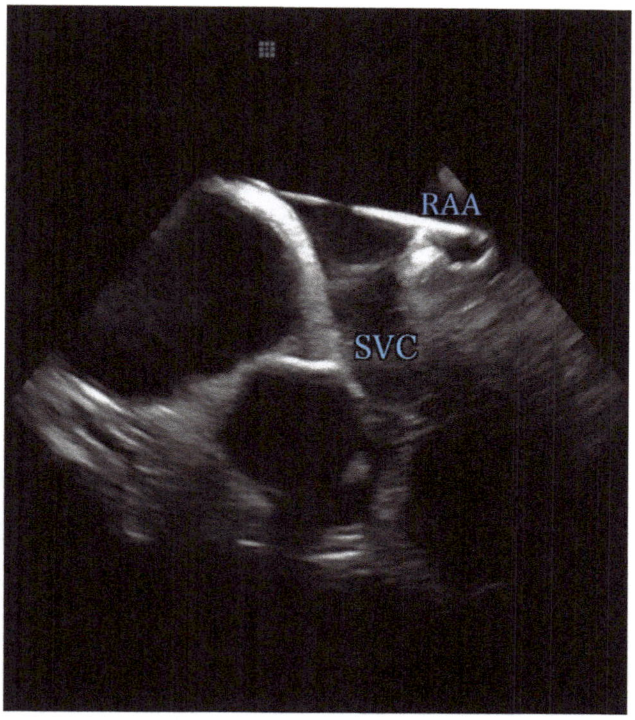

Figure 6.2 ICE visualization of exchange wire buckling in RAA.

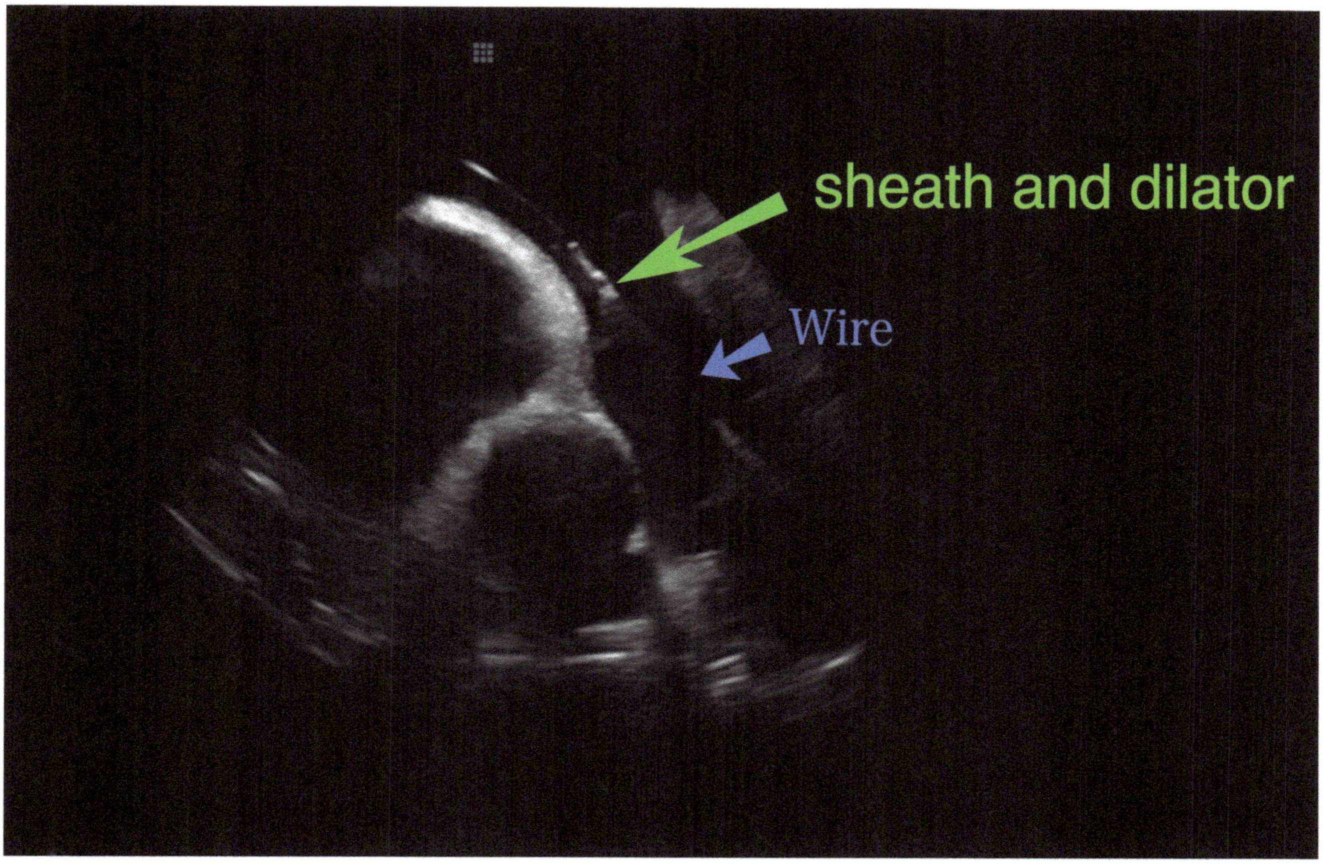

Figure 6.3 ICE visualization of long sheath advancing over exchange wire in superior RA and into SVC.

Needle Puncture

Once the sheath is visualized on ICE in the SVC, the wire is removed. The sheath should be carefully flushed. A Brockenbrough transseptal needle (BRK-1, Abbott) is advanced into the long sheath and flushed **Video 6.1**). Alternatively, a radiofrequency (RF)-enabled needle (Baylis Medical, Montreal, Canada) can be utilized as well. Once the needle is advanced the length of the sheath, the long sheath can then be slowly brought down from the SVC under ICE visualization until the sheath and needle are located at the intra-atrial septum (**Figure 6.4** and **Video 6.2**).

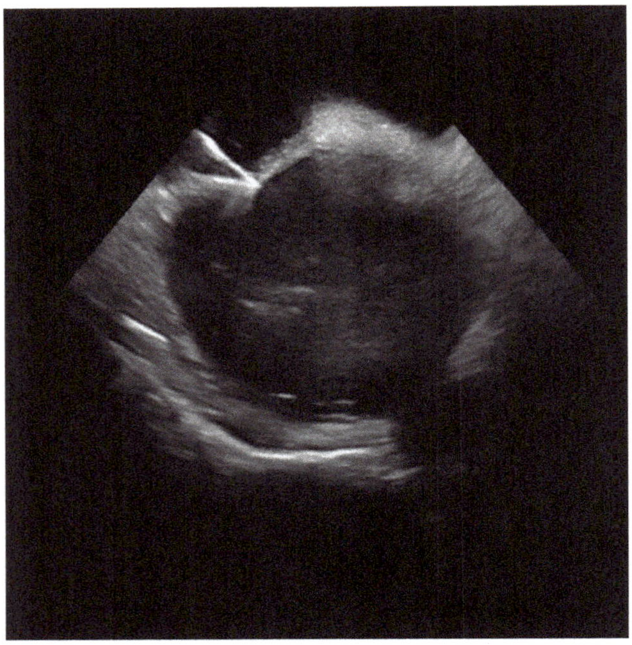

Figure 6.4 ICE visualization of sheath and needle positioned at the intra-atrial septum.

Positioning of the needle depends on the procedure being performed. A more posterior approach across the septum for atrial fibrillation ablation may be preferable, but if attempting to perform a PVC ablation or VT ablation in the left ventricle via transseptal approach, then a more anterior location on the fossa ovalis may be preferred. Heparin is given before transseptal puncture. ICE visualization allows for needle placement and direct visualization of tenting. Rotation of the ICE catheter posteriorly with clockwise moment assures that one is not too posterior.

Counterclockwise rotation anteriorly allows for movement away from the fossa and toward the aorta. Once positioning is confirmed on ICE, puncture with measured forward force is performed (**Video 6.3**). Injection of saline can confirm puncture into the LA. Advancement of an 0.032-inch-long wire into the left superior pulmonary vein under ICE visualization allows for a rail to be present for sheath advancement over the wire. The sheath can then be advanced over the wire into the LA visualized under ICE directly (**Figure 6.5**, **Figure 6.6**, and **Video 6.4**).

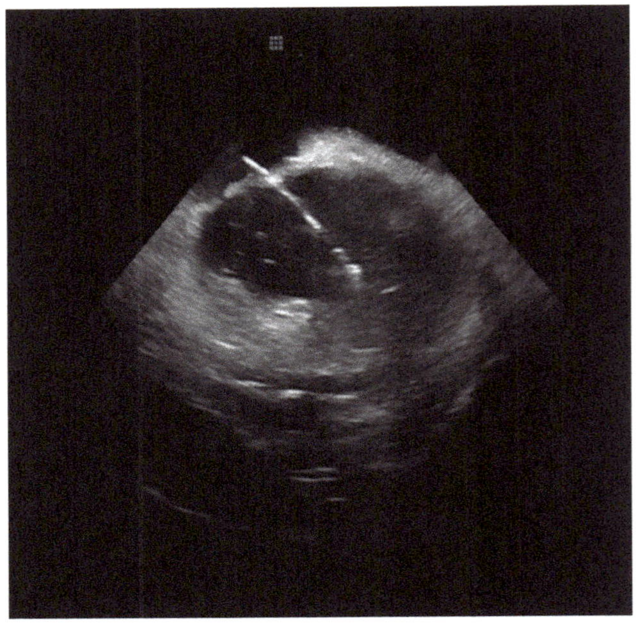

Figure 6.5 ICE visualization of sheath crossing over wire into the left atrium.

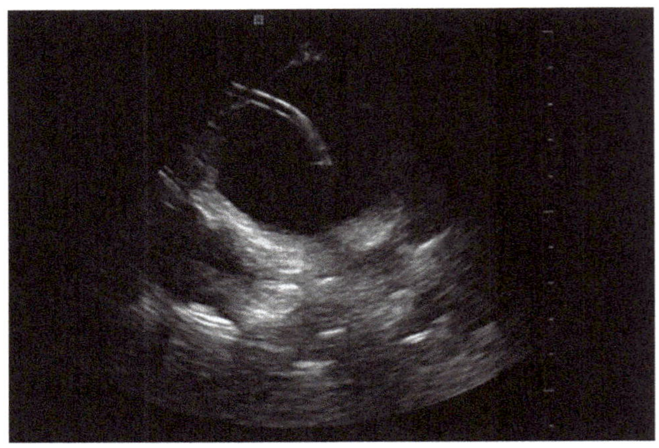

Figure 6.6 ICE visualization of sheath having crossed into the left atrium.

Challenges

The most common areas for difficulty and concern with fluoroscopy-free transseptal puncture are with visualization. When performing a standard transseptal puncture, the operator has several modalities to choose from, including fluoroscopy and ICE. The use of multiple modalities allows for some compensation when not visualizing the anatomy clearly in any single modality. While fluoroscopy does not demonstrate direct visualization of tissue, as ICE does, with respect to the contact with cardiac tissues, it does clearly show the location of radiopaque objects such as wires and sheaths. It is critical when performing this technique without fluoroscopy that wires are visualized. In addition, confirmatory movement of the wires and sheaths on ICE is critical to assure that another catheter is not misinterpreted as the wire. The importance of tactile feedback is also very important in performing a safe and successful procedure. Any resistance requires immediate cessation of movement and reevaluation of the clinical situation at hand.

Conclusions

Fluoroscopy-free transseptal puncture can be performed safely. Step-by-step procedure is key. It is an essential technique for an adult electrophysiologist given the need for transseptal access in the procedures most frequently performed.

References

1. Cournand A, Motley HL, Himmelstein A, Dresdale D, Baldwin J. Recording of blood pressure from the left auricle and the pulmonary veins in human subjects with intraauricular septal defect. *Am J Physiol.* 1947;150:267.
2. Ross J, Braunwald E, Morrow AG. Transeptal left atrial puncture; new technique for the measurement of left atrial pressure in man. *Am J Cardiol.* 1959;3:653–655.
3. Ross J, Braunwald E, Morrow AG. Left catheterization by the transeptal route: A description of the technique and its applications. *Circulation.* 1960;22:927–934.
4. Jaïs P, Haïssaguerre M, Shah DC, et al. A focal source of atrial fibrillation treated by discrete radio frequency ablation. *Circulation.* 1997;95:572–576.
5. Inoue K, Owaki T, Nakamura T, Kitamura F, Minamoto N. Clinical application of transvenous mitral commissurotomy by a new balloon catheter. *J Thorax Cardiovasc Surg.* 1984;87:394–402.
6. Baykaner T, Thosani AJ, Yasmeh B, et al. Safety and efficacy of zero fluoroscopy transseptal puncture. [Abstract B-PO02-126] *Heart Rhythm.* 2018;15(5 Suppl):S232.
7. Tardif JC, Vannan MA, Miller DS, Schwartz SL, Pandian NG. Potential applications of intracardiac echocardiography in interventional electrophysiology. *Am Heart J.* 1994;127:1090–1094.
8. Marrouche NF, Martin DO, Wazni O, et al. Phased-array intracardiac echocardiography monitoring during pulmonary vein isolation in patients with atrial fibrillation: Impact on outcome and complications. *Circulation.* 2003; 107:2710–2716.
9. Drago F, Silvetti MS, Di Pino A, Grutter G, Belivacqua M, Leibovich S. Exclusion of fluoroscopy during ablation treatment of right-sided accessory pathways in children. *J Cardiovasc Electrophysiol.* 2002;13:778–782.
10. Grubb N, Petzer E, Lang C, Colthart A, Elhag O. A zero fluoroscopy approach for electrophysiologic studies and catheter ablation for common supraventricular tachycardias. *Heart Rhythm.* 2006;3:S123.
11. Ebrille E, Caponi D, Siboldi A, et al. Single center experience of fluoroless AVNRT ablation guided by electroanatomic reconstruction in children and adolescents. *Pacing Clin Electrophysiol.* 2013;36(12):1460–1467.
12. Ferguson JD, Helms A, Mangrum JM, et al. Catheter ablation of atrial fibrillation without fluoroscopy using intracardiac echocardiography and electroanatomic mapping. *Circ Arrhythm Electrophysiol.* 2009;2:611–619.
13. Reddy VY, Morales G, Ahmed H, et al. Catheter ablation of atrial fibrillation without the use of fluoroscopy. *Heart Rhythm.* 2010;7:1644–1653.
14. Razminia M, Manankil MF, Eryazici PL, et al. Non-fluoroscopic catheter ablation of cardiac arrhythmias in adults: Feasibility, safety, and efficacy. *J Cardiovasc Electrophysiol.* 2012;23(10):1078–1086.
15. Sánchez JM, Yanics MA, Wilson P, Doshi A, Kurian T, Pieper S. Fluoroless catheter ablation in adults: A single center experience. *J Interv Card Electrophysiol.* 2016;45: 199–207.

Video Legends

Video 6.1 The transseptal needle is advanced into the long sheath. [00:03]

Video 6.2 The long sheath is then slowly brought down from the SVC under ICE visualization until the sheath and needle are located at the intra-atrial septum. [00:03]

Video 6.3 ICE imaging of transseptal puncture across intra-atrial septum. [00:03]

Video 6.4 The sheath is advanced over the wire into the LA visualized under ICE guidance. [00:03]

Video 6S Chapter summary and step-by-step procedures by Mansour Razminia. [10:49]

7

How to Maintain Safety With a Reduced Fluoroscopy Approach

José Osorio, MD; Gustavo X. Morales, MD

Introduction

Without safety, any improvement in technique and technology in the medical field cannot be widely adopted. Catheter ablation for cardiac arrhythmias has a good track record with respect to safety, and the continuing advancement of technology has contributed to make procedures more efficacious and safer.[1] Current fluoroscopy equipment has also evolved and exposes patients to lower absorptive doses of radiation compared to previous equipment, while preserving and improving image quality.

Reduction or even omission of fluoroscopy has only been allowed by the development of new technologies originally designed to be use in parallel with fluoroscopy; however, their synergistic use allows operators to rely on ionizing radiation less or even not at all.

The key to safely manipulating catheters in the intravascular space and cardiac chambers without fluoroscopy depends on: (1) live visualization of the catheter position and trajectory; (2) accurate recording of electrical signaling through the manipulated catheter; and (3) operators' tactile perception of uninterrupted catheter trajectory.

In non-fluoroscopic techniques, electroanatomic mapping (EAM) systems and intracardiac echo (ICE) are key elements for catheter visualization.

Diagnostic Catheter Manipulation and Positioning

As a diagnostic catheter enters the right atrium (RA), the operator is immediately alerted to the presence of electrophysiological signaling, prompting him/her to understand catheter orientation in the 2 traditional orthogonal views (right anterior oblique [RAO] and left anterior oblique [LAO]) within the EAM system. At first, the most challenging diagnostic catheter to position will be the coronary sinus (CS) catheter. The authors' laboratory uses multipolar, bidirectional deflective catheters that are gently manipulated by the operator while paying close attention to the electrophysiological signaling in the distal electrode. Guided by EAM and electrical signaling, the catheter is advanced into the CS. ICE can also identify the ostium (os) of the CS and confirm the presence of the diagnostic catheter inside it. The ICE catheter is rotated clockwise once the aortic valve and infundibular aorta are identified to direct the beam slightly posterior, and the CS os will be appreciated in the lower portion of the view (**Figure 7.1**).

Another technique that can be used to help safely position diagnostic catheters is to initially advance a contact-force sensor ablation catheter from the femoral vein to the RA guided in a similar way by EAM and electrophysiological signaling. A tactile sensation aided by contact-force live feedback can help safely and more

Fluoroscopy Reduction Techniques for Catheter Ablation of Cardiac Arrhythmias. © 2019 Mansour Razminia, Paul C. Zei, eds.
Cardiotext Publishing, ISBN: 978-1-942909-30-9.

confidently identify sensitive structures in the RA such as the CS os and body, right atrial appendage, and superior vena cava (SVC). Once the volumetric geometry of the structures has been identified, one can feel more confident to safely advance noncontact-force sensor diagnostic catheters.

Safety of Non-Fluoroscopic Ablation for Right-Sided Arrhythmias

Initial experience with non-fluoroscopic cardiac ablation was directed towards treatment of right-sided arrhythmias. In 2002, Drago et al. published their initial experience in 21 patients with Wolff-Parkinson-White (WPW) syndrome and right-sided accessory pathway, which were successfully treated with a single procedure in 19 patients with no reported complications, with minimal use of fluoroscopy.[2]

Subsequently, a series of publications consolidated the safety of non-fluoroscopic right-sided catheter ablations for supraventricular tachycardias, including atrioventricular nodal reentrant tachycardia (AVNRT), atrial tachycardia, and orthodromic reciprocating tachycardia using right-sided pathways.[3-5]

Although fluoroscopy was still utilized during these procedures in a number of patients, most procedures were indeed able to be performed safely without any fluoroscopy. Complications reported through these experiences were deemed unrelated to the non-fluoroscopic technique but rather related to the ablation procedure himself, such as transient AV block during AVNRT ablation.

One safety consideration for right-sided ablation is accurate identification and "tagging" of the position of the His bundle signal and to specifically understand its position compared to the site of ablation (**Figure 7.2**), thereby minimizing the risk of AV block due to inadvertent ablation too close to the His bundle or AV node. A second safety concern is avoiding ablation along the course of the right phrenic nerve while ablating the lateral wall of the RA. To mitigate this risk, 3-dimensional (3D) EAM systems have an advantage over fluoroscopy alone, as the operator can identify and tag sites where high-amplitude pacing result in phrenic nerve stimulation, thereby avoiding radiofrequency (RF) ablation in such sites to prevent right-sided diaphragmatic paralysis.[6]

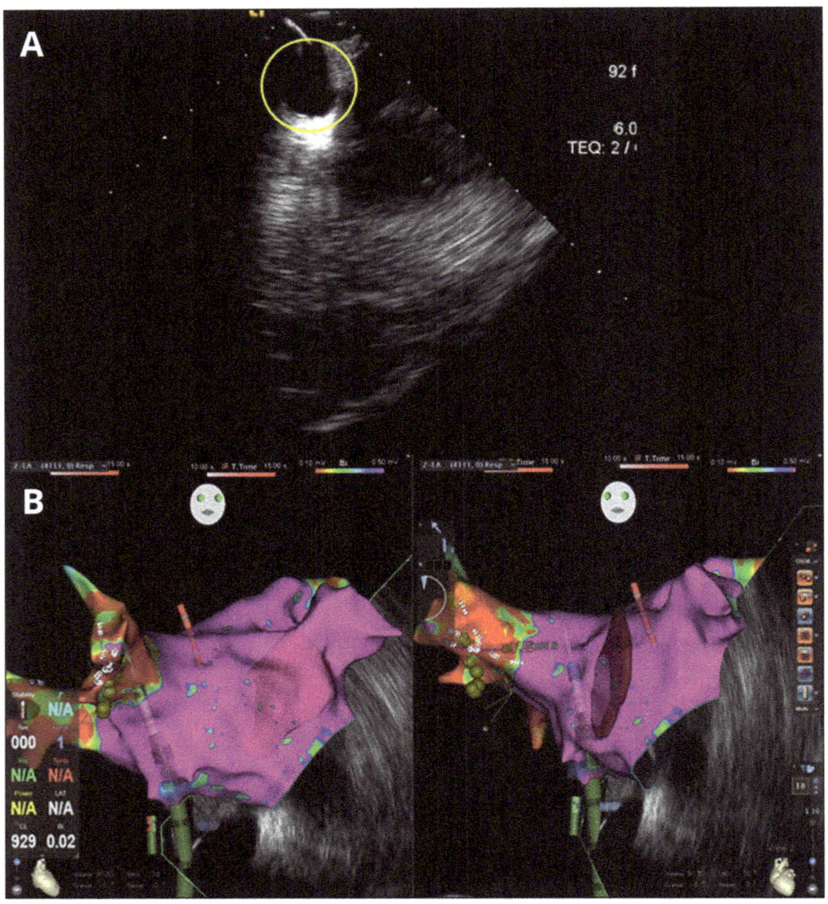

Figure 7.1 **A:** ICE image of the coronary sinus (CS) os (**yellow circle**). Appreciate the CS catheter inside the CS. **B:** EAM image in orthogonal views. Observe the ICE posteriorly directed to visualize the CS.

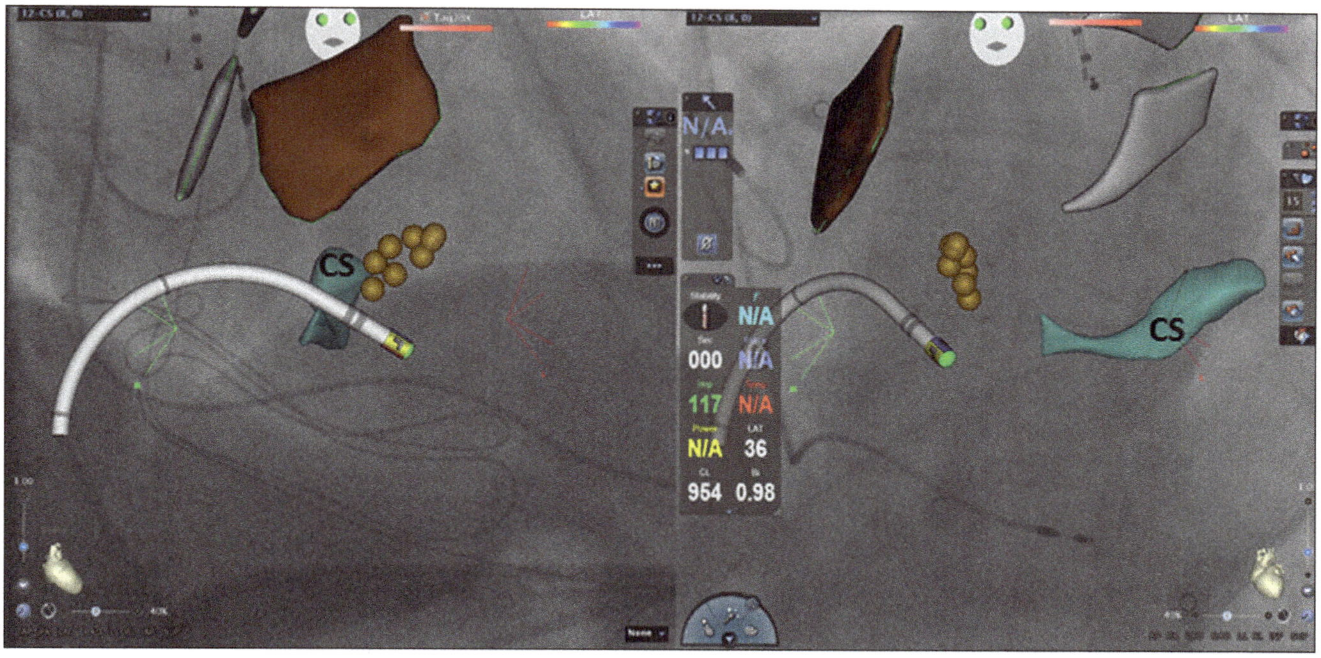

Figure 7.2 EAM image of the His cloud (**yellow points**). Ablation catheter (Abl) is positioned in the ara of the slow pathway at the base of the triangle of Koch. CS: coronary sinus.

Another common arrhythmia for which non-fluoroscopic technique has proven to be safe is typical cavotricuspid isthmus (CTI) dependent atrial flutter. Two separate studies have reported a non-fluoroscopic technique with minimal safety concerns.[7,8] In the authors' laboratory, most of the CTI ablations performed are in the setting of atrial fibrillation (AF), so therefore intracardiac echocardiography (ICE) visualization is available. ICE is extremely useful for understanding the anatomy of the CTI region and clearly superior to fluoroscopy, which relies only on the perception of catheter movement and at times the use of intravenous contrast to identify challenging anatomy along the CTI.[9] (Please refer to Chapter 11 for further details.)

Non-Fluoroscopic Transseptal Puncture

Since non-fluoroscopic EAM systems became widely available, operators have continued to decrease fluoroscopy exposure; however, for most operators, most of the reduction in fluoroscopy time is achieved through fluoroscopy reduction during catheter mapping and ablation after left atrial access is achieved. Transseptal access, for the vast majority of operators, continues to be a primarily fluoroscopy-guided procedure aided by intracardiac echocardiography. The most commonly used technique for transseptal access is the Brockenbrough (BRK) technique, which is guided by fluoroscopy.[10]

The first published experience of a transseptal access technique without the need of fluoroscopy was described by Clark et al. in 2008, where right atrial geometry was performed with an EAM system while transesophageal echocardiography was used to guide transseptal puncture.[11] With this technique, the operator was able to ablate left-sided accessory pathways successfully and safely.

Subsequently, in 2009, Ferguson et al. modified the technique to incorporate rotational ICE instead of transesophageal echocardiogram. They reported successful AF ablation using non-fluoroscopic, rotational ICE-guided transseptal puncture in 19 of 21 attempted cases with no reported complications. Rotational ICE currently is used infrequently, however.

The first description of phased-array ICE-guided transseptal puncture was not reported until 2010, when Reddy et al. published the results of 20 consecutive patients with paroxysmal AF where transseptal access was safely achieved.[12] This technique with phased-array ICE is the most commonly used technique.

There are several critical steps to maintain safety during non-fluoroscopic transseptal access:

1. While advancing the ICE catheter from the left femoral vein, one should be aware of the possibility of damaging the more fragile venous vessels. Therefore, real-time visualization of the iliac vein and inferior vena cava (IVC) is necessary to safely advance the ICE catheter. Not uncommonly, deflection of the ICE catheter is required to identify the true lumen of the vessel prior to advancing.

2. Once the superior portion of the IVC is reached, identification of the junction between the IVC and the RA clearly shows the site of entry where one should advance the ICE catheter. Keep in mind that in the vast majority of humans, the RA tends to be located slightly anterior to the IVC, and therefore a slight anterior tilt of the ICE (and other) catheters is typically required.

3. Once the ICE catheter is placed within the RA, the tricuspid valve should be identified using anterior deflection, positioning the ICE catheter such that the orifice of the tricuspid valve is located at the superior aspect of the narrowed section of the ultrasound-array field. Advancing the catheter through the tricuspid valve, releasing deflection, and turning clockwise, the left ventricle (LV) will be visualized in order to evaluate any preexisting effusion (**Figure 7.3**). Note that in the supine position, any free-flowing effusion will collect in a dependent fashion, typically within the epicardial space posterior to the LV base. If effusion is seen, baseline measurements of the effusions are taken to allow for serial interrogation of effusion size throughout the procedure.
4. To help understand the anatomy, the contours of the aortic valve and infundibular aorta and its long axis are typically delineated using CARTOSOUND (Biosense Webster, Irvine, CA), the module within the CARTO EAM system that allows integration of ICE imaging into the EAM. From there, a clockwise rotation of the ICE catheter is continued to mark with CARTOSOUND the following structures in respective order: Left atrial appendage, left pulmonary veins, and right pulmonary veins. This quick assessment and registration of the ultrasound anatomy allows one to rapidly identify the basic geometry of the left atrium, facilitating mapping and ablation catheter manipulation after obtaining left atrial access.
5. A posterior and rightward deflection of the ICE catheter opens a view of the junction between the SVC and RA. While in this view a long J-wire is advanced from the right femoral vein until identified by ICE entering the SVC (**Figure 7.4**).
6. Once the wire has been advanced to the SVC, the short femoral sheath is exchanged for the desired transseptal sheath. With the ICE catheter at all times visualizing in long axis the J-tip wire crossing the junction between the SVC and the RA, the transseptal sheath is advanced from the femoral vein over a fixed long wire until the sheath is clearly visualized by ICE entering over the wire to the SVC.

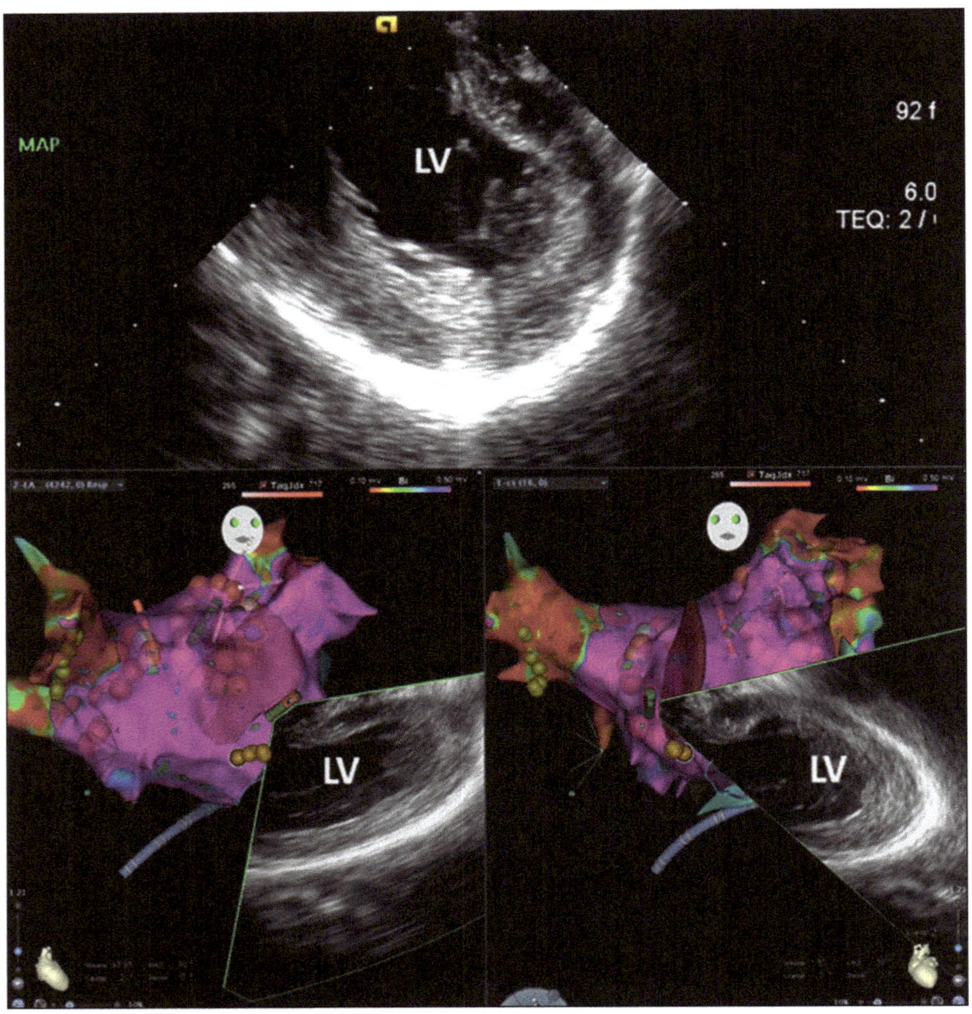

Figure 7.3 ICE image of the left ventricle (LV) showing the absence of pericardial effusion. EAM images in orthogonal projections, showing the position of the ICE catheter tip across the tricuspid valve into the right ventricle.

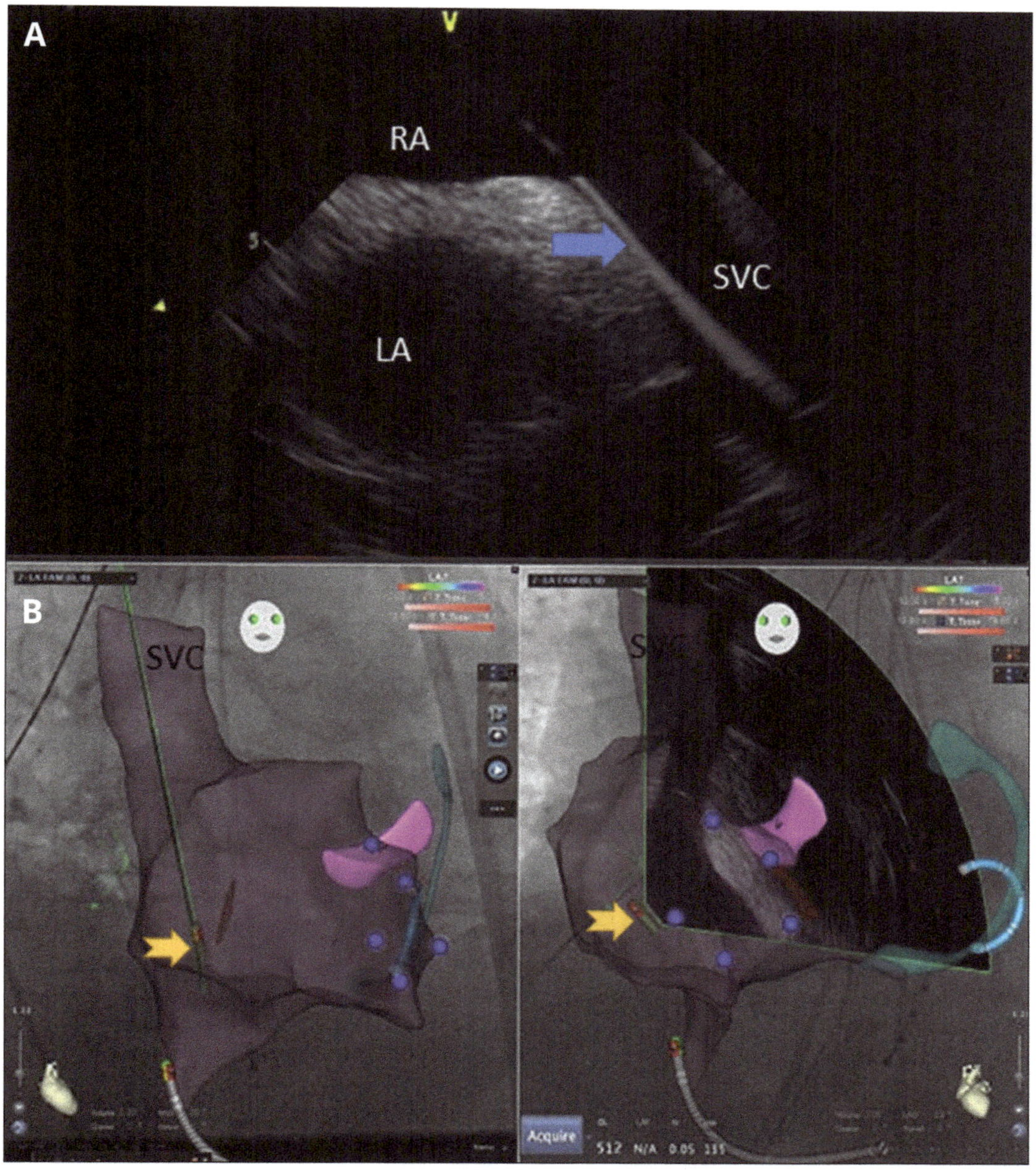

Figure 7.4 A: ICE image of the SVC and the guidewire (**blue arrow**) inserted from the right femoral vein into the SVC.
B: EAM image of the ICE catheter (**yellow arrow**) deflected posteriorly and rightward to direct the ICE beam towards the SVC. LA: left atrium; RA: right atrium; SVC: superior vena cava.

7. While fixing the sheath in the SVC, the long wire is removed, and saline is injected through the dilator of the long sheath. On ICE, bubbles are clearly visualized coming from cranial to caudal at the SVC–RA junction, confirming the location of the tip of the transseptal sheath within the SVC.

8. After inserting the BRK needle into the sheath dilator, rotation of the ICE probe may be needed to better visualize the tip of the dilator while pulling down the transseptal system towards the fossa ovalis (**Figure 7.5**). Another technique is to visualize the tip of the BRK needle with the EAM system. For this to occur, the proximal end of the needle needs to be connected to the anode of an alligator clip wire, and the cathode to an indifferent electrode in the body (which could be a wire inside the venous system). The tip of the BRK needle needs to be exposed carefully outside the sheath dilator to be visualized; in this way, the EAM system will identify the tip and allow the operator to visualize its trajectory while pulling down from the SVC to the fossa ovalis.

9. Once the transseptal sheath tip "drops" into the fossa ovalis, the ICE will determine the optimal site of puncture in the conventional fashion (**Figure 7.6**).

10. After transseptal access with the tip of the needle, saline is injected through the BRK needle to visualize microbubbles in the LA, confirming the location of the needle in the LA. Then, advancing the dilator and sheath to LA can be accomplished.

Another technique uses an atraumatic transseptal guidewire (SafeSept, Pressure Products, San Pedro, CA) to help "rail" the transseptal sheath across the septum.

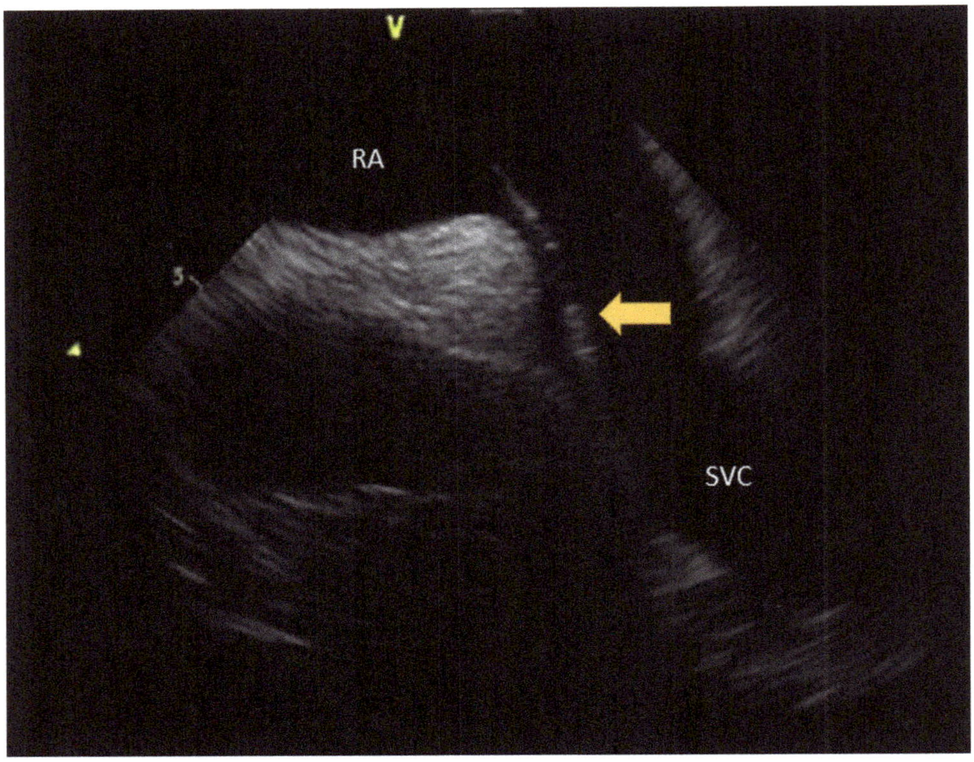

Figure 7.5 ICE image of the transseptal system (**yellow arrow**) while it is dragged down from the SVC to the fossa ovalis. RA: right atrium; SVC: superior vena cava.

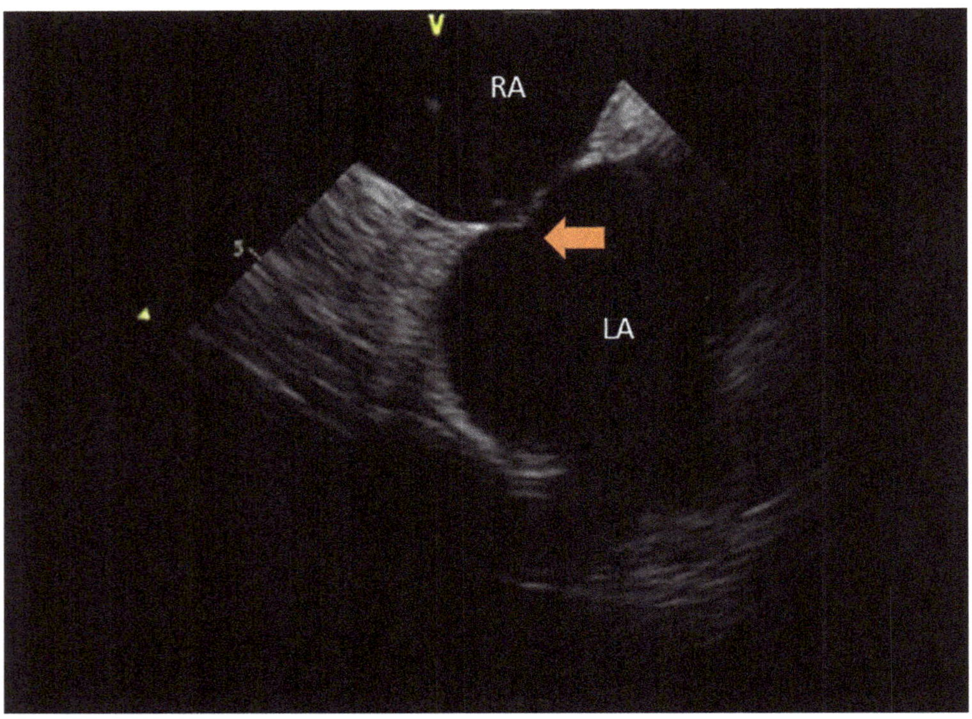

Figure 7.6 ICE image of the transseptal system (**orange arrow**) tenting the fossa ovalis, marking the ideal puncture site. LA: left atrium; RA: right atrium.

When double transseptal access is required, in the authors' laboratory, a single transseptal puncture is performed and a second LA access subsequently obtained through the same puncture site. The following technique is followed in our institution:

1. Once initial LA access has been obtained and the sheath and dilator are confirmed to be within the LA, a J-tipped wire is advanced, guided by ICE, into one of the left pulmonary veins. The sheath and dilator system are pulled back to the RA, keeping the wire in the left PV. If CARTOSOUND is available, tracing the site where the wire crosses the fossa ovalis can help identify the access location. Then, manipulating the ablation catheter in the right aspect of the fossa, guided by EMS and ICE, the ablation catheter is advanced into the LA via the already acquired transseptal puncture site (**Figure 7.7**).

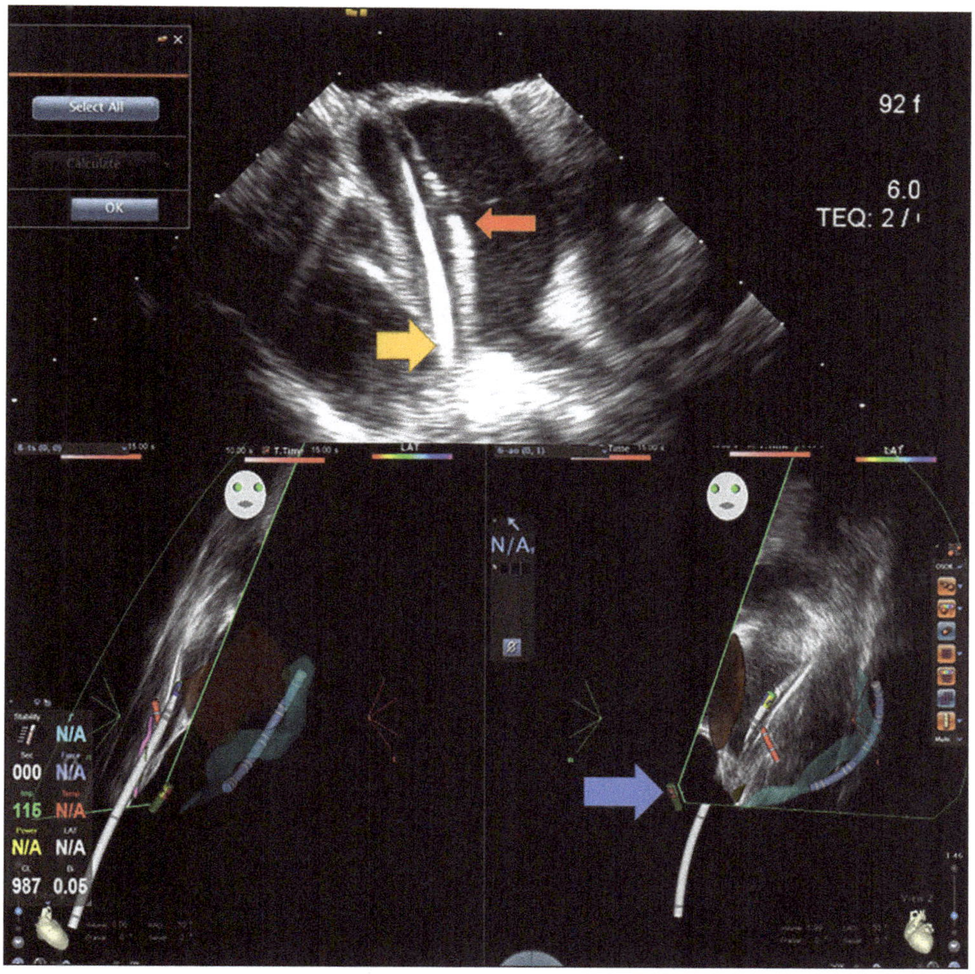

Figure 7.7 ICE image of the double transseptal access procedure. Observe the guidewire positioned in the left inferior pulmonary vein (**orange arrow**), and the ablation catheter (**red arrow**) just past the transseptal puncture site. The EAM orthogonal views images of the process.

2. After the ablation catheter and the guidewire are both securely in the LA, the sheath and dilator are advanced over the guidewire to the LA, enabling both transseptal sheath and ablation catheter manipulation in the LA.

Please see Chapter 6 for further details regarding transseptal puncture techniques.

Non-Fluoroscopic Technique for Left Atrial Arrhythmia Mapping and Ablation

The published literature of the role of non-fluoroscopic techniques in LA arrhythmias continues to grow. Left-sided accessory pathway-related arrhythmia ablations were the first to be reported with non-fluoroscopic techniques. In 2015, a series of 47 accessory pathways ablation without fluoroscopy was published. Twenty-one left-sided pathways were included. In all but 2 cases, the left-sided access was retrograde transaortic, which was achieved safely without the need for fluoroscopy. Acute success was achieved in all procedures, with only 2 left-sided pathways having clinical recurrence at 16 months follow-up. There were no complications related to the non-fluoroscopic procedures.[13]

The most challenging supraventricular arrhythmias for catheter ablation are clearly AF and atypical atrial flutters (aAFLs). Electro-anatomic mapping systems have successfully reduced the need for fluoroscopy to the point where in many institutions, fluoroscopy is not utilized. Several safety considerations are needed to successfully perform non-fluoroscopic AF ablations.

The first step after accessing the LA is to create an accurate 3D geometry of the LA, carefully identifying the os of all pulmonary veins (PVs) and the os of the left atrial appendage (LAA). ICE is extremely useful in this process, as it allows confirmation of the location of the multipolar mapping catheter in relation to the os of the PVs. It is customary in our laboratory to keep 2 orthogonal views in the EAM, including a RAO projection to maintain vigilance on the atrioventricular groove location, in order to avoid advancing the multipolar catheter through the mitral valve, where in particular, a circular mapping catheter may be entangled in the subvalvular apparatus.[14]

Once the LA geometry and voltage map have been created, we identify the trajectory of the phrenic nerve in the anterior antrum of the right PVs, by pacing from the tip of the ablator at high voltage (**Figure 7.8**). Once identified and tagged, the trajectory of the phrenic nerve can be avoided while applying RF energy.

Please refer to Chapters 13 and 14 for further details.

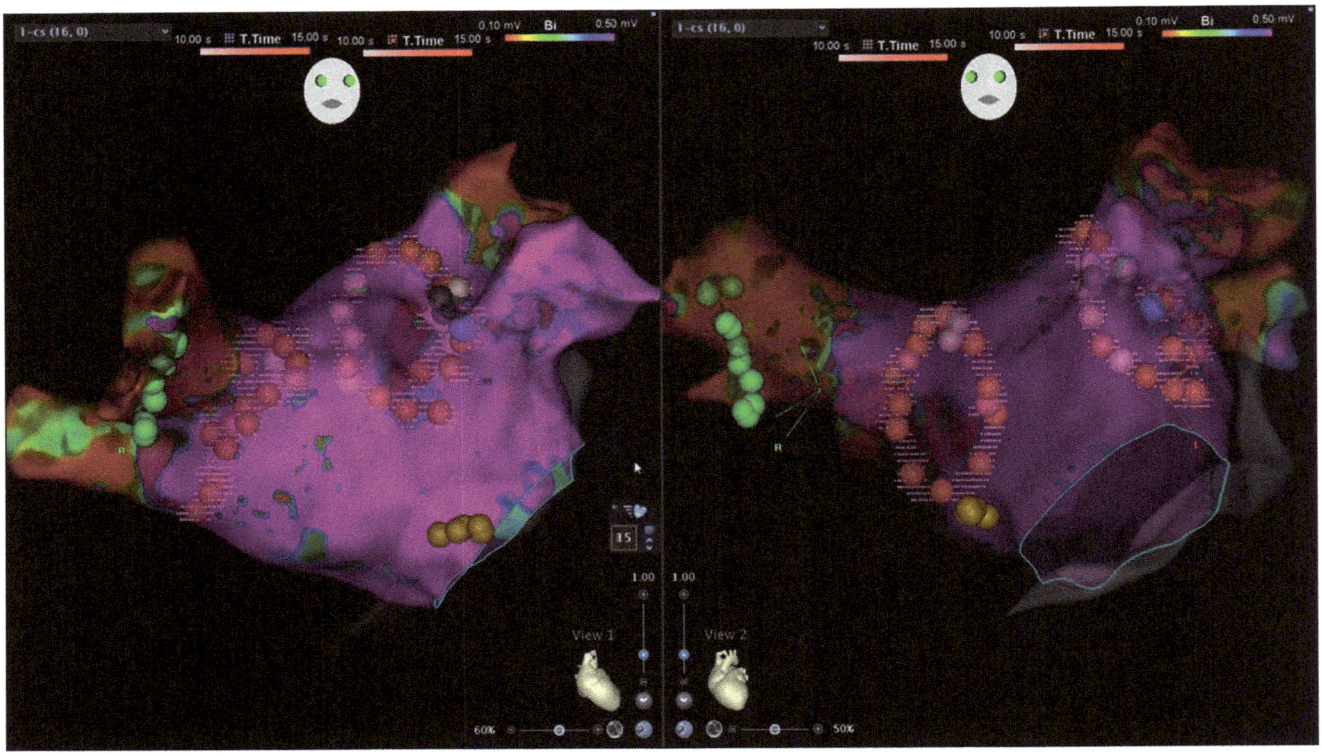

Figure 7.8 EAM system orthogonal views of the LA geometry reconstruction. Observe the **green tags** anterior to the right veins where the phrenic nerve was captured with high output pacing. The ablation lesions tags (**red dots**) are far away from the phrenic location tags.

Contact Force-Guided Non-Fluoroscopic Ablation and Safety

Although non-fluoroscopic catheter ablation of cardiac arrhythmias has been shown to be safe even prior to the advent of contact force-sensing catheters, we believe this new technology contributes to safer catheter navigation without fluoroscopy. Even with the use of fluoroscopy, high contact force can be inadvertently applied to the tissue during catheter manipulation. With the use of fluoroscopy, we can perhaps appreciate the bending of the most distal aspect of the catheter suggesting high contact; this is not possible with non-fluoroscopic navigation techniques, so inadvertent high pressure is a possibility. Real-time tissue-tip contact force measurements reassure the operator of the positioning and pressure exerted to the cardiac tissue without fluoroscopy.

One report of 30 patients, including 12 pediatric patients, using contact-force ablation catheters with the non-fluoroscopic technique described the ablation of right atrial (20 patients), left atrial (8 patients), and right ventricular outflow tract (2 patients) arrhythmias with no complications and no arrhythmia recurrence at 6 months.

The use of contact force catheters similarly likely improves safety during AF ablation. The safe and effective use of contact force sensor catheter during non-fluoroscopic ablation technique was evaluated in a randomized study.[15] Eight patients were randomized to CARTO- and ICE-guided AF ablation with a contact force catheter, where procedural characteristic and arrhythmia-free survival at 12 months were compared to traditional fluoroscopy-guided AF ablation techniques. No serious procedure-related complications were reported and no differences in arrhythmia-free survival at 12 months were found between the groups.

Non-Fluoroscopic in Ventricular Tachycardia

The published experience of reduced and non-fluoroscopic during ventricular tachycardia (VT) ablation procedures is scarce. Two technological tools have allowed making improvements in fluoroscopy reduction and safety during VT ablation.

Again, intracardiac echocardiography (ICE) helps to reduce fluoroscopy and safely navigate the cardiac chamber through:

1. The direct visualization of endocavitary structures (e.g., papillary muscles), which are currently not provided by any other real-time mapping system
2. The provision of detailed anatomical landmarks to improve the navigation of the ablation catheter

3. The monitoring of contact between the catheter tip and the ventricular tissue during pace mapping, activation mapping, and ablation[16]
4. The ability to identify early complications (e.g., pericardial effusion)

Two specific sites of arrhythmia origin where ICE can enhance safety in reduced fluoroscopy procedures are:

1. Coronary cusp VT, where the ICE can identify the tip of the ablation catheter in relation to the os of the coronary arteries, therefore helping to avoid inadvertent injury to those critical structures.
2. Papillary muscle VT, where EAM systems have limitation in acquiring detailed geometry of the intracavitary protrusion of the PM, therefore limiting the precise localization of such structures. ICE and the CARTOSOUND module can be quite helpful in determining the precise location and degree of contact of the catheter with the tissues in these regions, conferring safety and potentially enhancing effectiveness.[16]

A second technological tool useful to enhance safety in fluoroscopy reduction in ventricular tachycardia ablation procedures is the CARTOUNIVU module. This module allows the registration of still-frame fluoroscopic images to the CARTO system and superimposes the 3D map over the pre-acquired fluoroscopic image. See Chapter 4 for further details.

This tool was studied prospectively in 44 catheter ablation patients with ventricular tachycardia. Although these were not non-fluoroscopic procedures, CARTOUNIVU allowed a minimally fluoroscopic approach in approximately 50% of cases, mostly endocardial ablations.[17]

In our laboratory we find the best application of this technology in epicardial ventricular tachycardia ablation procedures. Although currently the technique of epicardial access relies fully on fluoroscopic guidance, CARTOUNIVU can register the coronary angiography images to help determine the anatomical relation between the ablation catheter and the major epicardial coronary branches. One important safety recommendation prior to applying RF energy in the epicardial space is to confirm the distance between the ablation catheter tip and any major epicardial arteries. This relies exclusively on fluoroscopic images and coronary contrast injection. Although this may work well with focal ablation of ventricular arrhythmias, not uncommonly ventricular arrhythmias require more extensive substrate modification to achieve success. Therefore, several coronary contrast injections in different fluoroscopic projections during the procedure, often with relocation of the ablation catheter along the intended target for arrhythmic substrate ablation, are required. CARTOUNIVU will subsequently enable visualization of the coronary angiographic images of the epicardial coronary arteries while applying RF energy to the epicardial surface without the need to repeat serial coronary angiography (**Figure 7.9**).

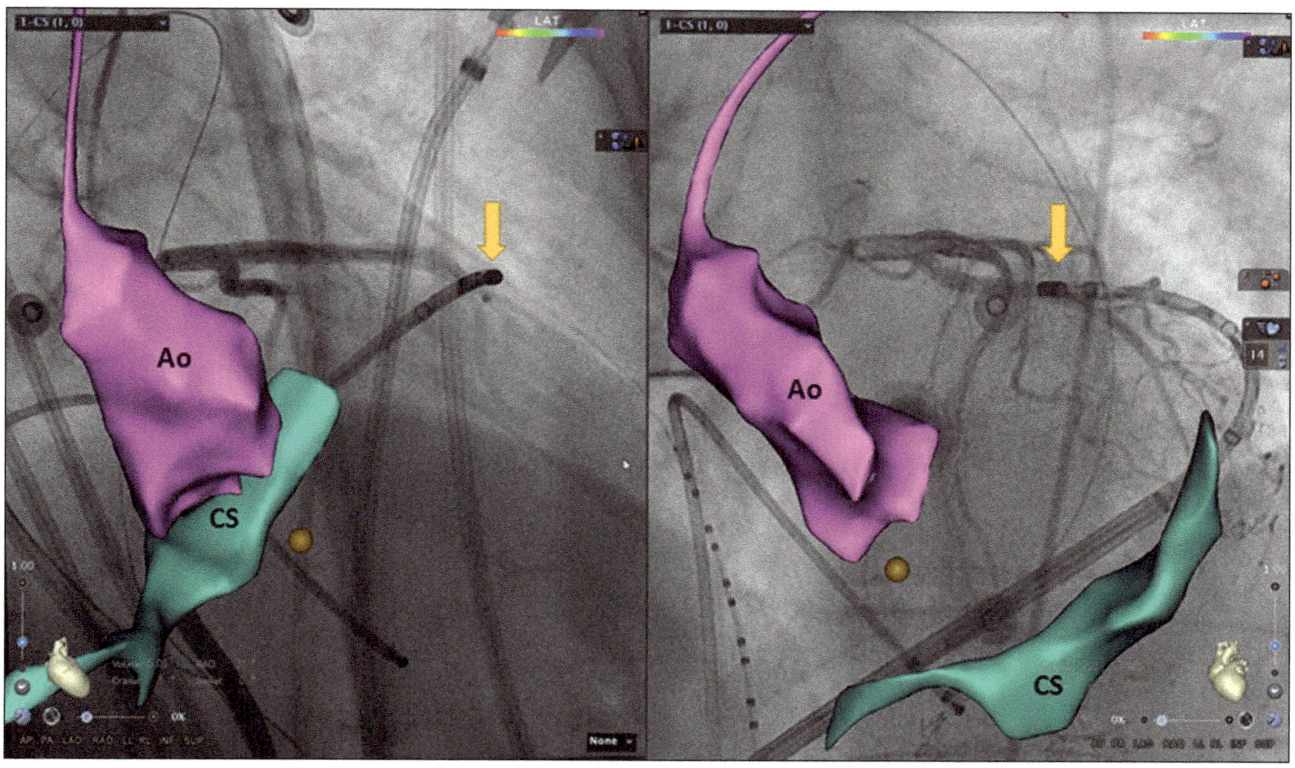

Figure 7.9 RAO and LAO views of CARTO mapping system with the CARTOUNIVU fluoroscopic acquisition during left coronary injection with the ablation catheter (**yellow arrow**) at the site of ablation in the epicardial space. Ao: aorta; CS: coronary sinus.

Conclusion

The safety of non-fluoroscopic techniques to ablate cardiac arrhythmias has been reported reasonably extensively in the literature. Technological tools such as EAM systems and ICE have contributed greatly to the safe development and application of non-fluoroscopic techniques to the full range of cardiac arrhythmias. Arrhythmias of all 4 heart chambers can be safely performed with non-fluoroscopic techniques provided certain safety tips such as the ones described in this chapter are strictly followed. In the future, the widespread adoption of non-fluoroscopic techniques and further technological development will allow operators to deliver these complex therapies safely.

References

1. Calkins H, Hindricks G, Cappato R, et al. HRS/EHRA/ECAS/APHRS/SOLAECE expert consensus statement on catheter and surgical ablation of atrial fibrillation. *Heart Rhythm.* Oct 2017;(14); No 10.
2. Drago F, Silvetti MS, Di Pino A, Grutter G, Bevilacqua M, Leibovich S. Exclusion of fluoroscopy during ablation treatment of right accessory pathway in children. *J Cardiovasc Electrophysiol.* 2002;13(8):778–782.
3. Tuzcu V. A non-fluoroscopic approach for electrophysiology and catheter ablation procedures using a three-dimensional navigation system. *Pacing Clin Electrophysiol.* 2007;30: 519–525.
4. Earley MJ, Showkathali R, Alzetani M, et al. Radiofrequency ablation of arrhythmias guided by non-fluoroscopic catheter location: A prospective randomized trial. *Eur Heart J.* 2006;27:1223–1239.
5. Alvarez M, Tercedor L, Almansa I, et al. Safety and feasibility of catheter ablation for atrioventricular nodal re-entrant tachycardia without fluoroscopic guidance. *Heart Rhythm.* 2009;6:1714–1720.
6. Schmidt B, Chun KR, Ouyang F, Metzner A, Antz M, Kuck KH. Three-dimensional reconstruction of the anatomic course of the right phrenic nerve in humans by pace mapping. *Heart Rhythm.* 2008 Aug;5(8):1120–1126. doi:10.1016/j.hrthm.2008.05.003
7. Razminia M, Manankil MF, Eryazici PL, et al. Non-fluoroscopic catheter ablation of cardiac arrhythmias in adults: Feasibility, safety, and efficacy. *J Cardiovasc Electrophysiol.* 2012 Oct;23(10):1078–1086.
8. Macias R, Uribe I, Tercedor L, Jimenez J, Barrio T, Alvarez MA. A zero-fluoroscopy approach to cavotricuspid isthmus catheter ablation: Comparative analysis of two electroanatomical mapping systems. *Pacing Clin Electrophysiol.* 2014; 37:1029–1037.
9. Bencsik G. Novel strategies in the ablation of typical atrial flutter: Role of intracardiac echocardiography. *Curr Cardiol Rev.* 2015;11:127–133.
10. Ross J Jr, Braunwald E, Morrow AG. Transseptal left heart catheterization: A new diagnostic method. *Prog Cardiovasc Dis.* 1960;2:315–318.
11. Clark J, Bockoven JR, Lane J, Patel CR, Smith G. Use of three-dimensional catheter guidance and trans-esophageal echocardiography to eliminate fluoroscopy in catheter ablation of left-sided accessory pathways. *Pacing Clin Electrophysiol.* 2008;31:283–289.
12. Reddy VY, Morales G, Ahmed H, et al. Catheter ablation of atrial fibrillation without the use of fluoroscopy. *Heart Rhythm.* 2010 Nov;7(11):1644–1653.
13. Scaglione M, Ebrille E, Caponi D, et al. Zero-fluoroscopy ablation of accessory pathways in children and adolescents: CARTO3 electroanatomic mapping combined with RF and cryoenergy. *Pacing Clin Electrophysiol.* 2015;38:675–681.
14. Sabar MI, Bajpai A, Momin A, Kaba RA. Circular mapping catheter entrapment in mitral valve apparatus requiring emergency surgery: A rarely reported complication of pulmonary vein isolation procedure for atrial fibrillation. *BMJ Case Rep.* 2017 Oct; 25;2017.
15. Bulava A, Hanis J, Eisenberger M. Ablation of atrial fibrillation using zero-fluoroscopy technique: A randomized trial. *Pacing Clin Electrophysiology.* 2015; 38:797–806.
16. Proietti R, Rivera S, Dussault C, et al. Intracardiac echo-facilitated 3D electroanatomical mapping of ventricular arrhythmias from the papillary muscles: assessing the 'fourth dimension' during ablation. *Europace.* 2017;19:21–28.
17. Cano Ó, Andres A, Osca J, et al. Safety and feasibility of a minimally fluoroscopic approach for ventricular tachycardia ablation in patients with structural heart disease. *Circ Arrhythm Electrophysiol.* 2016;9:e003706. doi:10.1161/CIRCEP.115.003706

8

How to Monitor Esophageal Temperature Without Fluoroscopy

Oliver D'Silva, MD; Hany Demo, MD; Theodore Wang, MD; Mansour Razminia, MD

Introduction

The prevalence of atrial fibrillation (AF) has risen and currently affects a growing portion of the U.S. population. In parallel with this increase in prevalence of disease has come an increase in ablation procedures for AF. As this procedure is becoming performed with increasing frequency, one of the remaining questions is how to optimize the procedure's safety, particularly with respect to the esophagus, to avoid the rare but potentially fatal complication of atrioesophageal fistula. Monitoring the esophageal temperature has been deemed to be one method to alert the operator and assist in guiding energy delivery during ablation of left atrial arrhythmias.[1,2] Traditionally, assessment of the location of the esophageal temperature probe was performed under fluoroscopic guidance. A non-fluoroscopic approach to esophageal temperature monitoring has been devised[3] and will be described in this section.

Procedure

There are several reported approaches to monitor the esophageal temperature without the use of fluoroscopy, 2 of which will be detailed in this section. In the first approach, a standard linear single-sensor probe (SSP) (Acoustascope, Smiths Medical ASD, Inc.) is used to monitor the temperature (**Figure 8.1**). In the second, a multisensor self-expandable probe (MSPs) CIRCA S-Cath MSP (CIRCA Scientific, LLC, Englewood, CO) (**Figure 8.2**) is used to monitor the esophageal temperature.

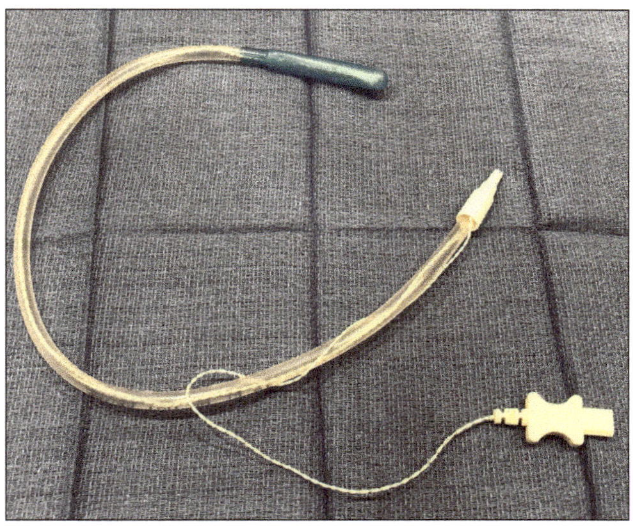

Figure 8.1 Standard linear single-sensor esophageal probe.

Fluoroscopy Reduction Techniques for Catheter Ablation of Cardiac Arrhythmias. © 2019 Mansour Razminia, Paul C. Zei, eds. Cardiotext Publishing, ISBN: 978-1-942909-30-9.

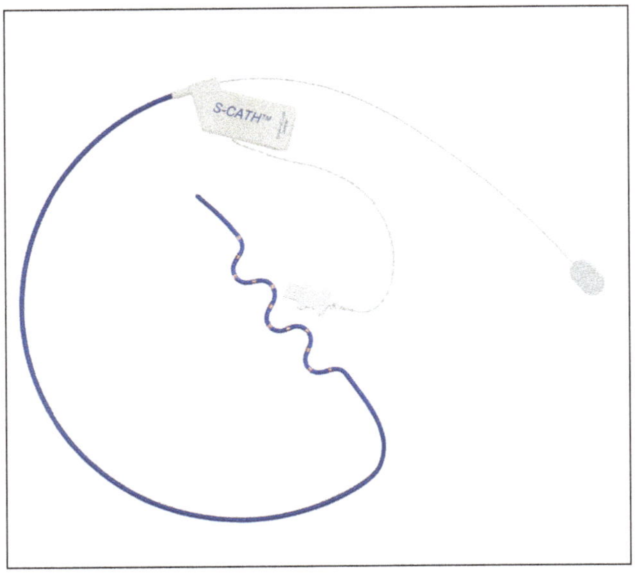

Figure 8.2 Multisensor self-expandable probe catheter, Circa S-Cath. (Reprinted with permission of CIRCA Scientific.)

Standard Linear Single-Sensor Probe

If an SSP probe is being used to monitor the esophageal temperature, the following steps are taken to place the probe prior to ablation and to adjust its position during ablation. First, using a scissor, a small cross-shaped slit is made in the outer covering of the distal end of the probe with care being taken to preserve the integrity of the probe (**Figure 8.3**). Next, gel is applied to the tip of a quadripolar catheter and it is inserted into the lumen of the probe. The quadripolar catheter is advanced such that its distal end aligns with the very distal tip of the esophageal stethoscope (**Figure 8.4**). The proximal end of the quadripolar catheter is then marked with a permanent marker (**Figure 8.5**). This marker helps the operator know the location of the tip of the quadripolar catheter relative to the tip of the probe; this is crucial to know precisely the location of the esophageal temperature probe. When the tip of the quadripolar catheter has exited the esophageal temperature probe, the quadripolar catheter tip may be visualized on the EnSite system (Abbott, Abbott Park, IL). In this fashion, the relative location of the temperature probe within the esophagus can be identified as the different pulmonary veins are isolated. To advance the temperature probe distally when ablating near the inferior pulmonary veins, the quadripolar catheter is withdrawn slightly such that the marker on the quadripolar catheter is seen 1 inch proximal to the proximal end of the esophageal temperature probe. At this point, the quadripolar catheter/temperature probe assembly may be advanced together without incurring the increased risk of perforation if the quadripolar catheter remained exposed to the esophageal lumen. After advancing the assembly, the quadripolar catheter is advanced slightly so that the marker aligns with the proximal end of the temperature probe. The temperature probe is then withdrawn minimally to unsheath the tip of the quadripolar catheter (**Figure 8.6**), revealing the relative location of the esophageal temperature probe. To delineate the course of the esophagus on the EnSite system relative to the LA and pulmonary veins, the temperature probe-quadripolar catheter assembly is withdrawn under electroanatomic mapping guidance while the tip of the quadripolar catheter is slightly exposed beyond the tip of the temperature probe (**Figure 8.7**).

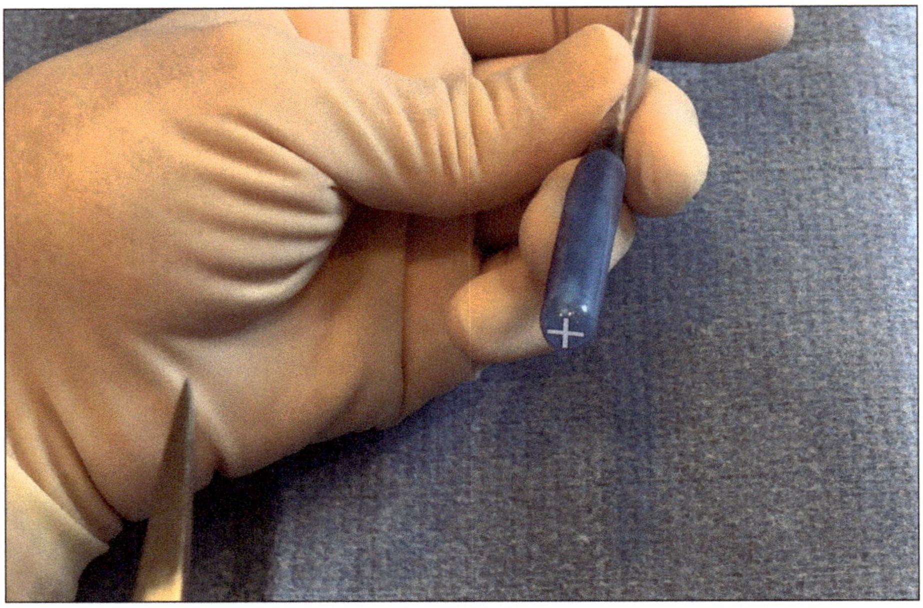

Figure 8.3 A small, cross-shaped slit is made in the outer covering of the distal end of the probe.

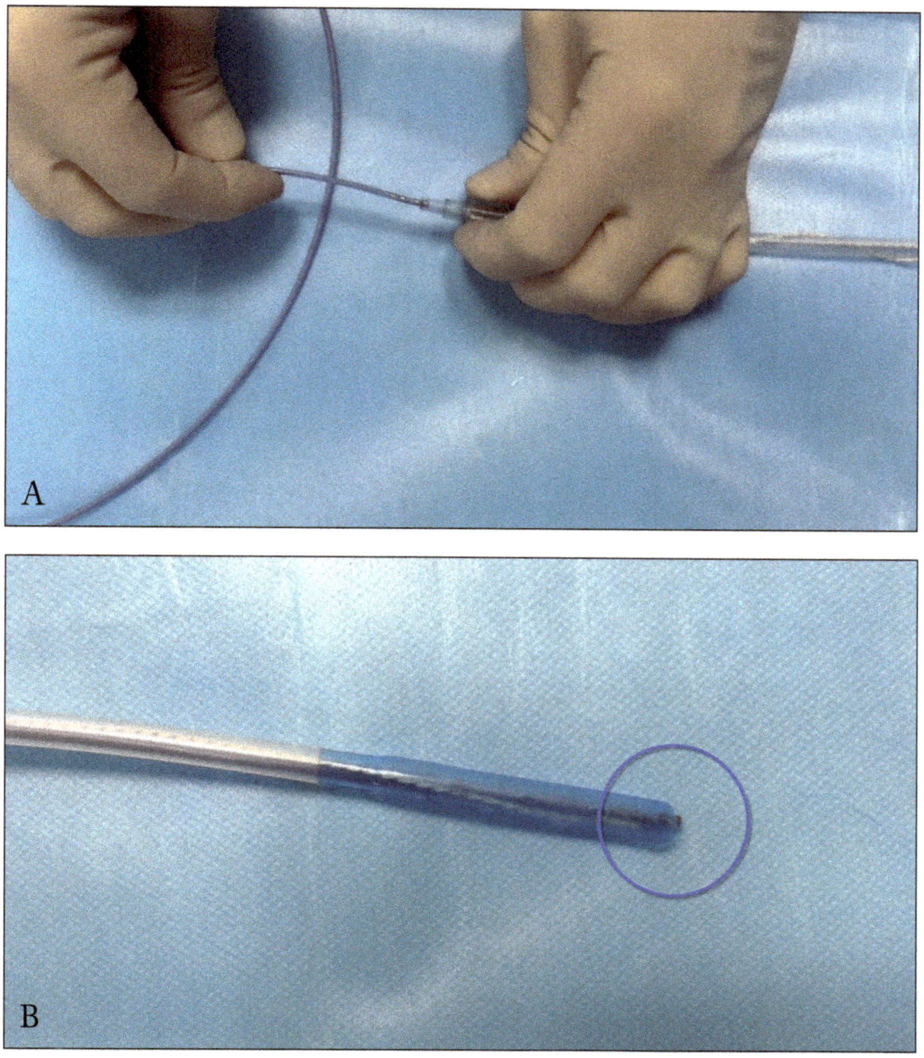

Figure 8.4 The quadripolar catheter is advanced through the esophageal stethoscope (**A**) such that the distal end aligns with the very distal tip of the esophageal stethoscope (**B**).

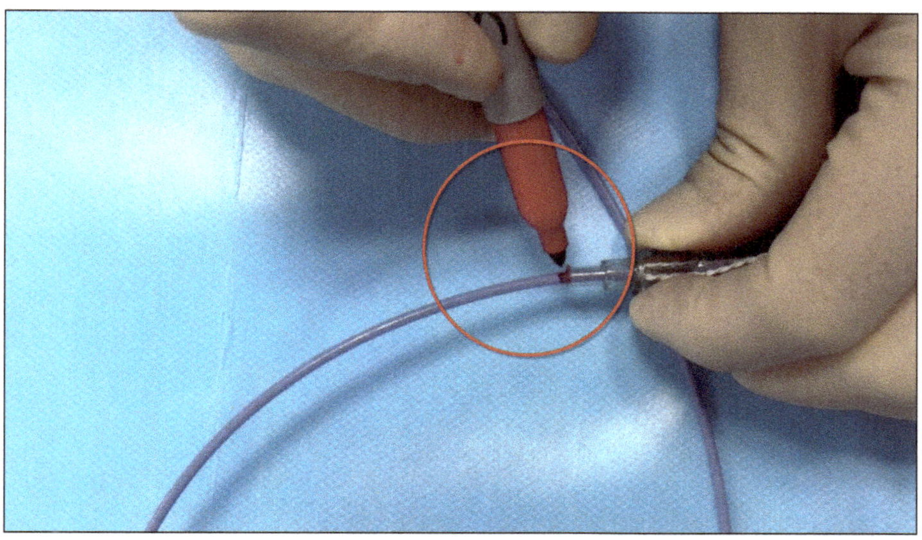

Figure 8.5 The proximal end of the quadripolar catheter is then marked with a permanent marker.

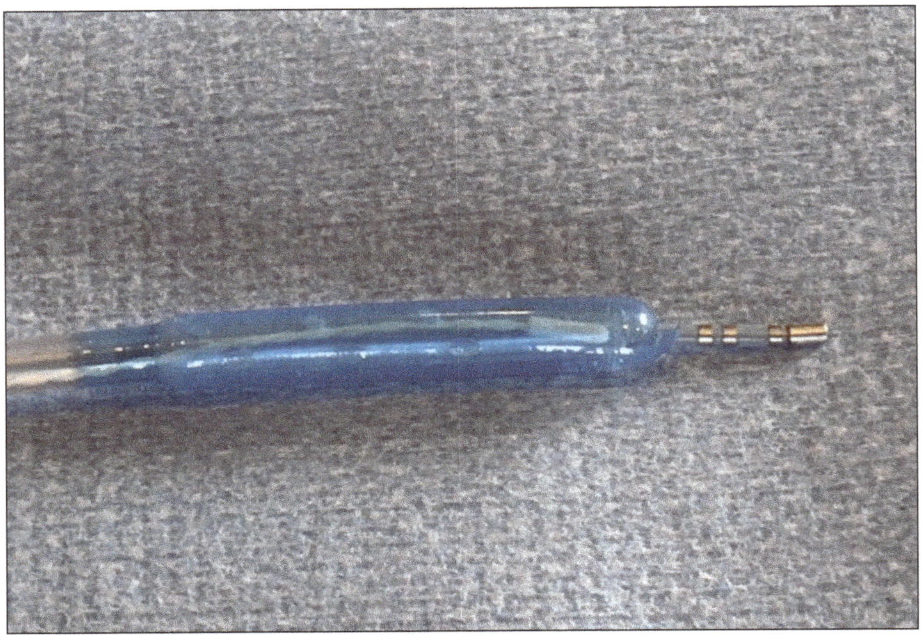

Figure 8.6 The temperature probe is then withdrawn minimally to unsheath the tip of the quadripolar catheter.

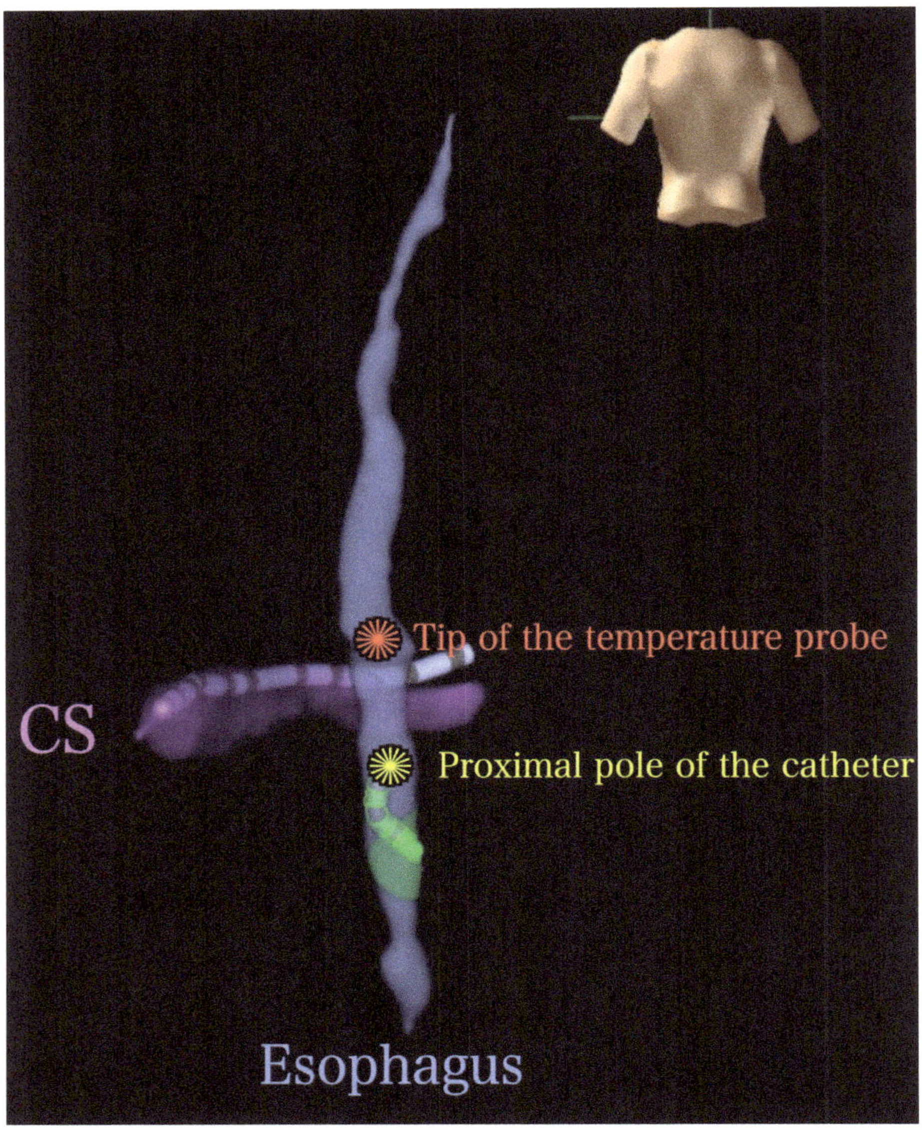

Figure 8.7 The esophagus course is delineated on the mapping system by withdrawing the temperature probe while the tip of the quadripolar catheter is exposed beyond the tip of the temperature probe.

An alternate strategy can be utilized with the CARTO system. A quadripolar catheter can be sutured near the tip of the temperature probe such that the relationship between them is fixed and known. The quadripolar catheter can then be visualized on the mapping system, and the 2 catheters moved as a unit. We emphasize keeping the quadripolar catheter at least 1 cm from the corresponding ablation site in the left atrium (LA) to avoid the theoretical risk of current sink to the catheter electrodes. Finally, other operators move the temperature probe via intracardiac echocardiographic (ICE) visualization of the esophagus.

Multisensor Self-Expandable Probes

If a multisensor, self-expandable probe is used to monitor the esophageal temperature, it is advanced into the esophagus under ICE guidance. The thermistors on the probe can be seen on ICE, with the most distal thermistor designated as "1" and the most proximal as "12" (**Figure 8.8**). From the home view, clockwise rotation is applied to the ICE catheter such that the left-sided pulmonary veins are visualized. To better visualize the esophagus, the ICE catheter is withdrawn minimally, and minimal left steer is applied. A slight amount of clockwise rotation is then applied such that the right inferior pulmonary vein (RIPV) is just coming into view. As the level of the RIPV often indicates a posterior location of the LA, this location is favored for visualizing the esophagus. In this view, the esophagus should be seen in a longitudinal view (**Figure 8.9**). At this point the probe is advanced into the esophagus. Once the sixth thermistor is seen at the level of the of the RIPV, the stylet for the probe is withdrawn and the serpentine shape of the temperature probe is seen under ICE (**Figure 8.10**). With the sixth thermistor at the level of the RIPV, the first thermistor is typically distal to the inferior border of the LA, and this method has been validated using fluoroscopy in our lab (**Figure 8.11**). The benefit of the multipolar temperature probe is increased sensitivity to temperature rises and the lack of need to adjust the temperature probe location in the esophagus as ablation is being performed.

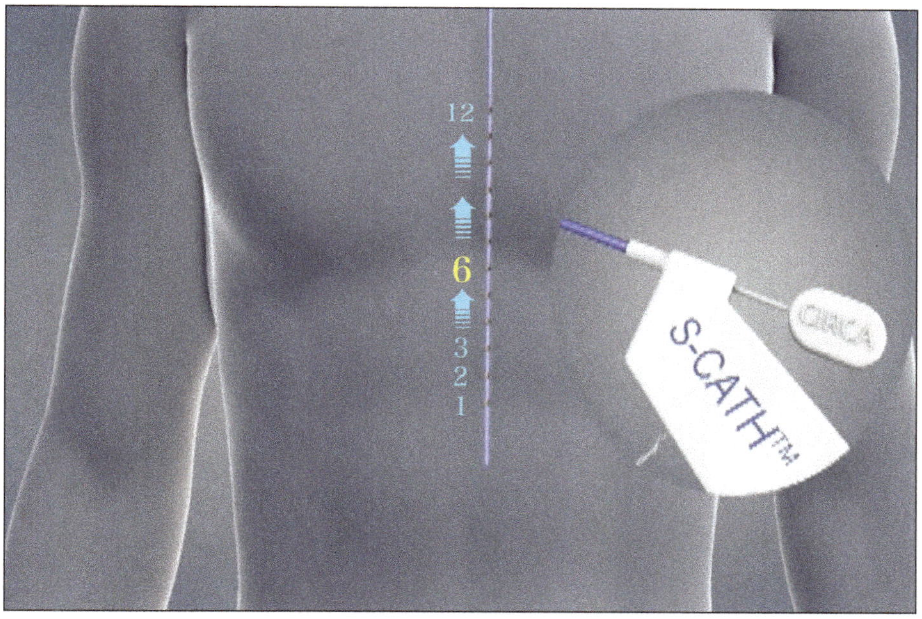

Figure 8.8 The Circa catheter with the most distal thermistor designated as "1" and the most proximal as "12." (Reproduced with permission of CIRCA Scientific.)

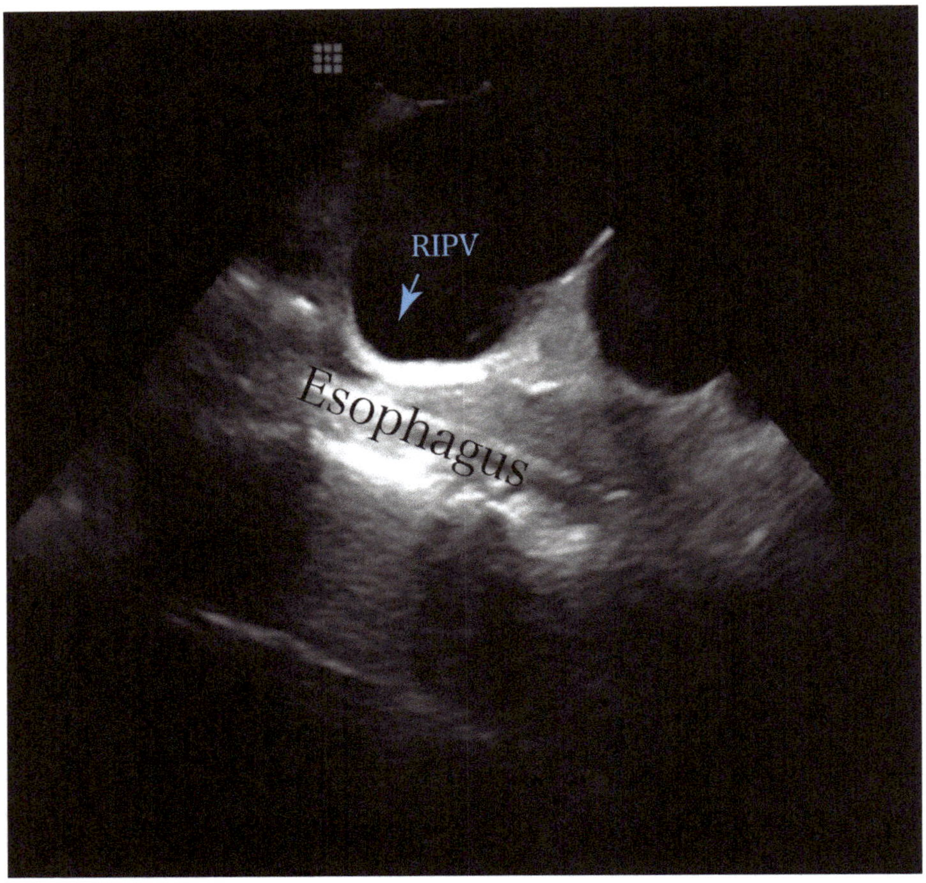

Figure 8.9 Longitudinal view of the esophagus with the right inferior pulmonary vein in view.

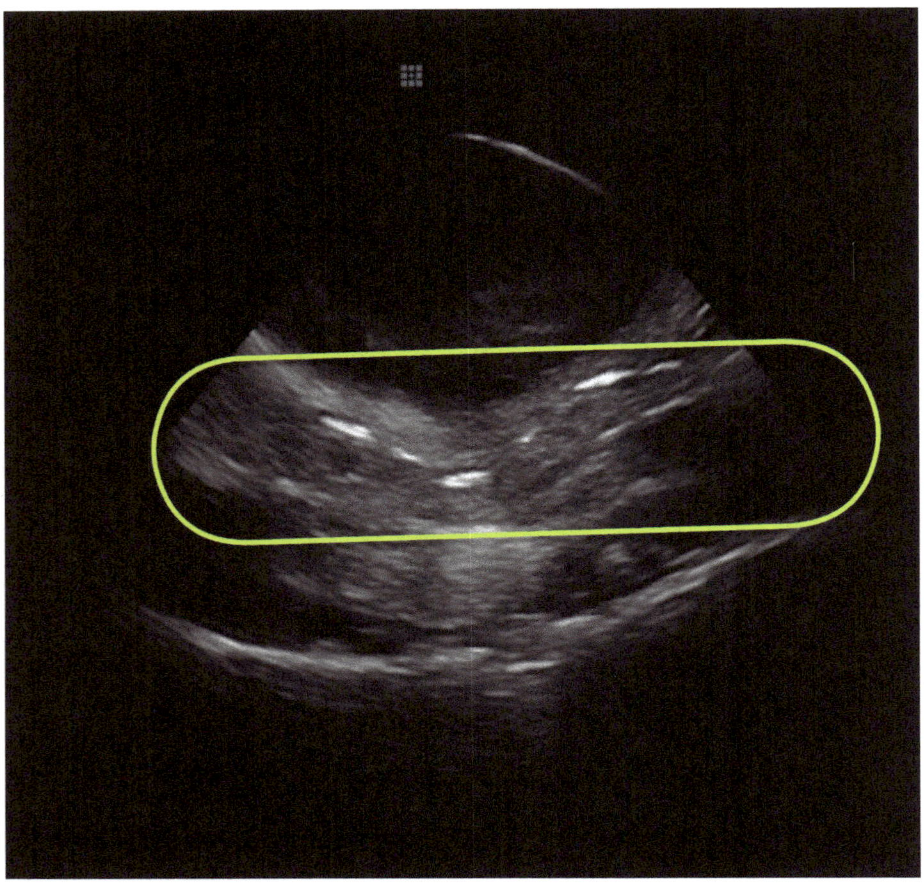

Figure 8.10 The stylet for the temperature probe is withdrawn, and the serpentine shape of the temperature probe is seen under ICE.

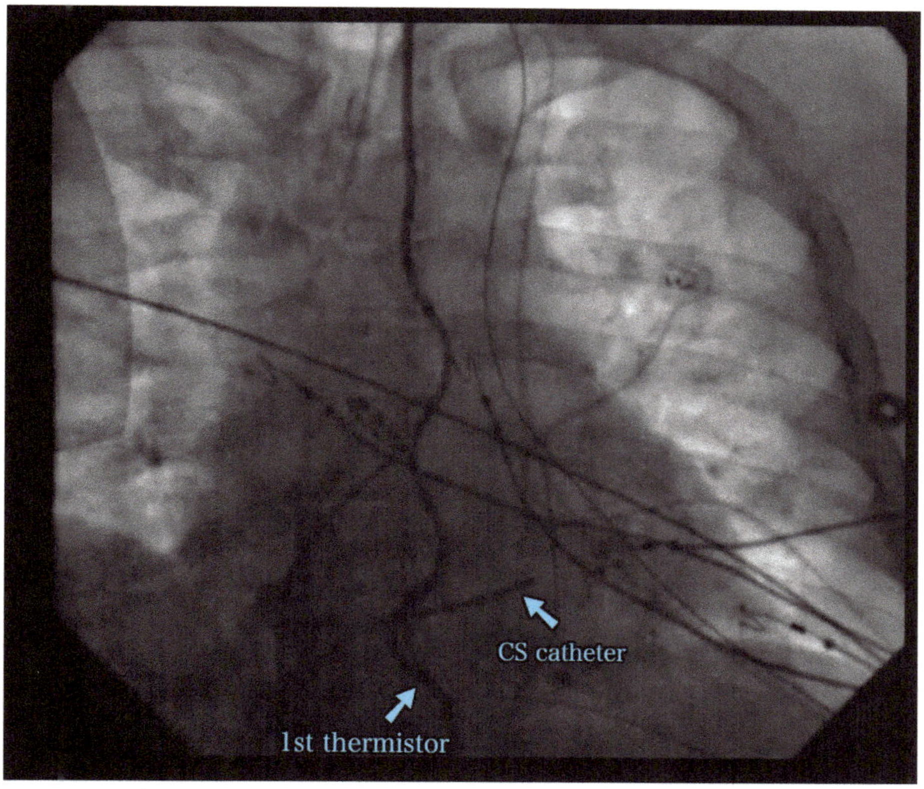

Figure 8.11 With the sixth thermistor at the level of the RIPV, the first thermistor is typically distal to the inferior border of the LA, and this method has been validated using fluoroscopy.

Advantages and Limitations

When compared to a traditional method of esophageal temperature monitoring using fluoroscopy, a fluoroscopy-free method of esophageal temperature monitoring offers an advantage of no harmful radiation being delivered to the patient, electrophysiology lab staff, and physicians. While the benefit of using esophageal temperature monitoring for reduction in esophageal injury is not absolutely clear at this point, it is one approach that can be undertaken without fluoroscopy. Other methods, such as the use of barium swallow or esophageal deviation, would necessitate the use of fluoroscopy.

A possible disadvantage of the fluoroscopy-free method of esophageal temperature monitoring is in the cost incurred by using a quadripolar catheter. Cost-effectiveness may be increased by resterilization and reuse of the quadripolar catheter. In our center, the quadripolar catheter is resterilized in a fashion similar to that of one being used to resterilize a transesophageal echocardiography probe.

Conclusion

The risk that radiation poses to patients and electrophysiology staff during catheter ablation procedures is significant and efforts should be made to try to eliminate unnecessary exposure whenever possible. While the amount of fluoroscopy used to monitor the location of the esophageal temperature probe may be not be very much, this stage of the procedure may have been a limiting factor for some operators to perform a truly fluoroscopy-free approach. Two approaches, one involving an SSP and another involving a multisensor, self-expandable probe can be performed without the use of fluoroscopy.

References

1. Perzanowski C, Teplitsky, Hranitzky PM, Bahnson TD. Real-time monitoring of luminal esophageal temperature during left atrial radiofrequency catheter ablation for atrial fibrillation: Observations about esophageal heating during ablation at the pulmonary vein ostia and posterior left atrium. *J Cardiovasc Electrophysiol.* 2006;17:166–170.
2. Redfearn DP, Trim GM, Skanes AC, et al. Esophageal temperature monitoring during radiofrequency ablation of atrial fibrillation. *J Cardiovasc Electrophysiol.* 2005;16: 589–593.
3. Sherzer AI, Feigenblum DY, Kulkarni S, et al. Continuous non-fluoroscopic localization of the esophagus during radiofrequency catheter ablation of atrial fibrillation. *J Cardiovasc Electrophysiol.* 2007;18:157–160.

Video Legend

Video 8S Chapter summary and step-by-step procedures by Mansour Razminia. [7:17]

Section 2

Ablation of Supraventricular Tachycardia

9

How to Ablate Atrioventricular Nodal Reentrant Tachycardia Using No Fluoroscopy

Nicholas H. Von Bergen, MD; Ian H. Law, MD

Introduction

Atrioventricular nodal reentrant tachycardia (AVNRT) is an arrhythmia that is well suited for radiation-free ablation. It is generally localized in an area easily accessible from the systemic venous circulation and is usually distant from coronary arteries and other structures that might prompt the use of angiography. Moreover, given the population with AVNRT (and supraventricular tachycardia [SVT] in general) presenting for catheter ablation tends to be younger, the likely benefits of fluoroscopy-free ablation is significant regarding lifetime risk of radiation-related complications. In this chapter, we will discuss the basic mechanism of AVNRT, an overview of AVNRT therapy, and describe a stepwise approach for a radiation-free ablation of AVNRT.

Background

AVNRT remains the most common mechanism of SVT in the pediatric and young adult population.[1,2] Patients typically describe a sudden-onset, sudden-termination arrhythmia with rates commonly over 200 bpm in the young.

The anatomic electrophysiologic mechanism of AVNRT is considered to be the result of a reentrant circuit involving 2 distinct conduction pathways, commonly termed the "fast" and "slow" pathways (**Figure 9.1**A and B). These pathways or inputs to the atrioventricular (AV) node were reported as early as 1956, when it was noted that a "jump" in the timing of the atrial and ventricular signals in canine hearts suggested dual AV nodal physiology.[3] Although there are examples of patients who have inducible AVNRT without the classic "jump," most electrophysiologists indeed ascribe the mechanism of arrhythmia to a dual pathway mechanism providing both an antegrade and retrograde limb of the reentrant circuit in the AV nodal area (Figure 9.1B).[4]

The earliest technique to cure patients of AVNRT was by surgical disruption of the perinodal area.[5] This was, understandably, associated with a relatively high risk of permanent AV block, and was replaced by transcatheter radiofrequency (RF) ablation in the late 1980s.[6,7] After initial ablations directed at the fast pathway, electrophysiologists quickly shifted from fast pathway to slow pathway ablations in the early 1990s, which forms the basis of the technique we use today.[8,9] Despite advances in ablation strategies, AVNRT continues to have relatively higher recurrences rates and an increased risk of AV nodal injury in comparison to other common reentrant arrhythmias after ablation.[10,11] This, in part, has prompted some physicians to shift from an anatomic guided ablation toward an ablation using voltage mapping, and occasionally propagation mapping, both of which will be described later in this chapter.

Fluoroscopy Reduction Techniques for Catheter Ablation of Cardiac Arrhythmias. © 2019 Mansour Razminia, Paul C. Zei, eds.
Cardiotext Publishing, ISBN: 978-1-942909-30-9.

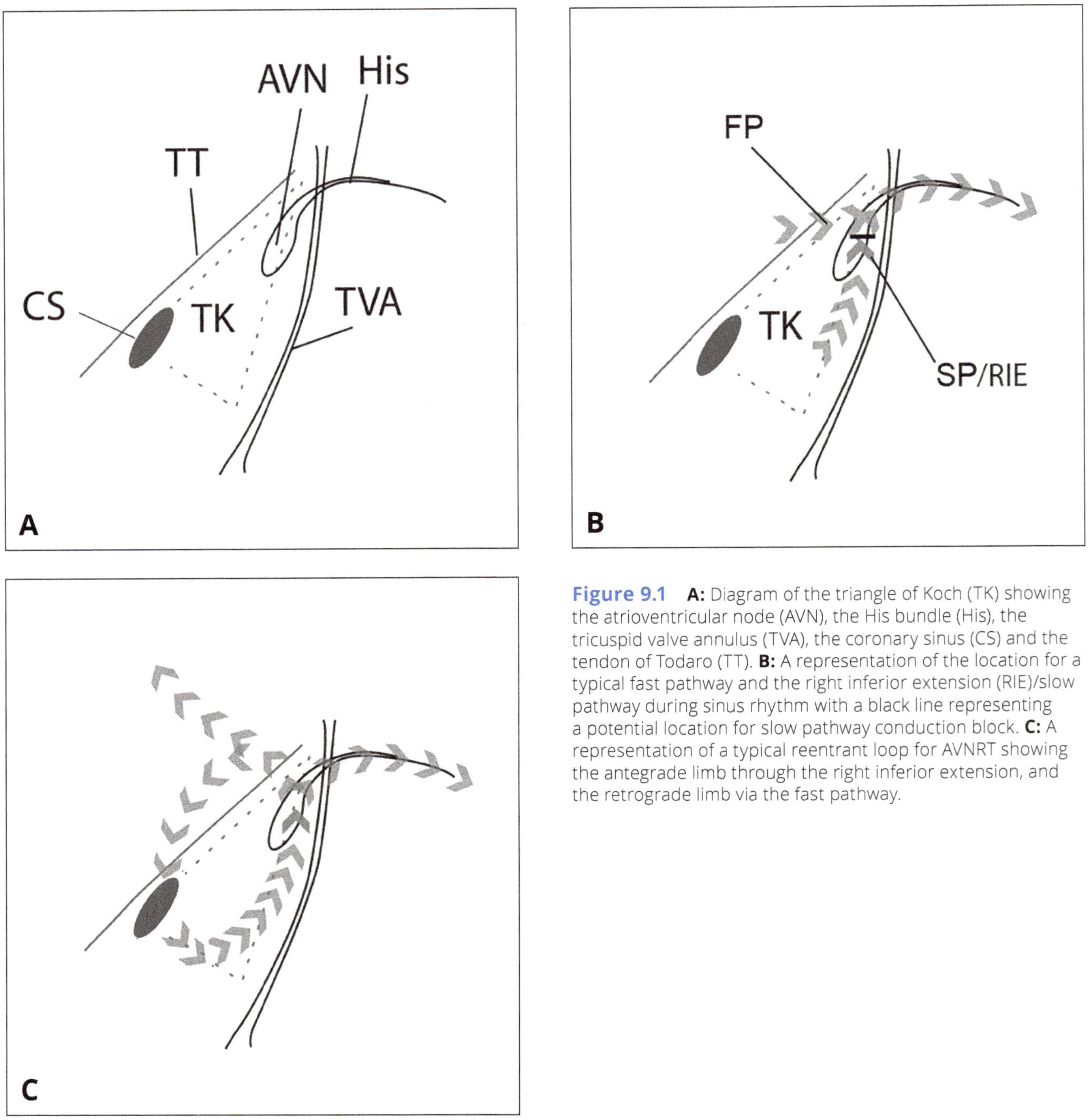

Figure 9.1 **A:** Diagram of the triangle of Koch (TK) showing the atrioventricular node (AVN), the His bundle (His), the tricuspid valve annulus (TVA), the coronary sinus (CS) and the tendon of Todaro (TT). **B:** A representation of the location for a typical fast pathway and the right inferior extension (RIE)/slow pathway during sinus rhythm with a black line representing a potential location for slow pathway conduction block. **C:** A representation of a typical reentrant loop for AVNRT showing the antegrade limb through the right inferior extension, and the retrograde limb via the fast pathway.

Mechanism of AVNRT

While there has been extensive investigation into AVNRT, there is no standard convention regarding the classification of AVNRT. AVNRT has been classified based on the speed of the antegrade and retrograde limb (i.e., slow/fast, fast/slow or slow/slow AVNRT), or based on its relative frequency of occurrence (i.e., typical or atypical AVNRT). It has also been described by the anatomic location of the antegrade and retrograde limbs (i.e., right inferior extension (RIE)/fast pathway vs. leftward extension). For the sake of clarity and accuracy, we will label AVNRT based on the location of both antegrade and retrograde conduction, with the most common "typical" AVNRT labeled as the RIE/fast pathway (FP) reentrant loop. This circuit is shown by the reentrant circuit in Figure 9.1C. Note that the reentrant circuit passes through the typical slow pathway area within the triangle of Koch (TK), which is defined by the central fibrous body (superior), the base of the CS (inferior), the tricuspid valve (ventricular), and tendon of Todaro (atrial).

The majority of AVNRT courses through the traditional slow pathway area in the lower to mid portion of the TK, referred to as the area of the RIE. However, authors have suggested involvement of other nodal inputs, such as in the left inferior septal extension (LIS) and, even less frequently, the left inferior lateral area (LILE) or other rare locations.[12-14] Fortunately, the antegrade limb typically courses through the RIE and the retrograde limb is dependent on the FP. Even when reentrant circuits do not utilize the FP, such as the traditionally labeled slow/slow AVNRT, a portion of the reentrant circuit will often include the RIE in its antegrade or retrograde limb. This allows successful ablation of most types of AVNRT with ablation in the RIE area. Therefore, the focus of our discussion on radiation-free ablation of AVNRT will target the typical RIE location, as this will be successful in the vast majority of cases. If this site is unsuccessful, then additional targets for ablation should be considered.

Stepwise Approach for a Radiation-Free Ablation of AVNRT

For a video exemplifying geometry creation utilizing electroanatomic mapping (EAM), including mapping, site selection, and ablation of AVNRT, please refer to **Video 9.1**.

After radiation-free access to the femoral veins as described in Chapter 5, a mapping catheter can be advanced to the heart while monitoring on the 3D mapping system. For initial geometry creation, a steerable multipole catheter may be used, which will eventually be placed into the CS, although utilizing the EnSite system (Abbott, Abbott Park, IL) requires proprietary catheters for map creation. If utilizing CARTO in its current iteration (CARTO3, Biosense Webster, Irvine, CA), an ablation catheter must be opened and utilized for initial EAM creation (Video 9.1). Once the catheter has reached the IVC/RA junction, atrial electrograms will be visible on the distal electrodes of the catheter. The operator can begin to obtain the geometry of the RA with advancement and gentle sweeps of the catheter through the RA while confirming the location by monitoring the atrial electrograms. The SVC can be accessed with advancement of the catheter while remaining right posterior lateral. Once the catheter passes from the RA to the SVC, loss of atrial signals will allow SVC identification. Once the SVC and IVC are identified, the basic geometry of the RA can be filled in with gentle clockwise and counterclockwise rotation of the catheter. During geometry creation, the His signals should be marked on the 3D map, typically near the 1–2 o'clock position of the tricuspid valve.

After RA geometry is obtained, the steerable catheter is advanced into the CS. From the femoral approach, this can be achieved with slow retraction and clockwise rotation of the steerable catheter that has been placed near 6 o'clock on the tricuspid valve. This will allow the catheter tip to dip leftward into the CS ostium (os), after which the operator can straighten and advance the catheter into the CS itself. From a jugular approach, a counterclockwise rotation on the catheter is needed to access the CS. Placement of at least 2 electrophysiology (EP) catheters—a coronary sinus catheter and a His catheter—is recommended (the authors use a combined His/RV catheter). Many centers also place a high right atrial electrophysiologic catheter. The His signal should be marked if not obtained during geometry creation (**Figure 9.2**).

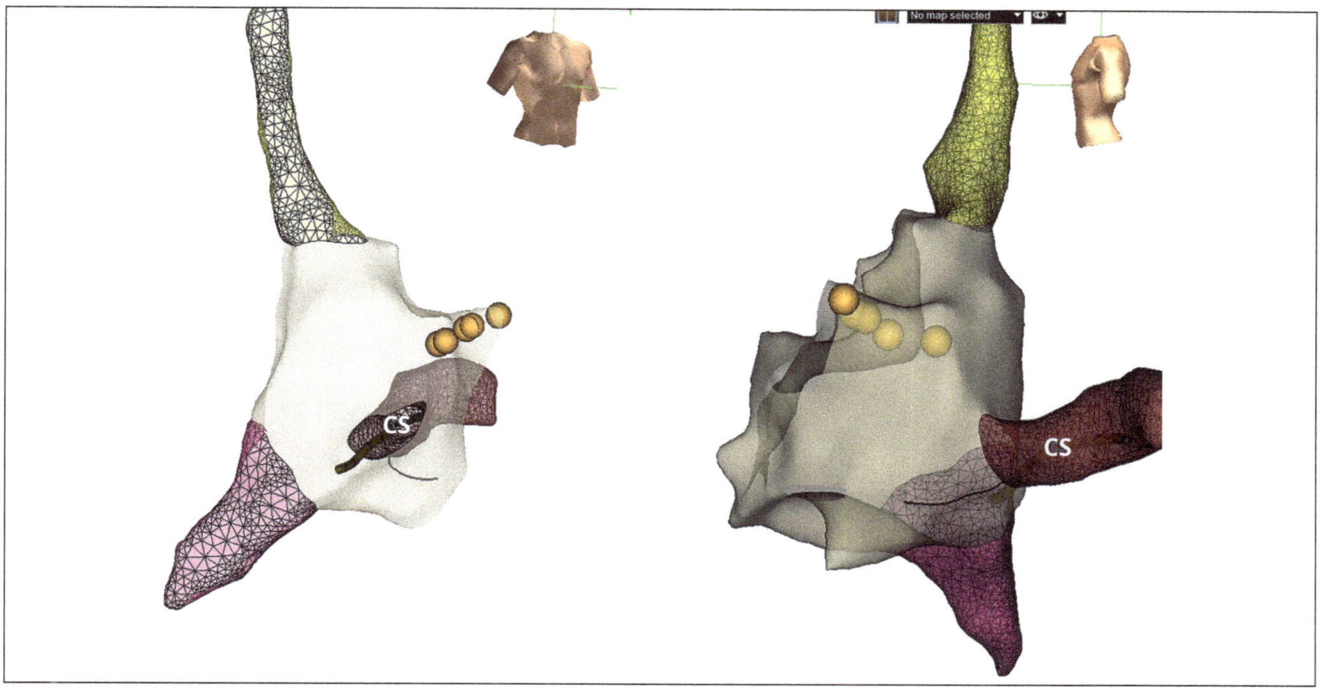

Figure 9.2 A 3D map of RA geometry with the His signals marked (**gold spheres**). Right anterior oblique and left lateral views are shown with the SVC, IVC, and CS in separate colors to assist with distinguishing landmarks.

If AVNRT is suspected or discovered during the EP testing, then careful attention to accurate delineation of the atrial septum and TK geometry is critical.

A baseline EP study should be performed with special attention towards determination of the AH/AV time indicating AH/AV jumps, inducibility of AV node echo beats, and inducibility of AVNRT. Another potential marker of AVNRT susceptibility is the A-A duration in comparison to the A-V duration at Wenckebach during rapid atrial pacing. Patients with inducible AVNRT are more likely to have an A-V duration that "crosses over" the A-A cycle length before Wenckebach. Stated differently, at the time of AV nodal Wenckebach during atrial pacing, the A-A duration (pacing cycle length) is shorter than the A-V time. This suggests the presence of a slow pathway. The absence of this finding during rapid atrial pacing following ablation can be an additional indicator of success.

If AVNRT is induced, the classic intracardiac electrograms for the most common RIE to FP (typical) AVNRT show overlapping atrial and ventricular signals with a VA interval typically less than 70 ms (**Figure 9.3**). Confirmation of AVNRT should be considered and may be different depending on the alternate arrhythmias the maneuvers are trying to exclude. These pacing maneuvers can include: ventricular overdrive pacing with a PPI > TCL and/or late atrial entrainment suggesting retrograde AV nodal conduction; adenosine block during ventricular pacing; parahisian pacing maneuvers to exclude a septal pathway; or a postventricular pacing AH response. These techniques (and others) will not be elaborated upon in this chapter and can be referenced in previous reviews.[2,14]

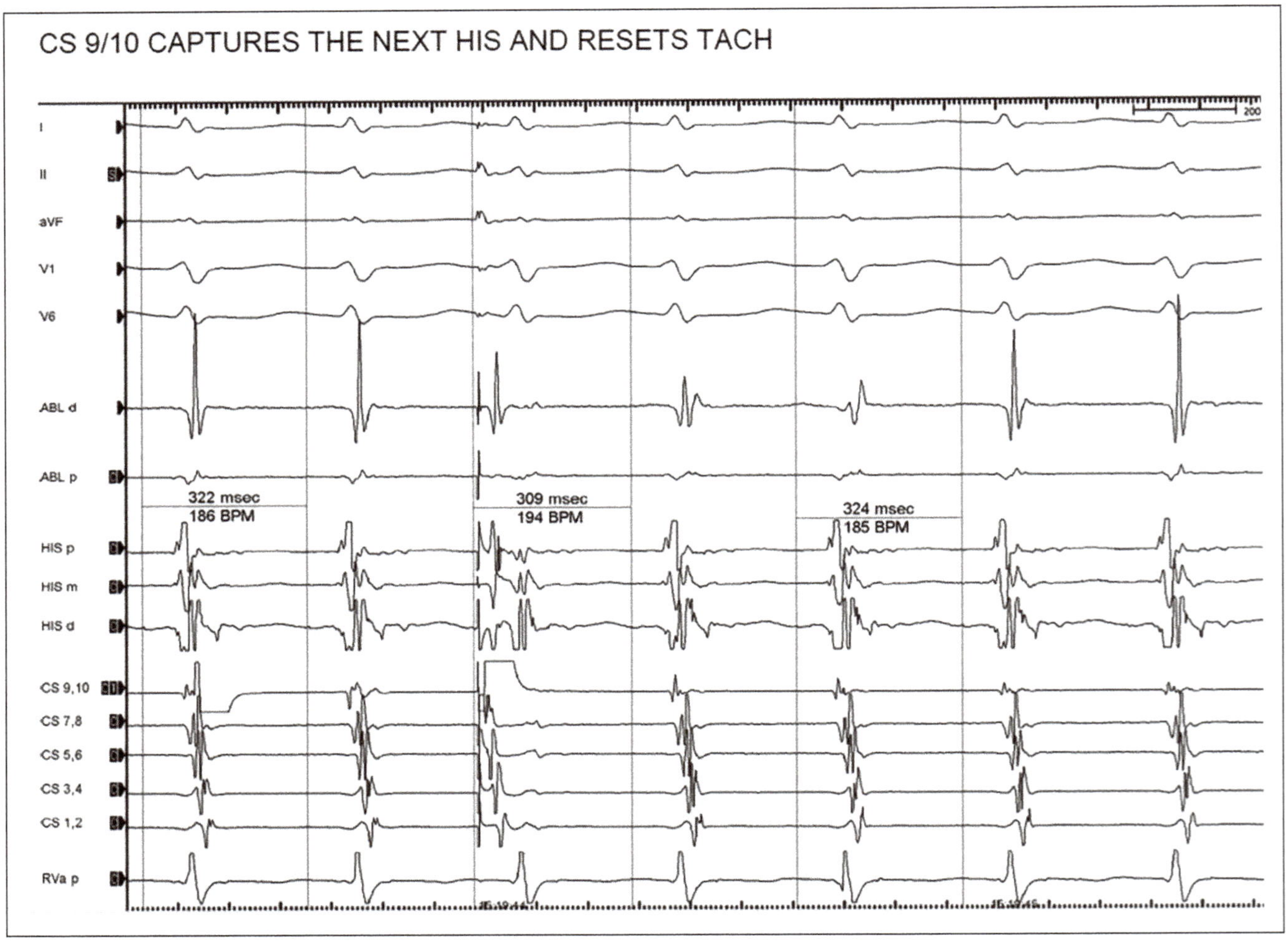

Figure 9.3 An example of AVNRT with antegrade limb entrainment at the proximal CS. Note the classic AVNRT appearance with overlapping atrial and ventricular signals. A single paced beat (third from left) from the proximal CS was placed just before the expected atrial signal. This nicely demonstrates advancing of the subsequent beat (pace-to-His timing 309 ms, in comparison to the tachycardia cycle length of 324 ms). Entrainment from this site could indicate either a left inferior extension (LIE) or a RIE, which can be distinguished with selective site pacing.

The appearance of typical RIE/FP AVNRT with confirmatory maneuvers is usually sufficient to consider a targeted ablation in the low TK in the RIE/typical slow pathway area. However, if the AVNRT is sustained and hemodynamically tolerated, it is often appropriate to map the circuit to confirm the typical RIE/FP reentrant loop. The earliest retrograde atrial activation can be easily mapped and as it is most commonly in the fast pathway area (Figure 9.1B). To determine the site of earliest antegrade activation and delineation of the reentrant loop, entrainment during AVNRT may be attempted. If the reentrant circuit's antegrade limb passes through the RIE, pacing in that area 10–40 ms in advance of the next atrial signal should advance the subsequent His (and A/V) signal slightly (Figure 9.3). The site advances the subsequent reentrant beat with the least premature entrainment (i.e., entrainment when pacing within 10-40 ms before the expected atrial electrograms, typically at or following the His signal) suggests the site of the antegrade limb.

If pacing in the RIE area and the subsequent AVNRT circuit is not advanced when pacing less than 40–50 ms earlier than the reentrant circuit, this may suggest an alternate antegrade limb, such as the LIE. In these cases, pacing the LIE or LILE extension via the CS catheter can be used to evaluate entrainment and should be compared to the RIE entrainment timing.

Once AVNRT is confirmed, a number of techniques for ablation of AVNRT can be considered. We will discuss 2 separate approaches, the traditional anatomic-based approach, and the voltage/propagation mapping technique, the latter is well-suited for and aided by 3D mapping.

The Anatomic Approach

An anatomic approach utilizes the previously generated 3D geometry of the right atrium and TK area for selection of the ablation site. See **Table 9.1** for a list of steps and Video 9.1. These steps can be used regardless of which type of ablation therapy is chosen. The operator must keep in mind the limitations of EAM. Mapping systems currently in use typically display the EAM as a fixed image, with manipulated catheters moving within that fixed map. However, the cardiac structures are, of course, constantly moving in real time due to both cardiac and respiratory motion. As a result, inherent inaccuracies in the "true" location of catheters, in particular the ablation catheter, with respect to the tissues of interest may be present. In addition, all mapping systems have an inherent refresh rate for the map images. There may as a result be small, but sometimes perceptible, delays in the movement of the catheters on the 3D map.

The traditional ablation site selection is based on AV ratios, slow pathway potentials, anatomic location and the response to therapy. Most practitioners place test ablations low in the TK (at the level of the lower portion of the CS os). An A:V ratio between 1:2 to 1:10 is typically chosen as a marker for an appropriate location within the TK. Physicians can also evaluate for a low amplitude elongated atrial signals which have been suggested to be the slow pathway potential of the antegrade limb in the RIE area.[6] Whether using RF or cryotherapy, test applications are placed while evaluating for a predictor of success such as loss of inducible AVNRT, loss of slow pathway conduction, or (if RF) junctional acceleration. This can be translated easily from a fluoroscopic approach to a radiation-free approach, even if operators have only limited comfort with the 3D mapping system.

Table 9.1 Stepwise approach for an anatomic guided ablation of AVNRT.

Create accurate geometry of the right atrium and TK area. Mark His location (Figure 9.2)

Place ablation catheter in anatomically appropriate area
- Typically begin low in the TK
- Consider evaluating for low amplitude, long duration atrial signals
- Identify A:V ratios areas of 1:10 to 1:2

Deliver test ablation applications to evaluate for effect (see RF vs. cryo discussion) with short-duration applications if no effect seen

If no effect with the test application
- Adjust catheter position and preform test application in next location, covering the low TK prior to advancing to locations closer to the His bundle.

Insurance applications should be placed at and around the site of successful ablation

Use appropriate end points with post ablation testing on and off isoproterenol

Using the anatomic approach, cryotherapy can be applied during AVNRT. We typically monitor intracardiac electrograms with both a live screen and a "triggered" screen that updates based on an atrial signal. This allows for accurate intracardiac electrogram monitoring for termination of the arrhythmia, if ablating with cryotherapy during SVT (often preceded by gradual slowing before termination), and of the AV nodal conduction after termination of the arrhythmia. If there is no slowing and termination of the AVNRT within 20 seconds of initiation of cryotherapy, terminating the application and moving to another target site is recommended. A short time to success has been suggested as an indication of a successful site, and a longer duration before slowing and termination may suggest only partial injury to the reentrant arrhythmia substrate.[15] Some physicians utilize cryomapping (to –30 degrees) with a 4-mm tip catheter. However, the 4-mm tip catheter has been shown to be associated with an increased risk of recurrence; therefore, use of a 6-mm cryocatheter may be preferable.[16-18]

Once the AVNRT has terminated, close monitoring of the AV nodal function is recommended during the full duration of the cryothermal application. Studies have suggested, and the authors support, an additional "freeze-thaw-freeze" application at the site of the first successful ablation. During each application, the operator continues to monitor for signs of potential AV node injury, as well as for recurrence of slow pathway conduction or inducible AVNRT by using occasional atrial and ventricular pacing maneuvers. If a single AV node echo beat is present after consolidation of lesions at the successful site, the authors typically attempt short test applications in new areas of the TK to eliminate the echo beat, with a full application and insurance application at the successful site of loss of the AV node echo. However, elimination of residual single echo beats has not been clearly demonstrated as necessary in more conventional RF ablation. If at any time there is evidence of PR prolongation, then the therapy is stopped, and one may consider not pursuing single echo beats.[19,20]

Due to slight increased risk of heart block during RF, applications are typically placed with lower power and the lesions are performed during sinus rhythm while monitoring for junctional acceleration and loss of inducible AVNRT after the lesions is placed. Once again, careful attention needs to be paid to (often retrograde) AV nodal conduction. The site selection for AVNRT is similar with both the RF and cryotherapy techniques utilizing the anatomic location, AV ratio and slow pathway potentials. It is important to note that accelerated junctional rhythms are not seen during cryothermal applications. Unlike cryotherapy, the RF catheter remains completely mobile during RF application, and therefore close attention to catheter movement, position, and potential build-up of torque, flex, or other mechanical tension that may result in sudden and unexpected catheter movement is critical. The ability to constantly monitor catheter position via the EAM system likely facilitates the safety aspect of this issue, as traditionally many operators using a fluoroscopy-based approach will continuously monitor catheter position fluoroscopy during RF application. This, of course, significantly adds to fluoroscopy time.

After ablation of the slow pathway, it is important to perform a full EP study on an isoproterenol infusion. In a large multicenter trial, the largest risk for recurrence was in those who did not undergo post testing with isoproterenol. Appropriate end points for RF ablation of AVNRT include lack of inducible AVNRT and only a single (or no) echo beat.[20]

Voltage and Propagation Mapping

In 2011, Bailin published "Direct visualization of the slow pathway in using voltage mapping for the ablation of AVNRT."[21] This landmark paper described the presence of low-voltage "bridges" as the target site for successful ablation of AVNRT. A subsequent study confirmed the presence of low-voltage areas as the site of successful ablation in pediatric patients.[22] This finding suggests that voltage mapping is a very useful adjunct in identifying the successful site of AVNRT ablation. In late 2017, with further refinement of the technique, it was noted that propagation mapping during sinus rhythm allowed further correlation with the site of successful ablation.[23] A prospective trial evaluating this technique is in progress at the time of this chapter publication. This technique will be described as we are encouraged by the initial successes seen by using propagation mapping with voltage mapping to identify successful sites of ablation.

After RA geometry creation, marking the His location and AVNRT confirmation, voltage mapping can be performed (**Figure 9.4**, Video 9.1). During sinus rhythm voltage points should be obtained throughout and around the TK, including the atrial septum from the areas around the His potentials to below the coronary sinus. A catheter with relatively close spacing and/or high-density electrodes should be used to assist with mapping of the area of the TK. With current mapping system technologies, several options for high-density electrode mapping catheters are available and may be considered, although utilizing these catheters adds significant cost to the procedure. We often obtain additional points around the right atrium to fill in the propagation-wave progression.

After this, voltage points are excluded if they did not occur during sinus rhythm. In particular, premature atrial complexes, junctional beats or catheter-induced artifact should be discarded. We strive to obtain at least 35 data points reflected on the surface in the area of the TK with current 3D mapping systems. If there is inadequate point density, further points can be collected. The aforementioned newer mapping systems provide more rapid acquisition of data points and verification, which may further speed the process and greatly improve signal density.

Next, the propagation wave during sinus rhythm can be visualized as it progresses through the TK using the points collected during the voltage point collection (**Figure 9.5**). Again, if there are atrial signals that are inconsistent with timing (such as a premature atrial complex), they should be excluded to allow accurate timing of the atrial signals during sinus rhythm.

Once electrogram accuracy is confirmed, the atrial wave collision can be evaluated and marked. Typically, during sinus rhythm the atrial wave front proceeds from the sinus node towards the fast pathway area. The atrial wave front then slowly progresses through the superior TK, while quickly conducting posterior to the tendon of Todaro and around the CS os to the low TK area. These separate wave fronts (slow progression from high in the TK, and more brisk progression from low in the TK) usually collide near the level of the CS in the TK. This site can be anatomically tagged and, in concert with low-voltage signals, appears to more accurately identify the successful site of ablation (Figure 9.5).[23]

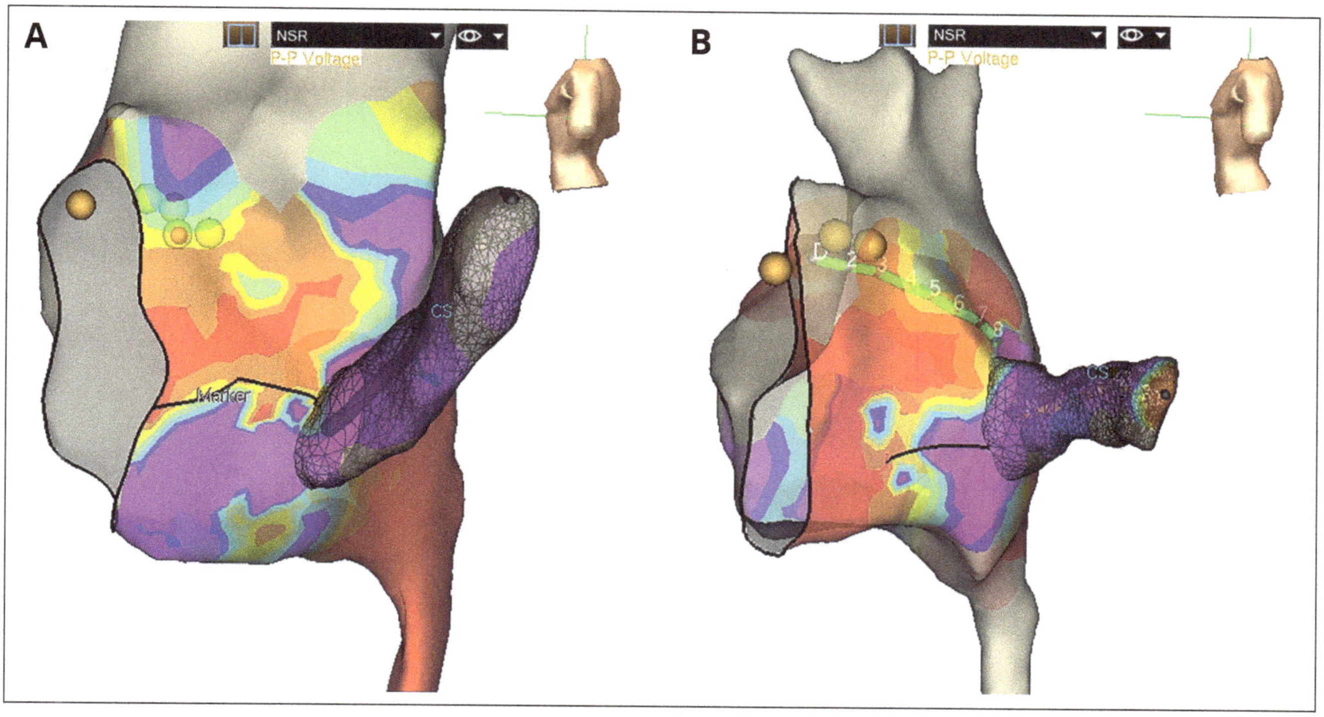

Figure 9.4 Two examples of voltage maps of the TK from separate patients. In both images, a left-lateral view of the RA is shown with the coronary sinus progressing towards the right side of the page. The His signals have been marked by the **yellow/orange spheres**. The colors represent atrial voltages with the low voltage (**red**) set at 0.1 mV and the higher voltage (**purple**) set at >2 mV. Note the low-voltage area through much of the low to mid TK. In both images, the site of the propagation wave collision was also labeled as a **black line** progressing from the CS towards the TV (discussed later).

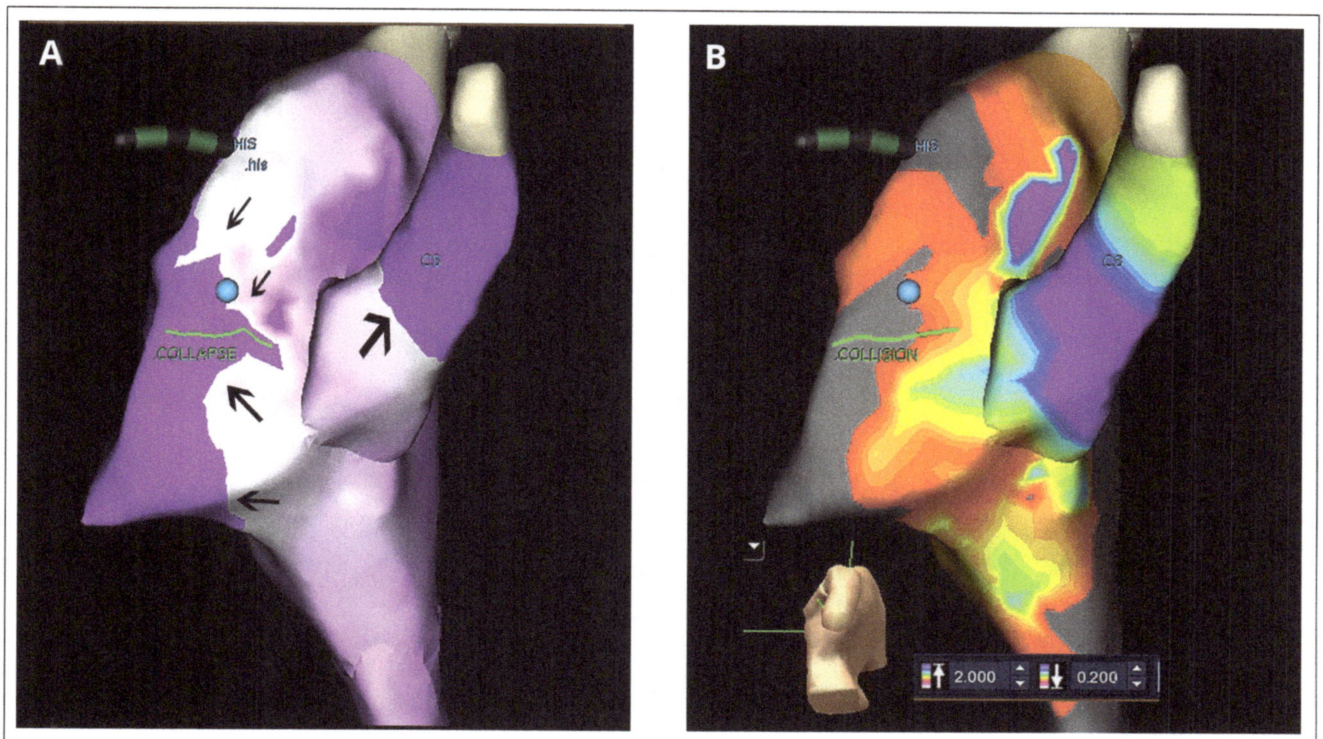

Figure 9.5 **A:** An example of a propagation wave. The **bright white** represents the leading edge of the atrial depolarization wavefront, and the **transparent white** represents the sites that the wavefront has passed. The **purple** indicates nondepolarized tissue. **Arrows** are used to indicate direction of wavefront progression, and a **green line** labeled "collision" is drawn where the 2 wavefronts collide. This is marked on the 3D map for assistance of AVNRT ablation localization. **B:** The voltage map, with the propagation wave collision site marked, can now be used to determine the site of ablation, typically at or slightly superior to the wave collision, at a low-voltage site, near the ventricular side of the TK. The **blue sphere** represents the successful cryoablation site over a low-voltage area in this patient.[23] (Reprinted with permission from Van Aartsen A, Law IH, Maldonado JR, Von Bergen NH. Propagation mapping wave collision correlates to the site of successful ablation during voltage mapping in atrioventricular nodal reentry tachycardia. *J Innov Cardiac Rhythm Manag.* 2017;8(9):2836–2842.)

We mark the site of wave collision on the map and evaluate for a low-voltage signal (< 0.5 mV, often closer to 0.0.05 to 0.3 mV) at or just superior to the wave collision. This allows us to choose a target for ablation, typically first choosing a site near the ventricular end of the TK. Once again, we typically ablate during SVT using cryotherapy, or during sinus (or atrial pacing) using RF as discussed in the anatomic approach above. Care needs to be taken to closely monitor AV nodal and fast pathway conduction. Once the successful site is determined, then ablations proceed as discussed in the above anatomic guidance section, incorporating a "freeze thaw freeze" application and consolidation lesions around the successful site when cryotherapy is utilized. A step-by-step chart for the voltage and propagation mapping technique is included (**Table 9.2**).

Table 9.2 Stepwise approach for, and voltage and propagation map-guided ablation of, AVNRT. Also see Video 9.1 for a tutorial.

Create an accurate geometry of right atrium and TK area. Mark His location (Figure 9.2 and Video 9.1)
Obtain atrial voltage and timing points during sinus rhythm (with multipole catheter) (Figure 9.4 and Video 9.1)
• Confirm atrial signals accuracy of timing and amplitude, delete ectopic/junctional beats
Evaluate propagation wave collision and mark wave collision on map (Figure 9.5A)
Select site of ablation over a low-voltage area (typically 0.1 to 0.5mv), at or slightly superior to the wave collision (Figure 9.5B and Video 9.1)
• Confirm adequate safety, distant from His signals
• Consider incorporation of "traditional" slow pathway circuits (anatomic location, AV ratio, low amplitude signals)
Deliver test ablations to evaluate for effect (see RF vs. Cryo discussion) terminating therapy if no effect on the arrhythmia or arrhythmia substrate is seen early in the application
If no effect with the initial test application
• Adjust catheter position and preform test application in next location, covering the low TK prior to locations closer to the His bundle. We preferentially select low-voltage sites near the wave collision first
Insurance applications should be placed at and around the site of successful ablation (Video 9.1)
Repeat testing on and off isoproterenol with use of appropriate end points

Conclusion

Atrioventricular nodal reentrant tachycardia is an arrhythmia that is well-suited for a radiation-free procedure. Radiation-free 3D mapping techniques as described here can improve both short- and long-term success for ablation of this arrhythmia.

References

1. Goyal R, Zivin A, Souza J, et al. Comparison of the ages of tachycardia onset in patients with atrioventricular nodal reentrant tachycardia and accessory pathway-mediated tachycardia. *Am Heart J.* 1996;132(4):765–767.
2. Ko JK, Deal BJ, Strasburger JF, Benson DW, Jr. Supraventricular tachycardia mechanisms and their age distribution in pediatric patients. *Am J Cardiol.* 1992; 69(12):1028–1032.
3. Moe GK, Preston JB, Burlington H. Physiologic evidence for a dual A-V transmission system. *Circulation.* 1956; 4(4):357–375.
4. Tai C-T, Chen S-A, Chiang C-E, et al. Complex electrophysiological characteristics in atrioventricular nodal reentrant tachycardia with continuous atrioventricular node function curves. *Circulation.* 1997;95(11):2541–2547.
5. Pritchett EL, Anderson RW, Benditt DG, et al. Reentry within the atrioventricular node: Surgical cure with preservation of atrioventricular conduction. *Circulation.* 1979;60(2):440–446.
6. Haïssaguerre M, Warin JF, Lemetayer P, Saoudi N, Guillem JP, Blanchot P. Closed-chest ablation of retrograde conduction in patients with atrioventricular nodal reentrant tachycardia. *N Engl J Med.* 1989;320(7):426–433.
7. Kunze KP, Geiger M, Schläter M, Kuck KH. Catheter-induced modulation of impulse conduction of the atrioventricular node by radio-frequency current. *Dtsch med Wochenschr.* 1988;113(35):134–31348.
8. Haïssaguerre M, Gaita F, Fischer B, et al. Elimination of atrioventricular nodal reentrant tachycardia using discrete slow potentials to guide application of radiofrequency energy. *Circulation.* 1992;85(6):2162–2175.
9. Jackman WM, Beckman KJ, McClelland JH, et al. Treatment of supraventricular tachycardia due to atrioventricular nodal reentry by radiofrequency catheter ablation of slow-pathway Conduction. *N Engl J Med.* 1992;327(5): 313–318.
10. Hanninen M, Yeung-Lai-Wah N, Massel D, et al. Cryoablation versus RF ablation for AVNRT: A meta-analysis and systematic review. *J Cardiovasc Electrophysiol.* 2013; 24(12):1354–1360.
11. Siebels H, Sohns C, Nurnberg JH, Siebels J, Langes K, Hebe J. Value of an old school approach: Safety and long-term success of radiofrequency current catheter ablation of atrioventricular nodal reentrant tachycardia in children and young adolescents. *J Interv Card Electrophysiol.* 2018.
12. Inoue S, Becker AE. Posterior extensions of the human compact atrioventricular node: A neglected anatomic

feature of potential clinical significance. *Circulation.* 1998; 97(2):188–193.
13. Katritsis DG, John RM, Latchamsetty R, et al. Left septal slow pathway ablation for atrioventricular nodal reentrant tachycardia. *Circ Arrhythm Electrophysiol.* 2018;11(3): e005907.
14. Katritsis DG, Josephson ME. Classification, electrophysiological features and therapy of atrioventricular nodal reentrant tachycardia. *Arrhythm Electrophysiol Rev.* 2016; 5(2):130–135.
15. Kaltman JR, Tanel RE, Wegrzynowicz B, et al. Time and temperature profile of catheter cryoablation of right septal and free wall accessory pathways in children. J *Cardiovasc Electrophysiol.* 2008;19(4):343–347.
16. Sandilands A, Boreham P, Pitts-Crick J, Cripps T. Impact of cryoablation catheter size on success rates in the treatment of atrioventricular nodal re-entry tachycardia in 160 patients with long-term follow-up. *Europace.* 2008;10(6):683–686.
17. Chanani NK, Chiesa NA, Dubin AM, Avasarala K, Van Hare GF, Collins KK. Cryoablation for atrioventricular nodal reentrant tachycardia in young patients: predictors of recurrence. *Pacing Clin Electrophysiol.* 2008;31(9):1152–1159.
18. Das S, Law IH, Von Bergen NH, et al. Cryoablation therapy for atrioventricular nodal reentrant tachycardia in children: A multicenter experience of efficacy. *Pediatr Cardiol.* 2012.
19. Eckhardt LL, Leal M, Hollis Z, Tanega J, Alberte C. Cryoablation for AVNRT: Importance of ablation endpoint criteria. *J Cardiovasc Electrophysiol.* 2012;23(7):729–734.
20. Stern JD, Rolnitzky L, Goldberg JD, et al. Meta-analysis to assess the appropriate endpoint for slow pathway ablation of atrioventricular nodal reentrant tachycardia. *Pacing Clin Electrophysiol.* 2011;34(3):269–277.
21. Bailin SJ, Korthas MA, Weers NJ, Hoffman CJ. Direct visualization of the slow pathway using voltage gradient mapping: A novel approach for successful ablation of atrioventricular nodal reentry tachycardia. *Europace.* 2011;13(8): 1188–1194.
22. Malloy L, Law IH, Von Bergen NH. Voltage mapping for slow-pathway visualization and ablation of atrioventricular nodal reentry tachycardia in pediatric and young adult patients. *Pediatr Cardiol.* 2014;35(1):103–107.
23. Van Aartsen A, Law IH, Maldonado JR, Von Bergen NH. Propagation mapping wave collision correlates to the site of successful ablation during voltage mapping in atrioventricular nodal reentry tachycardia. *J Innov Card Rhythm Manag.* 2017;8:2836–2842.

Video Legend

Video 9.1 A step-by-step video tutorial for AVNRT ablation utilizing voltage and propagation wave collision mapping. [7:43]

10

How to Ablate Accessory Pathways Using No Fluoroscopy

Raman L. Mitra, MD

Accessory pathways that lead to symptomatic atrioventricular reentry tachycardia (AVRT) or a rapid ventricular response during atrial fibrillation (AF), as in Wolff-Parkinson-White (WPW) syndrome or concealed atrioventricular bypass tracts, frequently affect younger patients. For many years, radiofrequency (RF) catheter ablation has been shown to be an effective treatment but traditionally has required fluoroscopy.[1] Non-fluoroscopic ablation is desirable in such patients to avoid radiation exposure, in particular to the gonads and thyroid in this generally younger patient population. This approach also offers an option to avoid maternal and fetal radiation for pregnant women with symptomatic arrhythmias. Finally, there are clear benefits to the physician and staff by reducing the need to wear heavy lead shielding which is associated with orthopedic issues after long term use.

As with all accessory pathway ablations, examination of the 12-lead electrocardiogram (ECG) during tachycardia and sinus rhythm is critical, since this will usually allow localization of a manifest pathway (WPW) if present and even with a concealed pathway, some clues to the location may be gleaned from the RP interval, as well as the axis and morphology of the P wave during tachycardia.[2-4] The electrocardiographic findings may help to plan for the ablation in several ways, including anticipating the likelihood of whether transseptal puncture or retrograde aortic approach may be needed; the potential need for longer stabilizing or steerable sheaths; the possibility of needing a cryocatheter with a suspected parahisian pathway or a Mahaim pathway; and assessment of potential damage to collateral structures such as the atrioventricular node, coronary arteries and veins, or valves.

There are several common requirements for a non-fluoroscopic approach for ablation procedures, regardless of the type of arrhythmia:

1. The ability to gain safe access to the heart via the femoral venous or arterial system.
2. For left-sided pathways, phased-array intracardiac echocardiography (ICE) to delineate the cardiac chambers, valves, and vessels and create a sound map of the heart (2-, 3-, or 4-chamber), and obtaining transseptal access.
3. Obtaining accurate respiratory gating and periodically assessing that this has not changed during the case.
4. Creation of an electroanatomic volumetric and voltage map that is merged or combined with the sound map.
5. Choice and placement of diagnostic catheters.
6. Pacing maneuvers, electrogram analysis, and stimulation protocols to determine the location and properties of the accessory pathway.

Fluoroscopy Reduction Techniques for Catheter Ablation of Cardiac Arrhythmias. © 2019 Mansour Razminia, Paul C. Zei, eds.
Cardiotext Publishing, ISBN: 978-1-942909-30-9.

7. Choosing the best type of ablation catheter (irrigated vs. nonirrigated RF, or cryocatheter) and anatomic approach to the pathway.

8. Choosing the appropriate power level for ablation, monitoring of impedance and force (when contact force is used), and monitoring of AV and VA conduction.

9. Assessing the results of ablation.

As in all non-fluoroscopy procedures, careful attention must be paid to safe access and delivery of catheters and sheaths to the heart, particularly in the presence of tortuous vascular anatomy or stenosis to avoid inadvertent vascular perforation or dissection in the abdomen. One of the most effective ways to avoid such complications is to use long, soft-tipped J-wires over which longer sheaths are deployed allowing delivery of the catheters to the inferior vena cava (IVC) just below the right atrium (RA). Alternatively, a multielectrode catheter may be used to create vascular geometry using electroanatomic mapping (EAM) systems providing a "road map to the heart." Close attention to catheter electrogram monitoring is critical to recognize when the catheter has reached the right heart as well as location within the heart. There are two main systems available to create EAMs: CARTO (Biosense Webster, Irvine, CA) and EnSite (Abbott, Abbott Park, IL). The former has the advantage of full integration of the ICE images with the EAM as well as visualization of the shaft and curvature of the ablation catheter. The latter has the advantage of being open access and catheter agnostic, allowing use of less expensive diagnostic catheters to create an initial EAM prior to choosing more expensive mapping and ablation catheters.

The availability of contact force catheters has also made non-fluoroscopic access to the heart safer since the catheters may be advanced based on force measurements as opposed to tactile sense alone. Additionally, the assessment of the degree of force during ablation is invaluable to create an adequate lesion and minimize perforation risk. Since accessory pathways are along the atrioventricular groove where the contact with the annulus cannot be gauged by fluoroscopy alone, contact force and electrogram morphology provide complementary data to effectively ablate the accessory pathway.[5] In the remainder of this chapter, examples will be provided illustrating the technical approach to ablate accessory pathways in different locations as opposed to diagnostic maneuvers to explain the underlying mechanism of the tachycardia, which is beyond the scope of this text. None of the cases shown utilized fluoroscopy.

The author's initial approach is to place a long sheath (for the ICE catheter, Biosense Webster's SOUNDSTAR), a short 8-Fr for the decapolar coronary sinus (CS), or a duodecapolar catheter for the RA and CS. For the ablation catheter, an SL0 or SR0 sheath (Abbott) is inserted into the right femoral vein and may be used for right-sided pathways. The same sheaths may be used to gain transseptal access if a left-sided pathway is present. Sometimes, the ICE catheter is initially omitted for a suspected right-sided pathway. In general, all left-sided pathways are ablated via a transseptal approach and rarely within the CS, which may require fluoroscopy and contrast venography for any suspicion of CS vascular anomalies.[6-8] When a left-sided pathway is suspected, a 5-Fr sheath is placed in the right femoral artery, which can later be upsized in case a retrograde aortic approach is needed.

It is essential to perform respiratory gating in non-fluoroscopic procedures to assure accurate creation of the non-fluoroscopic map as well as localization of ablation lesions. This can be done very easily by placing the ICE catheter or ablation catheter into the right hepatic vein, which transduces the right hemidiaphragm excursion well or across the tricuspid valve in the right ventricular outflow tract.

The next step is to create a volumetric map of the superior vena cava (SVC), RA, IVC, and CS. This is usually performed with the ablation catheter; however, alternatively, this can be performed with a multi-electrode catheter such as a PentaRay (Biosense Webster) or a decapolar catheter. The choice is somewhat dependent on the EAM system used (CARTO or EnSite). **Figures 10.1**, A–C show examples of using a decapolar diagnostic catheter with the EnSite system, advancing from the right femoral vein to the RA. The venous anatomy is created as the catheter is advanced in the IVC. Once the tip of the catheter reaches the RA, atrial electrograms are recorded. The catheter is then advanced to the SVC and is swept around the RA and eventually placed within the CS. This is performed with a simultaneous right anterior oblique (RAO) and left anterior oblique (LAO) view. All regions where the His bundle is recorded are tagged with yellow dots. Figure 10.1C shows placement of a duodecapolar catheter without fluoroscopy once the map is created.

Figure 10.2A shows the pre-excited 12-lead ECG of a patient with WPW syndrome and orthodromic AVRT due to a right parahisian accessory pathway. Pre-excitation was intermittent and the location of the pathway was determined both based on mapping of intermittent pre-excitation as well as from earliest retrograde conduction during orthodromic tachycardia and RV pacing. Figure 10.2B shows the position of the catheters for ablation of this pathway. The associated video (**Video 10.2**) shows 3D rotation prior to initiation of cryoablation. Using color, transparency, and 3D rotation are important tools to position catheters and tag important electrograms.

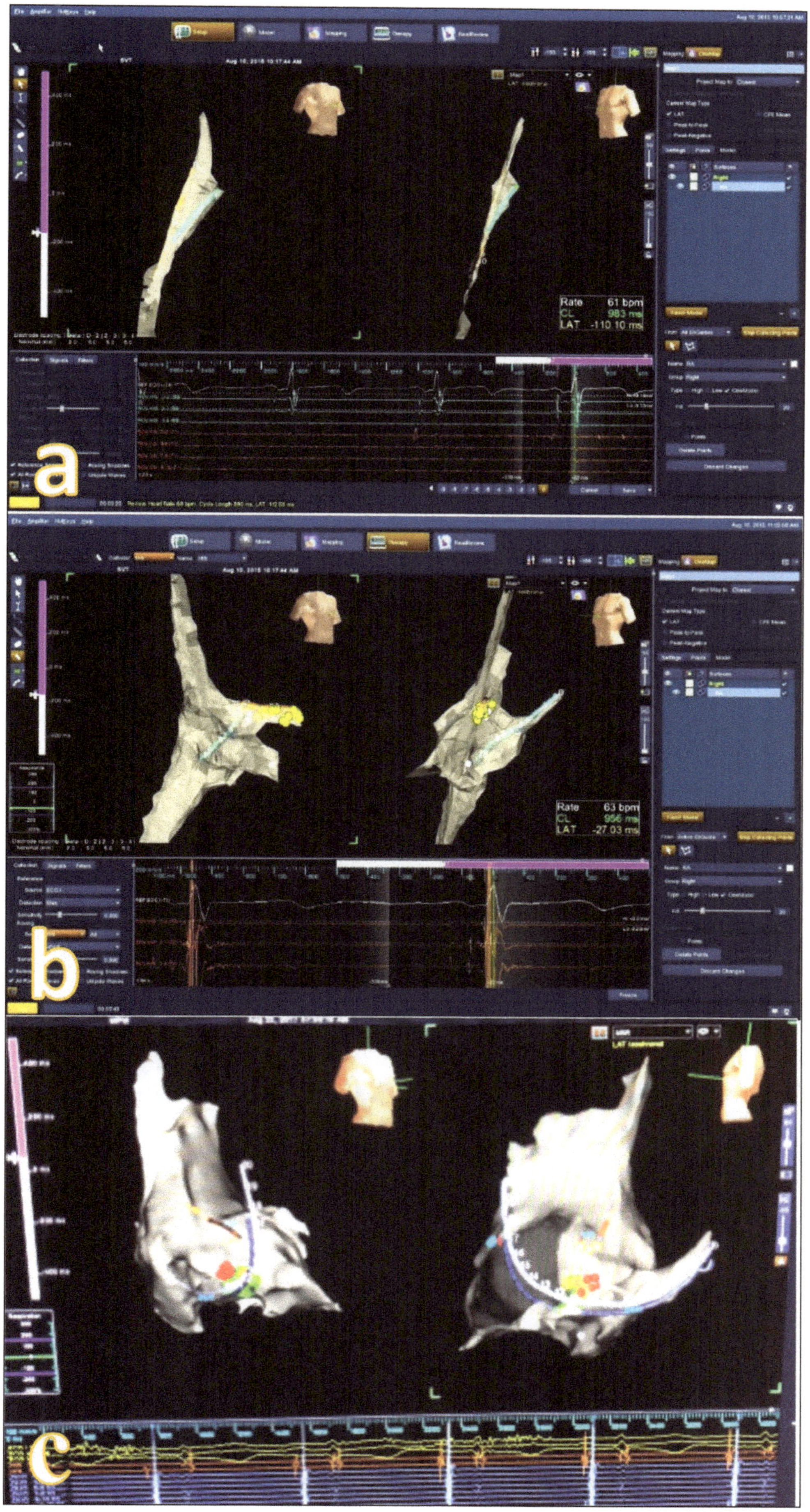

Figure 10.1 **A:** A decapolar catheter is advanced via the right femoral vein to delineate the course of the right femoral vein. **B:** Creation of an EAM of the right atrium with **yellow dots** delineating the His bundle region and decapolar navigated into the coronary sinus. **C:** Placement of a duodecapolar catheter in the coronary sinus. (**Video 10.1**)

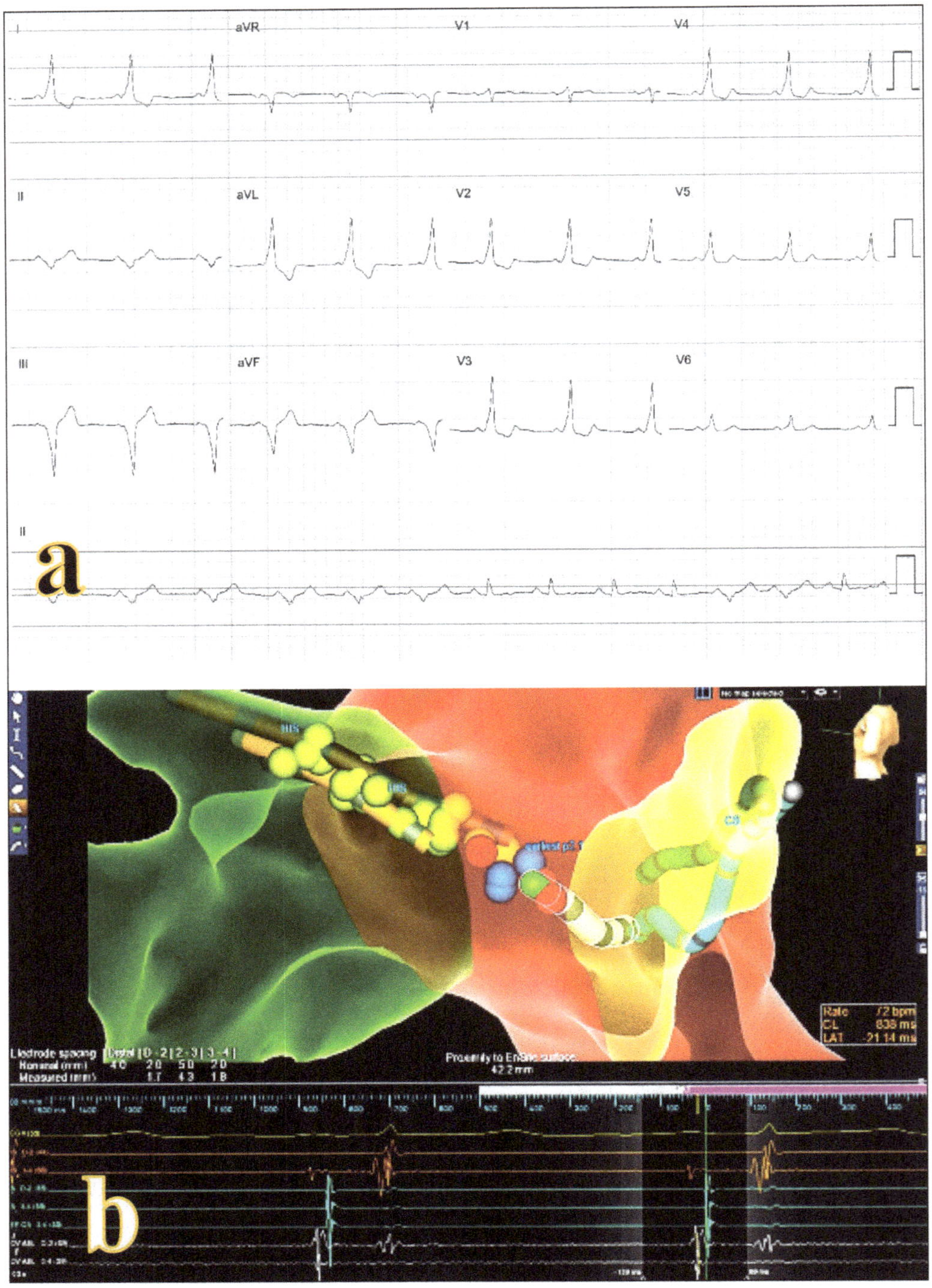

Figure 10.2 **A:** WPW with a pre-excited ECG due to a right parahisian pathway. **B:** Position of catheters using transparency in a left posterolateral view to ablate the right parahisian pathway of Figure 10.2. **Yellow dots** show His cloud and the His catheter is **orange** at the RA (**red**) right ventricle (**green**) junction. The decapolar catheter (**blue**) is shown in the CS (**yellow**). What appears to be a second CS catheter was a saved image of the original CS placement to make sure that the CS has not moved during the case. The real time CS catheter shows an inferior deflection at electrodes 7-8 due to pacing electrode selection, which is seen with EnSite. A 4-mm cryocatheter (Medtronic Inc., Minneapolis, MN) was used for ablation due to the proximity to the compact AV node. The **red dot** was used to mark the most proximal region of His bundle recording. The **blue dots** represent the ablation points. Note the use of transparency and color to delineate structures, catheters, and key electrogram sites. The pathway was ablated without affecting AV nodal conduction despite a very small intermittent His bundle deflection on the second beat seen on the ablation catheter electrogram. Note the larger A to V ratio on the ablation catheter compared to the His bundle catheter (Video 10.2).

Left-sided accessory pathways require either a transseptal or retrograde aortic access. Traditionally these approaches have been felt to require fluoroscopy for safety. The advent of ICE has largely obviated the need for fluoroscopy for transseptal access and in fact even in labs that use fluoroscopy for transseptal access, ICE is used adjunctively. ICE is also helpful for retrograde aortic approaches and can define the aortic valve and ascending aorta accurately. For these types of cases, the author finds the CARTO system most useful due to its full integration of ICE maps with EAMs and contact force in real time and the ability to visualize the proximal curve of the ablation catheter as opposed to just the distal electrodes.

Figure 10.3 stepwise illustrates the creation of the initial ICE and non-fluoroscopic maps of the left atrium (LA), IVC, RA, SVC, and CS and ultimately achieving transseptal or retrograde aortic access to the LA and left ventricle (LV). Initially the ICE catheter is used to create a sound map of the LA including mitral annulus and pulmonary veins for reference (Figure 10.3A). This is followed by using the ablation catheter to create a volumetric map of the right-sided structures (Figure 10.3B). The transseptal site can be seen on ICE and tagged on the map (Figure 10.3C). The CS catheter can then be placed using the map created (Figure 10.3D). For left-sided pathways, distal CS placement is often critical in order to bracket the earliest ventricular electrogram during pre-excitation during sinus rhythm or earliest retrograde atrial electrogram tachycardia/RV pacing. At times, resistance due to tortuosity or a valve of Vieussens may be encountered as a catheter is advanced into the CS which may increase the risk of CS perforation. Steerable contact force catheters are useful to create the CS volumetric map as shown in Figure 10.3E. Once this hybrid (sound and catheter volumetric) map is created, transseptal puncture is performed under ICE guidance and pressure guidance.

In cases where retrograde aortic access is required, the proximal ascending aorta and aortic valve are added to the ICE map. These images can be obtained from with the ICE catheter in the right ventricular outflow tract. The contact force ablation catheter is then advanced up the abdominal aorta and to the aortic arch. The ICE map and catheter volumetric map are then merged to render the entire aortic valve, root and arch. The ablation catheter is then prolapsed into the left ventricle in the RAO projection as is typically done under fluoroscopy and further mapping may be performed (**Video 10.3F**).

The ECG of a patient with WPW syndrome and orthodromic tachycardia is shown in the upper panel of **Figure 10.4**A. This is suggestive of a left posteroseptal pathway and based on the very negative and wide delta wave in lead II, the possibility of the pathway traversing the coronary sinus was considered.[6-8] The initial approach was transseptal as shown in Figure 10.4B. Initially, pre-excitation was eliminated; however, after 10 minutes, orthodromic SVT recurred even prior to return of pre-excitation as shown in Figure 10.4C. Repeat ablation finally eliminated both antegrade and retrograde conduction, and there was no return of pre-excitation or orthodromic SVT 1 hour after the last lesion on isoproterenol.

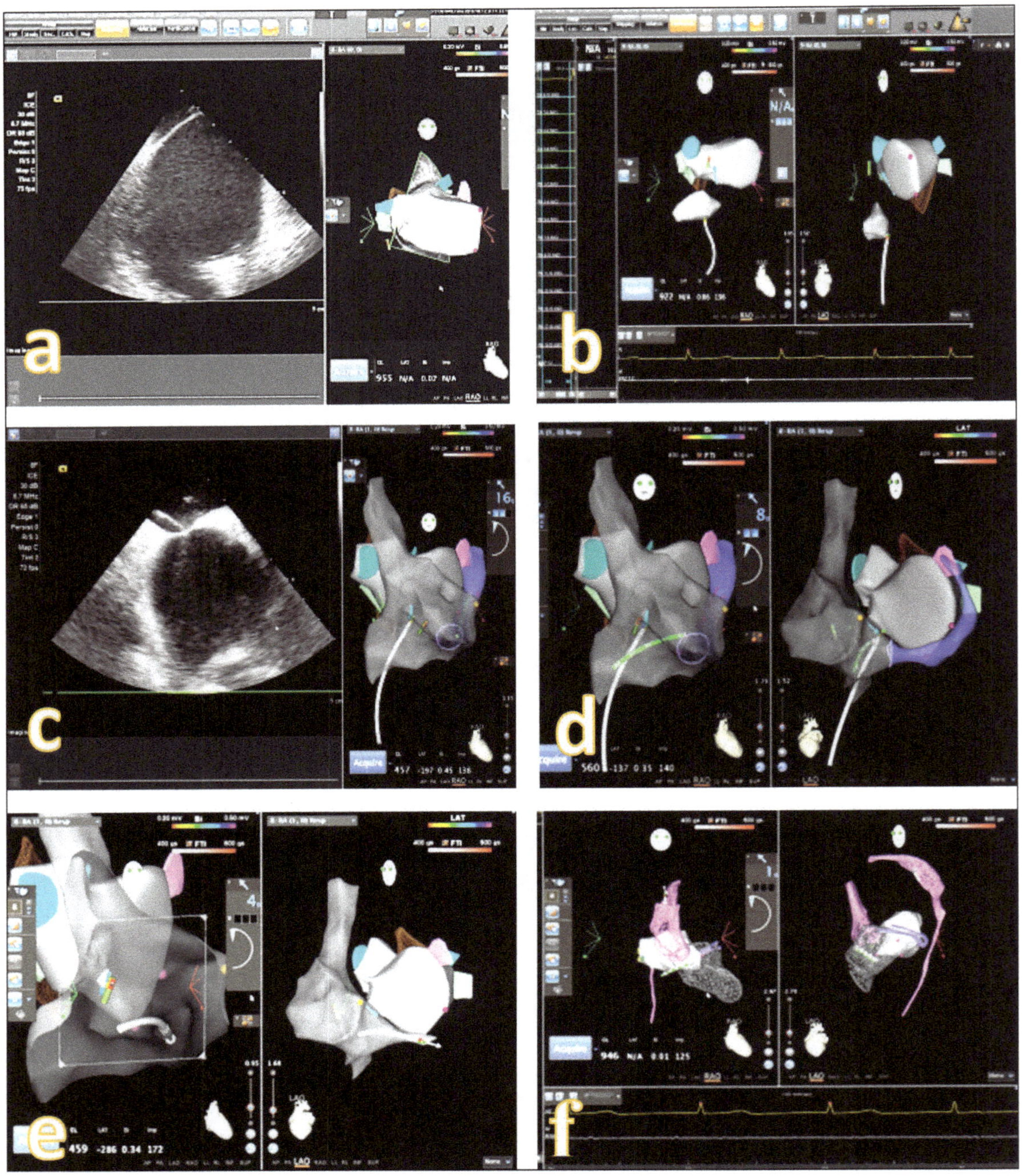

Figure 10.3 **A:** ICE image and sound map of the left atrium. **Video 10.3A**
B: Using SmartTouch catheter in the IVC to create volumetric map of the IVC, RA, SVC, and CS. The **red dots** represent the mitral annulus recorded on ICE. The pulmonary veins (**blue** and **green**) are shown coming off the LA. The ablation catheter starts at the IVC and is advanced under force guidance and curved and swept in the RA to create the volumetric map. The esophagus can be seen behind the LA in **brown**. **Video 10.3B**
C: Transseptal site on ICE, marked in **blue** on RA septum with integrated ICE and EAM. **Video 10.3C**
D: Placing of CS catheter. **Video 10.3D**
E: RAO and clipping plane and LAO with contact force SmartTouch catheter entering CS os with 4 g of force. **Video 10.3E** illustrates how the contact force is used to safely navigate the catheter to the distal CS and create the CS volumetric map.
F: Non-fluoroscopic technique for retrograde aortic access. LV (**meshed grey**) and ascending aorta (**meshed pink**), which is then merged with catheter map of the descending aorta and arch as the catheter is advanced. The catheter is then prolapsed into the left ventricle (Video 10.3F).

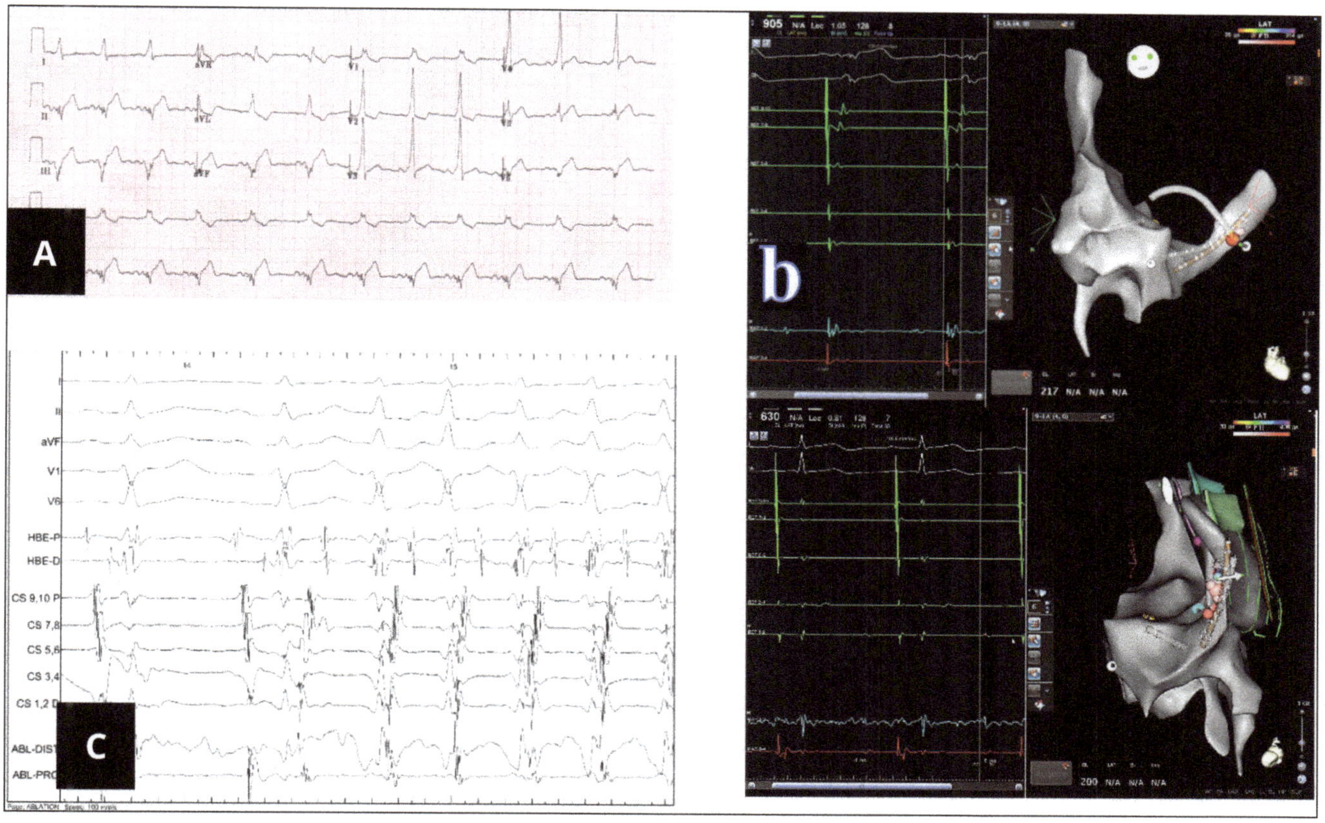

Figure 10.4 **A:** 12-lead ECG showing WPW with a left posterior bypass tract suggesting fiber traversing the coronary sinus based on negative delta waves in leads II and V6. **B:** Upper panel shows preablation electrograms (**blue**) during pre-excitation and electroanatomic images of initial transseptal catheter position for ablation (**red dot**). Due to proximal electrode on the shaft, the curvature of the transseptal ablation catheter is seen. The SVC, right atrium, and CS and CS catheter are clearly defined. Bottom panel shows post-ablation loss of pre-excitation which required multiple lesions (**pink dots**) as seen in a left lateral angulation. **C:** After the early RF lesions, pre-excitation was eliminated but spontaneous orthodromic SVT still occurred during sinus (second beat) indicating remaining concealed bypass tracts in this location and required further ablation in this region.

The patient returned with symptoms of palpitations 1 year later and the ECG showed recurrent pre-excitation similar to that previous to the first ablation. The approach for the second ablation was to map the coronary sinus based on the initial ECG suggesting an epicardial pathway and consistent with the difficulty to ablate the pathway on the initial procedure. **Figure 10.5**A and B show the electrograms and EAM seen in the coronary sinus. The catheter impedance was 150 ohms. Delivery of 10 W through the saline irrigated catheter eliminated the remaining WPW fibers in under 3 seconds as shown in Figure 10.5C. The patient has subsequently done well without recurrence.

Figure 10.6 shows that a similar approach may be taken for ablation of concealed left-sided pathways. Loss of retrograde conduction is seen during ventricular pacing during ablation of a left posterior pathway via transseptal access.

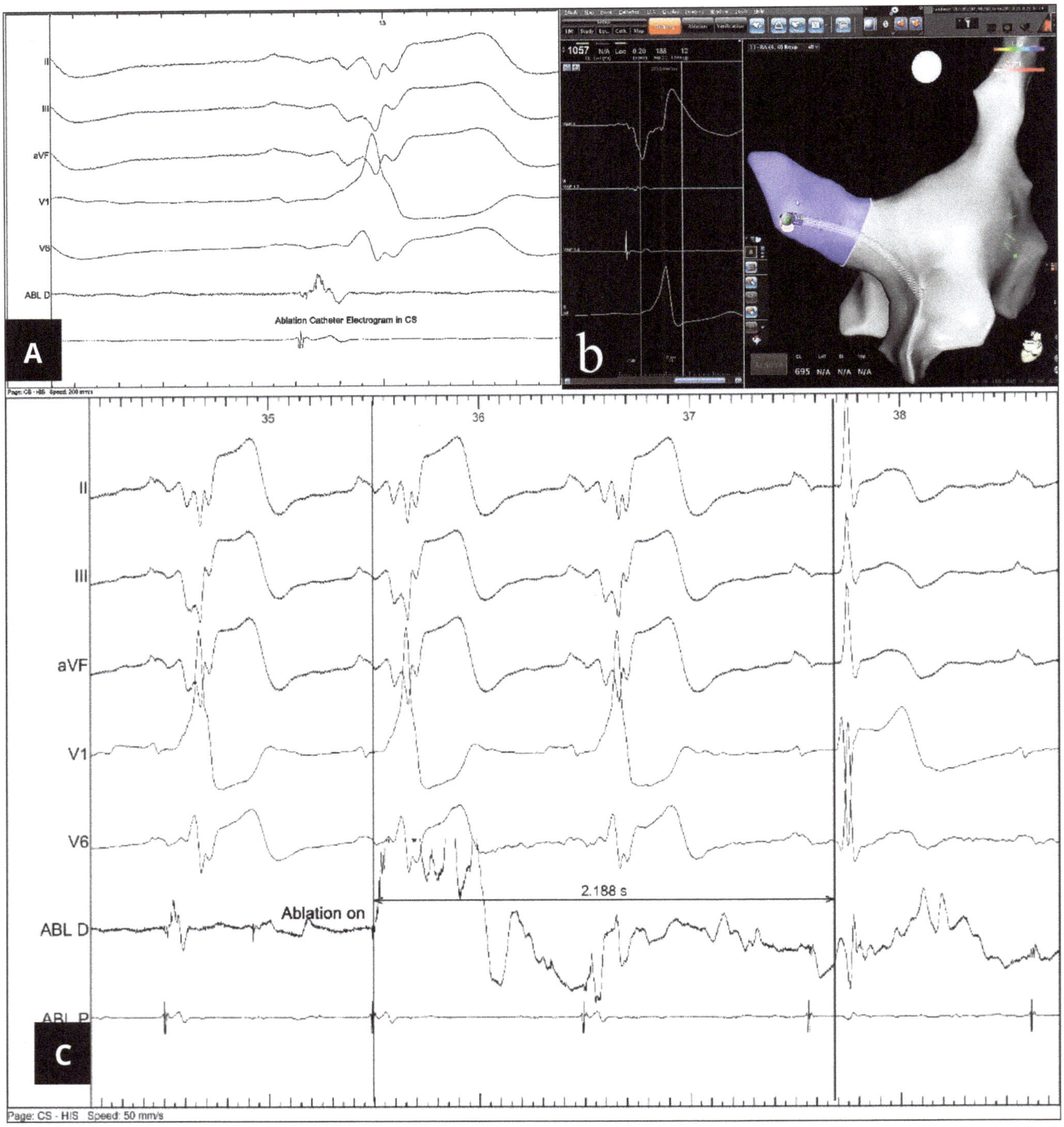

Figure 10.5 **A:** Electrogram from the coronary sinus showing continuous atrioventricular activity with possible bypass tract potential. **B:** Non-fluoroscopic map from a posteroanterior view showing the ablation catheter in the CS corresponding to the electrogram in Figure 10.5A. **C:** A 10-W lesion through the saline irrigated catheter eliminated pre-excitation within 2 seconds as seen in the lower panel.

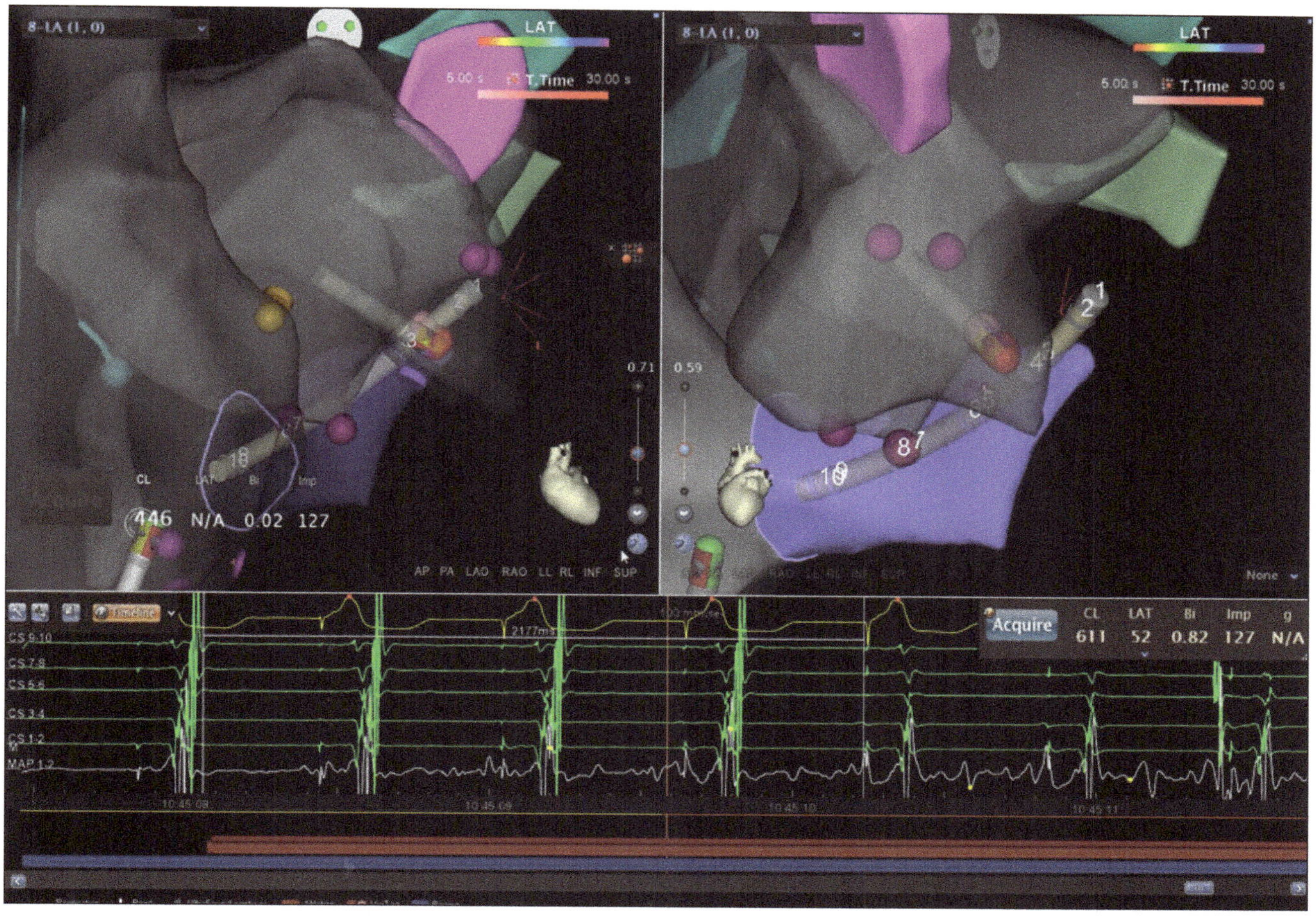

Figure 10.6 Ventricular pacing during RF ablation of a concealed left posterolateral bypass tract shows loss of retrograde conduction. AP views are on left, and LA on right. Coronary sinus shown in **blue** with CS decapolar catheter. Left atrial appendage from sound map in **pink**; left superior pulmonary vein is blue and left inferior pulmonary vein is **green**. Mitral annulus points are **magenta** and His bundle points **yellow**. Real-time position of ablation catheter is lower RA (**green tip**) and replay mode of CARTO shows position of ablation catheter (**red tip**) during loss of retrograde conduction through bypass tract while ventricular pacing during ablation.

In our lab, a total of 29 patients with accessory pathways have undergone catheter ablation over the last over the last three years. **Table 10.1** shows the patient profile. No fluoroscopy was used in any patient. No complications occurred including hemopericardium, heart block or damage to the AV conduction system, or vascular complications. Only one patient required a repeat procedure due to an epicardial coronary sinus pathway that was successfully ablated within the coronary sinus as described above. All other patients have had no recurrence of WPW nor recurrent arrhythmias. These results support the concept that accessory pathway ablation may be performed effectively and safely with no fluoroscopy.

Once an understanding of safe and effective mapping and ablation using ICE and EAM tools currently available is achieved, the same principles of electrophysiological mapping and ablation traditionally utilized can be incorporated successfully into a zero-fluoroscopy approach.

Table 10.1 Characteristics of patients undergoing catheter ablation for accessory pathways between 8/2015 and 8/2018.

• Total patients	29
• Male/Female	17/12
• Mean Age	35
• Median Age	33
• WPW	9
• Left-sided	21
• Transseptal	20
• Parahisian	2
• Cryocatheter	2
• CS ablation	1
• Retrograde aortic and transseptal	1
• Fluoroscopy dose	0

References

1. Jackman WM, Wang XZ, Friday KJ, et al. Catheter ablation of accessory atrioventricular pathways (Wolff-Parkinson-White syndrome) by radiofrequency current. *N Engl J Med.* 1992;324:1605–1611.
2. Arruda MS, McClelland JH, Wang X, et al. Development and validation of an ECG algorithm for identifying accessory pathway ablation site in Wolff-Parkinson-White syndrome. *J Cardiovasc Electrophysiol.* 1998;9:2–12.
3. Milstein S, Sharma AD, Guiraudon GM, et al. An algorithm for the electrocardiographic localization of accessory pathways in the Wolff-Parkinson-White syndrome. *Pacing Clin Electrophysiol.* 1987;10:555–563.
4. Rostock T, Sydown K, Steven D, et al. A new algorithm for concealed accessory pathway localization using T wave subtracted retrograde P-wave polarity during orthodromic atrioventricular reentrant tachycardia. *J Interven Card Electr.* 2008;22:55–63.
5. Guletta, S, Tsiachris D, Della Bella P. Catheter ablation of an anteroseptal accessory pathway guided by contact force monitoring technology and precise electroanatomic mapping. *Europace.* 2014;16:825.
6. Lesh MD, Van Hare G, Kao AK, Scheinman MM. Radiofrequency catheter ablation for Wolff-Parkinson-White syndrome associated with coronary sinus diverticulum. *Pacing Clin Electrophysiol.* 1991;14:1479–1484.
7. Takahashi A, Shah DC, Jaïs P, Hocini M, Clementy J, Haïssaguerre M. Specific electrocardiographic features of manifest coronary vein posteroseptal accessory pathways. *J Cardiovasc Electrophysiol.* 1998;10:1015–1025.
8. Sun Y, Arruda M, Otomo K, et al. Coronary sinus-ventricular accessory connections producing posteroseptal and left posterior accessory pathways: Incidence and electrophysiological identification. *Circulation.* 2002;106:1362–1367.

Video Legends

Video 10.1 Placement of a duodecapolar catheter in the coronary sinus. [00:29]

Video 10.2 **Yellow dots** show His cloud and the His catheter is **orange** at the RA (**red**) right ventricle (**green**) junction. The decapolar catheter (**blue**) is shown in the CS (**yellow**). What appears to be a second CS catheter was a saved image of the original CS placement to make sure that the CS has not moved during the case. The real time CS catheter shows an inferior deflection at electrodes 7-8 due to pacing electrode selection, which is seen with EnSite. A 4-mm cryocatheter (Medtronic Inc, Minneapolis, MN) was used for ablation due to the proximity to the compact AV node. The **red dot** was used to mark the most proximal region of His bundle recording. The **blue dots** represent the ablation points. Note the use of transparency and color to delineate structures, catheters, and key electrogram sites. The pathway was ablated without affecting AV nodal conduction despite a very small intermittent His bundle deflection on the second beat seen on the ablation catheter electrogram. Note the larger A to V ratio on the ablation catheter compared to the His bundle catheter. [00:40]

Video 10.3A ICE image and sound map of the left atrium. [00:02]

Video 10.3B Using SmartTouch catheter in the IVC to create volumetric map of the IVC, RA, SVC, and CS. The **red dots** represent the mitral annulus recorded on ICE. The pulmonary veins (**blue** and **green**) are shown coming off the LA. The ablation catheter starts at the IVC and is advanced under force guidance and curved and swept in the RA to create the volumetric map. The esophagus can be seen behind the LA in **brown**. [1:17]

Video 10.3C Transseptal site on ICE, marked in blue on RA septum with integrated ICE and EAM. [00:37]

Video 10.3D Placing of CS catheter. [1:19]

Video 10.3E RAO and clipping plane and LAO with contact force SmartTouch catheter entering CS os with 4 g of force. Illustrates how the contact force is used to safely navigate the catheter to the distal CS and create the CS volumetric map. [00:14]

Video 10.3F Non-fluoroscopic technique for retrograde aortic access. LV (**meshed grey**) and ascending aorta (**meshed pink**), which is then merged with catheter map of the descending aorta and arch as the catheter is advanced. The catheter is then prolapsed into the left ventricle. [2:02]

11

How to Ablate Typical Atrial Flutter Using No Fluoroscopy

Saurabh Shah, MD

Introduction

Of all cardiac radiofrequency ablation procedures, ablation of the cavotricuspid isthmus (CTI) for atrial flutter (AFL) is perhaps the least daunting, and may therefore be recommended as a starting point for the operator new to fluoroscopy-free ablation. Nearly universally, preparation requires the substitution of fluoroscopy with technologies such as intracardiac echocardiography (ICE) and a three-dimensional (3D) electroanatomic mapping (EAM) system (EnSite/CARTO/Rhythmia).[1-8] Rarely, radiofrequency ablation of AFL-CTI without fluoroscopy has been accomplished without ICE or EAM using intracardiac electrograms (EGM). However, the requirement of stable catheter–tissue contact along an anatomically variable ablation target renders the routine use of this approach unlikely to succeed. Technologies such as MediGuide also facilitate zero fluoroscopy use but only after prerecording 2D cinefluoroscopy.[9] Magnetic resonance imaging-(MRI-) guided ablation of AFL-CTI are reported but remain investigational and widely unavailable.[10]

Techniques discussed in this chapter are readily applicable and consistently eliminate exposure for patient or operator to radiation from fluoroscopy. This chapter guides the reader through standard techniques with variations and tips in how to successfully ablate AFL-CTI without fluoroscopy. Instruction on negotiating common challenges and a video link follow.

Standard Technique, Variations, and Challenges

Prior to the Procedure

Upon confirming AFL-CTI clinically and an indication for its ablation, obtain informed consent and prepare the consented patient for non-fluoroscopic ablation as follows:

1. Maintain oral anticoagulation with warfarin or a direct oral anticoagulant (DOAC) through the day of the procedure. In patients at higher risk from intraprocedural bleeding, hold DOAC 12 to 24 hours prior to the procedure. *Variation:* Substitute a short course of dabigatran for other DOACs starting 3 days prior to the procedure if the specific antidote idarucizumab is readily available at your institution. The recently available drug andexanet alfa should facilitate uninterrupted apixaban and rivaroxaban use when it becomes widely available.

2. Suspend antiarrhythmics (except amiodarone) 5 half-lives prior to procedure on a case-by-case basis depending on the need for arrhythmia inducibility.

3. Omit preprocedural transesophageal echocardiogram if you do not suspect a lapse in therapeutic anticoagulation within the prior 4 weeks or if the patient presents in sinus rhythm.

Fluoroscopy Reduction Techniques for Catheter Ablation of Cardiac Arrhythmias. © 2019 Mansour Razminia, Paul C. Zei, eds.
Cardiotext Publishing, ISBN: 978-1-942909-30-9.

4. Perform a preprocedural anesthesia risk evaluation to determine the safety of procedural moderate conscious sedation to achieve sufficient analgesia and patient cooperation. Consider extremity restraints and deep sedation with propofol, dexmedetomidine, or similar agents to limit patient movements from destabilizing the EAM geometry critical for fluoroscopy-free ablation.

In the Electrophysiology Lab

The operator and staff do not require the use of radiation shielding garments at any point during the procedure. However, staff should maintain a fluoroscope in disabled or standby mode remote from the field. The procedure is undertaken via the following steps:

1. Apply mapping system patches and recording system leads. The author's team defaults to the EnSite EAM paired with a 9-Fr ViewFlex ICE catheter. Other options, including the CARTO or Rhythmia EAMs and Siemens 8-Fr Acuson ICE catheter with or without navigation (CARTO SOUNDSTAR), are acceptable alternatives requiring some adjustments discussed below.
2. Obtain bilateral femoral vein access under ultrasound guidance as described in Chapter 5 of this textbook. Rarely, right internal jugular vein (IJV) ultrasound guided access is required when lower extremity access is limited.
3. Insert the following sheath introducers for the listed catheters:
   - Right femoral vein:
     - 8-Fr - roving/ablating catheter
     - 7-Fr - duodecapolar catheter to tricuspid valve annulus
     - 6-Fr - steerable multipolar (8 or 10) catheter to proximal coronary sinus (CS)
   - Left femoral vein:
     - 10-Fr (20 cm to 30 cm length to allow sheath in the low IVC) - ViewFlex ICE
     - *Variation:* 9-Fr standard length sheath if using the 8-Fr Acuson ICE

   If desired, fewer sheaths and catheters may be used. Performing AFL-CTI ablation without ICE and relying primarily on the mapping system is a reasonable approach.

   Tip: To position longer sheath in low IVC, gently advance a ~150-cm, 0.035-inch standard J-wire through the introducer needle until atrial or ventricular ectopy is seen or baseline wander noted on the recording system's surface ECG leads. Typically, the wire has been advanced sufficiently when the back end of the wire nears the patient's feet. Resistance to wire advancement prior to this indicates passage into a tributary vein. In this case, withdraw the wire a short distance and redirect it with rotation and needle reorientation. Shorter length (10 to 15 cm) introducer sheaths may suffice and have the advantage of shorter wire. However, the 9-Fr ViewFlex ICE catheter lacks the ease of maneuverability necessary to negotiate sharp left common iliac vein-inferior vena cava junction. *Challenges:* IVC filters pose a challenge still negotiable without the use of fluoroscopy. Numerous filter types have been crossed safely using fluoroscopy.[11] Given the concern for thrombus dislodgment and filter migration we require the patient has been chronically anticoagulated and the implant in place >6 months. To reduce the number of crossings of the IVC filter, IJV access is used to position a single duodecapolar catheter capable of lateral TV annulus and coronary sinus recording. Via each of 2 femoral accesses a straight-tipped wire is advanced cranially across the IVC filter until intracardiac ectopy is seen. To limit the number of times the IVC filter is crossed, long sheaths are carefully passed over the wire. Abdominal ultrasound visualization of the IVC filter is possible and may aid visualization of each step. Curved long sheaths are straightened out over a dilator and wire during removal.
4. Introduce the ICE catheter to the mid-to-low right atrium (RA) first. Tweak the turn knobs to navigate out of tributary veins and over prominent Eustachian ridges.

   Challenges: Pacemaker or ICD leads do not pose an insurmountable challenge for fluoroless ablation. We require the leads have been implanted for at least 6 weeks for fluoroless ablation. Visualize and record baseline lead position under ICE. Avoid catheter–lead entanglement by passing around leads rather than through its loops. Often, directing catheter tips toward the low lateral RA immediately upon atrial entry from the IVC avoids catheter-lead entanglement. Catheter deflections are released prior to removal from the RA. Pre- and post-procedure device interrogation are recommended, and revisualization of pacing lead locations to confirm they are unchanged at case end is a good idea.
5. Record baseline images from the home view (**Figure 11.1**) in the right atrium of the CTI anatomy and also of surrounding structures. *Tip:* From the RA, pan clockwise/overhand direction about 180 degrees from the laterally located crista terminalis or pectinate muscle, past the home view containing tricuspid

valve (TV) and CTI; then onto the aortic knob, left atrial appendage and interatrial septum assessing for a patent foramen ovale. Flex anterior or posterior to optimize images. Pay attention to challenging anatomy in the CTI in the form of a long TV to IVC distance (> 4 cm), deep bottle-necked pouches (**Figure 11.2**), and/or prominent Eustachian valves (**Figure 11.3**) or ridges.[12] Challenging CTI anatomy impacts the choice of ablation catheter and the use of additional long sheaths or catheter maneuvers (**Figure 11.4**). *Variation:* When using CARTO SOUNDSTAR, also collect tightly spaced contours of the CTI anatomy.

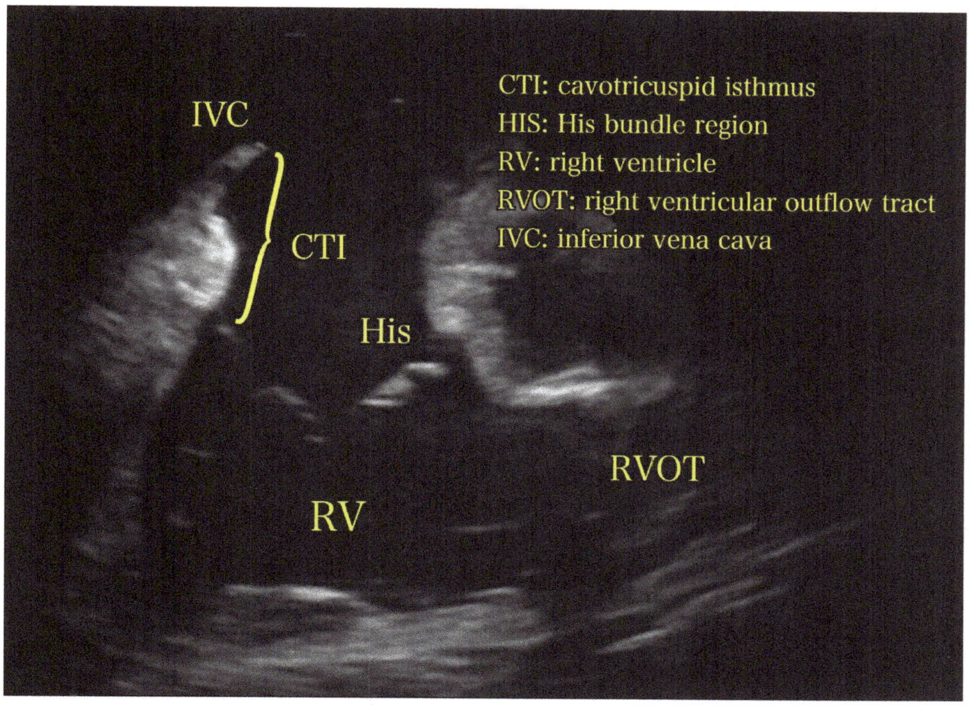

Figure 11.1 Pertinent cardiac anatomic structures are identified by ICE in the home view.

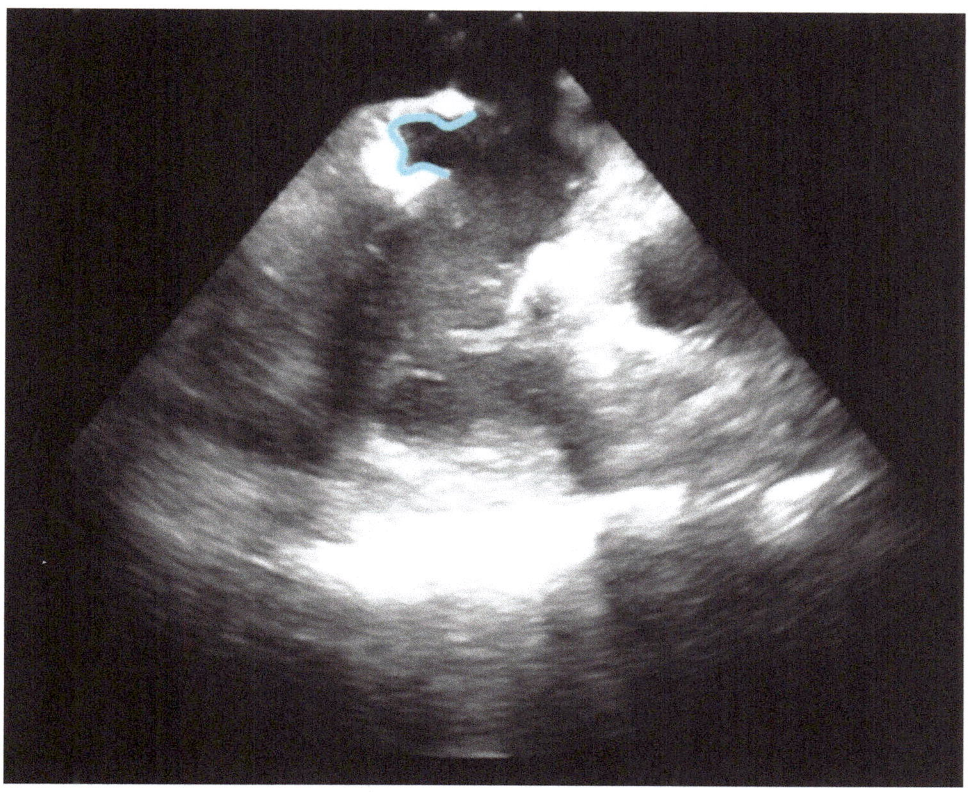

Figure 11.2 Patient with prior tricuspid valve annuloplasty has a complex CTI with bottleneck-shaped pouch.

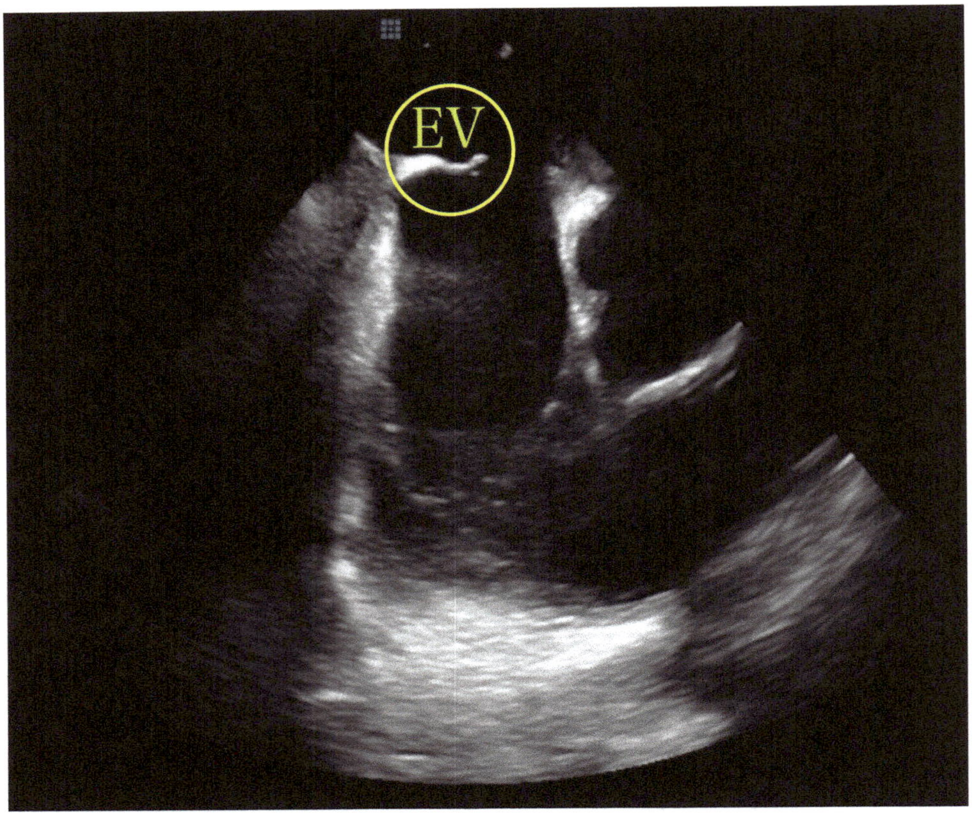

Figure 11.3 Prominent Eustachian valve (EV) makes for challenging access to the proximal CTI.

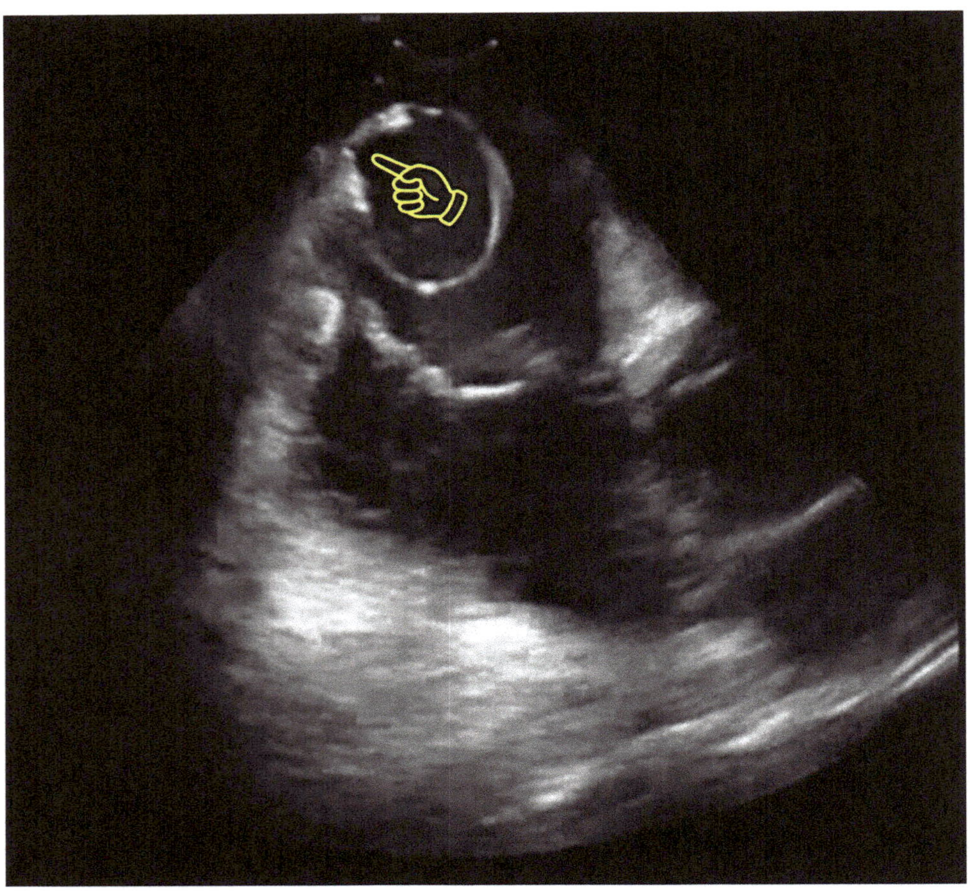

Figure 11.4 Use of U-curve on ablation catheter facilitates ablation at base of a prominent Eustachian valve, an otherwise difficult area to reach.

6. Record baseline images from the right ventricle (RV) of baseline pericardial effusion and left atrial appendage thrombus. Return to home view by withdrawing ICE to the low RA in the plane of the CTI. *Tip:* To obtain baseline RV images flex the ICE catheter anteriorly, maintaining visualization of the TV until orthogonal to the plane of the valve and parallel to the floor of the RV. Advance the ICE 1 to 2 centimeters past the valve and partly release flexion for low RV outflow tract images. Pan about 180 degrees slowly, recording the presence of the baseline maximal pericardial effusion typically seen in the initial left atrial views. Catheter-induced ventricular ectopy is common and transient. Panning further visualizes the left atrial structures.

7. Introduce mapping catheters, collecting venous geometry from the IVC to SVC and creating a right atrial shell focused around the CTI. *Tip:* When using the EnSite EAM, first introduce the steerable multielectrode coronary sinus catheter into the body. Collect venous geometry in orthogonal views while gently advancing the catheter toward the right atrium, avoiding branch vessels. Alternatively, advance the catheter in a prolapsed orientation to better retain within the IVC. Initial appearance of EGMs along the catheter's most cranial bipoles indicates proximity to the RA endocardium in the IVC. EGMs may be missed if advanced too rapidly past the RA. From the RA level slowly withdraw the catheter until loss of all EGMs and tag this position as IVC in the EAM. Gently advance the catheter directing it slightly rightward and posterior toward the SVC. Upon loss of all EGMs tag this position SVC. Avoid catheter trajectory anteriorly deep into the RA appendage or leftward across a patent foramen ovale and into a pulmonary vein. Maintain a high degree of suspicion and use ICE to confirm catheter location. From the SVC withdraw catheter into the RA and continue to collect right atrial geometry, tagging the bundle of His as you maneuver the catheter into the proximal coronary sinus using EGMs, biplane view in the EAM, and ICE guidance. Once stably positioned in the coronary sinus, perform respiratory compensation in the EAM to spatially stabilize subsequent geometry. At this point, EAM reference can switch from external to the coronary sinus catheter if required for stability. Next, insert the duodecapolar catheter into the body and maneuver it to the right atrium using the existing geometry and adding any new geometry from this catheter. In the RA, curl the catheter tip toward the free wall, advancing and twisting it until seated along the tricuspid valve annulus from lateral CTI to septum. *Variation:* When using CARTO first advance a navigation-enabled catheter, typically the ablating catheter, to create geometric shell. Extracardiac field of view with CARTO or Rhythmia is restricted in comparison to EnSite. When difficulty is encountered outside of the range of view, advance catheter in parallel with ICE visualization or use longer sheaths to bypass regions blind to the EAM.

8. Select an ablation catheter based on CTI anatomy visualized on ICE. We select a non-irrigated 8-mm tip ablation catheter for long and/or smooth CTI. The presence of pouches or heavy trabeculation justifies the use of an irrigated-tip ablation catheter. The ability to visualize catheter–tissue contact and edema formation during ablation under ICE obviates the need for routine use of a contact force measuring catheter. There is no technical disadvantage in using one, however. *Challenges:* Longs sheaths such as SR0, RAMP, or steerable types require ICE to confirm coplanar alignment of the long sheath with the ablation catheter. To calibrate a catheter's reach outside of the sheath, combine ICE visualization with the use of the sheath detection features of the EAM including catheter shaft distortion.

9. After confirming AFL-CTI by usual methods, ablate the CTI, dragging the catheter continuously from tricuspid annulus to inferior vena cava under EGM, EAM, and ICE guidance until sustaining bidirectional block. *Tip:* An assistant can be invaluable for continuous ICE catheter handling during ablation. Titrate ablation duration and power not only using EGM diminution and impedance drop but also ICE visualization. Use ICE to gauge intermittency of catheter contact, especially at the mobile TV annulus and adjust accordingly. Catheter visualization during patient movement or large respiratory variation can sometimes be an insurmountable issue on EAM for which ICE can help compensate. Use ICE to orient the catheter in complex anatomy such as pouches and prominent Eustachian ridges. Direct ablation catheter–tissue contact and postablation tissue changes seen by ICE (**Figure 11.5**) complement other findings to confirm lesions. Visualization of steam pops and surveillance for pericardial effusions are an additional important role for ICE.

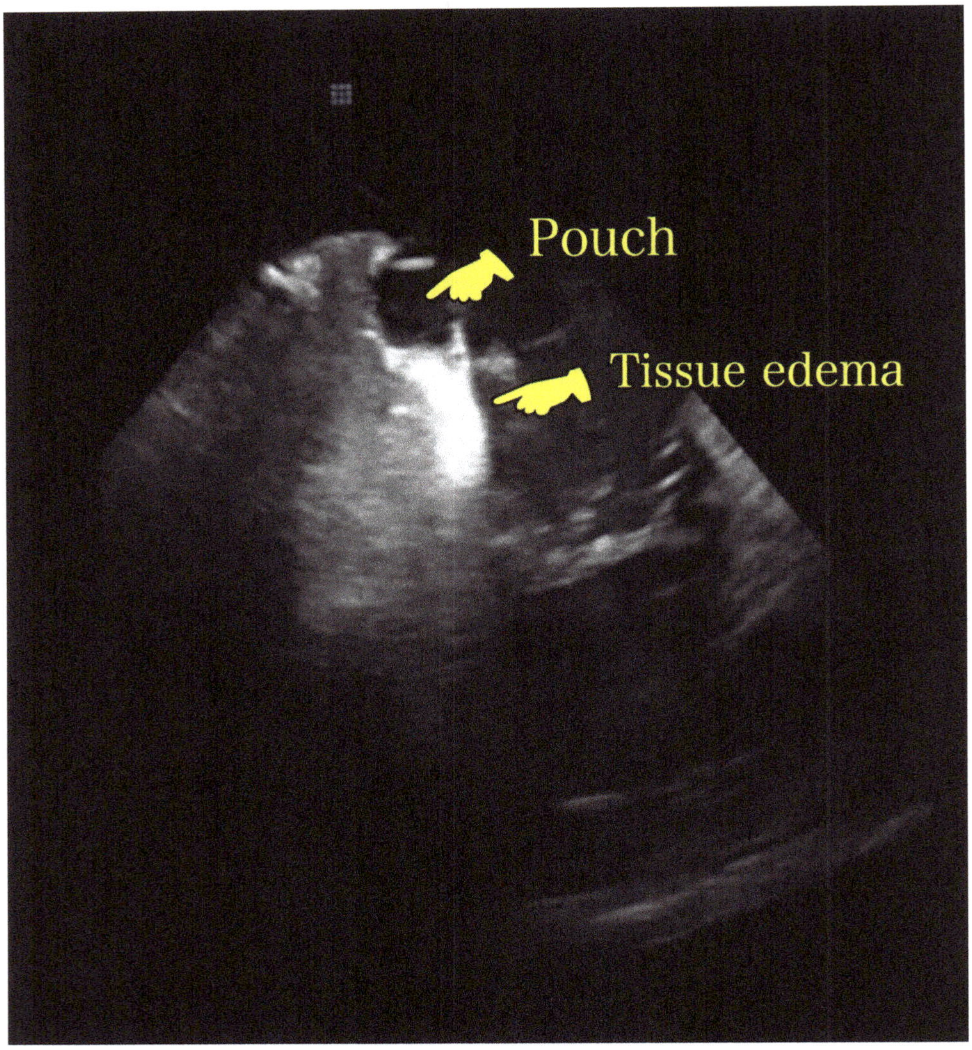

Figure 11.5 Echogenic appearance of edematous cavotricuspid isthmus tissue indicates the path of ablation.

Conclusion

With planning, the routine ablation of AFL-CTI without fluoroscopy can be performed successfully. Furthermore, it can be argued that eliminating fluoroscopy improves safety and efficacy through the required use of ICE and EAM—technologies that not only overlap with fluoroscopic guidance but augment the information offered by fluoroscopy alone. Fluoroscopy use for AFL-CTI ablation likely will soon become a thing of the past.

References

1. Leonelli FM, Tomassoni G, Richey M, Natale A. Usefulness of three-dimensional non-fluoroscopic mapping in the ablation of typical atrial flutter. *Ital Heart J.* 2002;3:360–365.
2. Ormaetxe-Merodio JM, Martinez-Alday JD, Arcocha-Torres MF, et al. Fluoroscopy free ablation of the cavotricuspid isthmus: Results of a pilot multi-center study. *Eur Heart J.* 2008;29 Suppl 1:743 (Abstract).
3. Pachòn M, Arias MA, Castellanos E, Puchol A. No fluoroscopy for cavotricuspid isthmus-dependent right atrial flutter ablation. *Heart Rhythm.* 2009;6:433–434. Epub 2008 July 24.
4. Àlvarez M, Tercedor L, Herrera N, et al. Cavotricuspid isthmus catheter ablation without the use of fluoroscopy as a first-line treatment. *Cardiovasc Electrophysiol.* 2011;22: 656–662.
5. Razminia M, Manankil MF, Eryazici PL, et al. Non-fluoroscopic catheter ablation of cardiac arrhythmias in adults: Feasibility, safety, and efficacy. *J Cardiovasc Electrophysiol.* 2012;23:1078–1086.
6. Macias R, Uribe I, Tercedor L, et al. A zero-fluoroscopy approach to cavotricuspid isthmus catheter ablation: Comparative analysis of two electroanatomical mapping systems. *Pacing Clin Electrophysiol.* 2014;37:1029–1037.
7. Fernandez-Gomez JM, Morina-Vazquez P, Morales Edel R, et al. Exclusion of fluoroscopy use in catheter ablation procedures: Six years of experience at a single center. *J Cardiovasc Electrophysiol.* 2014;25:638–644.
8. Merino J. Tools or toys? The 20-year anniversary of the non-fluoroscopic mapping system dilemma. *Rev Esp Cardiol.* 2017;70:690–693.

9. Sommer P, Wojdyla-Hordynska A, Rolf S, et al. Initial experience in ablation of typical atrial flutter using a novel three-dimensional catheter tracking system. *Europace.* 2013;15:578–581.
10. Chubb H, Williams S, Whitaker J, et al. Cardiac electrophysiology under MRI guidance: An emerging technology. *Arrhythm Electrophysiol Rev.* 2017 Jun; 6(2):85–93.
11. Jez J, Starek Z, Lehar F, Wolf J, Novak M. Complex electrophysiology intervention in a patient with an inferior vena cava filter. *Cor et Vasa.* 2015;57(5):e341.
12. Bencsik G. Novel strategies in the ablation of typical atrial flutter: Role of intracardiac echocardiography. *Curr Cardiol Rev.* 2015;11(2):127–133.

Video Legends

Video 11S Chapter summary and step-by-step procedures by Mansour Razminia. [5:35]

12

How to Ablate Atrial Tachycardia and Atypical Flutter Using No Fluoroscopy

Dan Alyesh, MD; Sri Sundaram, MD

Introduction

Use of fluoroscopy has been necessary to visualize cardiac structures and catheters within the body. But fluoroscopy has been associated with negative effects on patients and staff in the electrophysiology (EP) laboratory. Staff are subject to the long-term effects of radiation exposure as well as orthopedic injury from the use of heavy, protective lead aprons.[1] With the recent improvements in intracardiac echo (ICE), 3D anatomic mapping systems, and ablation catheters, it is now possible to complete a complex, left atrial ablation procedure without the use of fluoroscopy.

Catheter ablation of drug-refractory, symptomatic atrial fibrillation (AF) has been shown to effectively improve quality of life and reduce arrhythmia burden.[2-6] While ablation of paroxysmal atrial fibrillation has achieved a high rate of success with one procedure, ablation of persistent AF with a single procedure has not been as successful. Recurrences in persistent AF patients can manifest as atypical atrial flutters (aAFL), which can be quite symptomatic and difficult to treat medically.[7-9] These arrhythmias are more common if linear ablation lesion sets were performed during the index procedure.[10-13] Ablation of aAFL can be challenging with limited success and long procedural times.[14-16] With lengthy procedure times and the challenge of identifying the critical isthmus, prolonged fluoroscopy times are common in ablation of aAFL. With the harmful effects of radiation, reducing fluoroscopy use has become critical with ablation of aAFL. In this chapter, we describe the modifications we make to the traditional procedure to allow for a non-fluoroscopic case.

Access to the Left Atrium

Achieving access to the left atrium (LA) is one of the challenges of non-fluoroscopic ablation. This chapter will describe the authors' process, as it may be different than the common practice of many operators. First, venous access to the femoral veins is obtained via the standard modified Seldinger technique. Ultrasound visualization of the femoral vein is performed to avoid accessing the femoral artery. In addition, the access needle does not advance beyond the posterior margin of the vein, decreasing the likelihood of a retroperitoneal hematoma.

After access, the coronary sinus (CS) catheter is introduced via the left femoral vein, and the 3D mapping system is used to track the movement of the catheter into the heart. Use of a "generic" mapping catheter currently is feasible only on the EnSite (Abbott, Abbott Park, IL) mapping system; a proprietary magnet-enabled ablation catheter is required for initial mapping whilst utilizing the CARTO (Biosense Webster, Irvine, CA) system. A 3D map is made of the right atrium (RA), the superior portion of the right ventricle, and the interatrial septum. After these structures have been identified, the location of

Fluoroscopy Reduction Techniques for Catheter Ablation of Cardiac Arrhythmias. © 2019 Mansour Razminia, Paul C. Zei, eds.
Cardiotext Publishing, ISBN: 978-1-942909-30-9.

the coronary sinus ostium (os) can be identified, and a catheter can be advanced into the CS. An ICE catheter is then introduced via a sheath from the left femoral vein and advanced to visualize the RA, interatrial fossa, LA, pulmonary vein ostia, and aortic valve. Should any concerns arise in the case, we also assess the baseline presence of pericardial fluid as a reference point. A guidewire is then introduced from the right femoral vein and followed with ICE into the superior vena cava (SVC). We advance an SL1 sheath (Abbott) over the guidewire into the SVC. A BRK-1 needle (Abbott) is then introduced through the sheath and advanced until it is about 2 cm from the distal end of the dilator. While visualizing the interatrial septum with the ICE catheter, the dilator, sheath, and needle apparatus is withdrawn until it falls into the fossa ovalis. Using the ICE catheter, the ideal fossa location is identified. For radiofrequency ablation, a posterior fossa location is visualized and for cryoablation, a more anterior location is identified. After the appropriate location has been visualized, the BRK-1 needle is advanced and the septum punctured. Saline is infused through the needle tip and creates micro-bubbles in the LA, which can be visualized on ICE. This confirms the location of the puncture. The dilator is then advanced minimally into the LA. The needle is withdrawn, and a stiff guidewire is introduced into the LA and advanced into a left-sided pulmonary vein under ICE guidance. The sheath and dilator apparatus is then advanced over the guidewire. By advancing over a guidewire, the sudden forward progression of the dilator and sheath apparatus as it crosses the septum can be directed away from the posterior wall of the LA or the LAA. If a second access to the LA is needed, this process is repeated. We typically use the Agilis NxT steerable sheath (Abbott) for the second access.

Equipment

Fluoroscopy-free procedures have become achievable because of the advancement of the equipment used in electrophysiology. The authors' EP laboratory predominantly uses the EnSite Precision mapping system (Abbott). We prefer this system because of the ability to track the movement of catheters from the access sheath to the heart. In addition, the advanced data collection ability of the system is of benefit with ablation of aAFLs. With the EnSite Precision mapping system, there is no maximum number of data points that can be taken per case. However, we typically obtain approximately 75,000 data points per case using a multipolar mapping catheter. This heightened resolution allows for better identification of the area of interest for ablation. In addition, the cost per case in the hospital system is significantly less with this mapping system. Other operators have reported a similar process with other 3D anatomic mapping systems such as CARTO (Biosense Webster) and Rhythmia (Boston Scientific, Chattuck, MA).[17,18]

For ICE imaging, the authors use the ViewFlex ICE catheter (Abbott), but have also used the AcuNav Ultrasound ICE catheter (Biosense Webster). Both of these ICE catheter systems are be comparable. For mapping, the most efficient way to obtain the anatomy and activation is with a multipolar catheter. For de novo procedures in the LA, we typically use a decapolar circular mapping catheter, which can then be advanced to the pulmonary veins to evaluate for activity. The recently introduced Advisor HD Grid Mapping Catheter, Sensor Enabled (Abbott) has become our catheter of choice for aAFL as it has greater number of electrodes that are closely spaced and can detect data in multiple planes, including perpendicular wavefronts. In addition, the catheter has a less traumatic surface and is more pliable than other multipolar, high-density catheters.

3D Anatomic Mapping System

The 3D mapping system is set up with a coronary sinus (CS) electrogram as the mapping reference. The usual setup has been described previously.[19] The CS reference electrogram was selected based on the amplitude and consistency.[20] A detailed explanation of the exact set up and data acquisition methods have been described in detail previously.[21,22] Briefly, 3 major setting changes are made for aAFL when using the Precision mapping system:

1. The absolute peak (Abs peak) is used rather than the onset to determine the timing of the electrical activity. This allows for rapid collection of data points within the LA and minimizes the need for the operator to review the collected data. This, in turn, can lead to quicker procedure times.

2. The Precision mapping system is set to display all mapping points with only 8 isochronal color bands in the following activation pattern: white → red → orange → yellow → green → light blue → dark blue → purple. Interpretation of the map is simplified with this limited color palette. Each color band represents equally spaced timing. Therefore, large and wide color bands represent fast conduction, while tightly spaced color bands represent slow conduction. The color sequence must follow this order. With only 8 colors to analyze, following the sequence of activation is simplified (**Figures 12.1–12.3**).

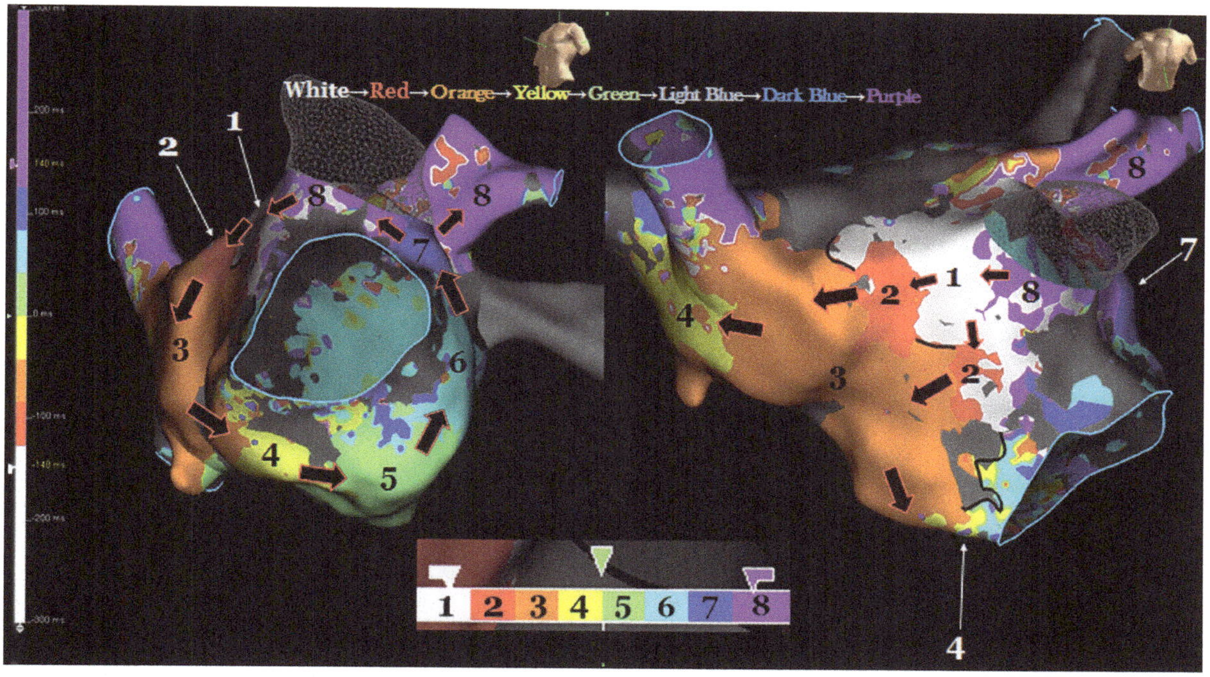

Figure 12.1 Left atrium seen from a left lateral view on the left and an anterior view on the right. The tachycardia progresses from White → Red → Orange → Yellow → Green → Light Blue → Dark Blue → Purple. The color scheme shows a counterclockwise rhythm around the mitral valve. This arrhythmia was terminated with ablations in the area of the **white region** (area 1) and the **red region** (area 2).

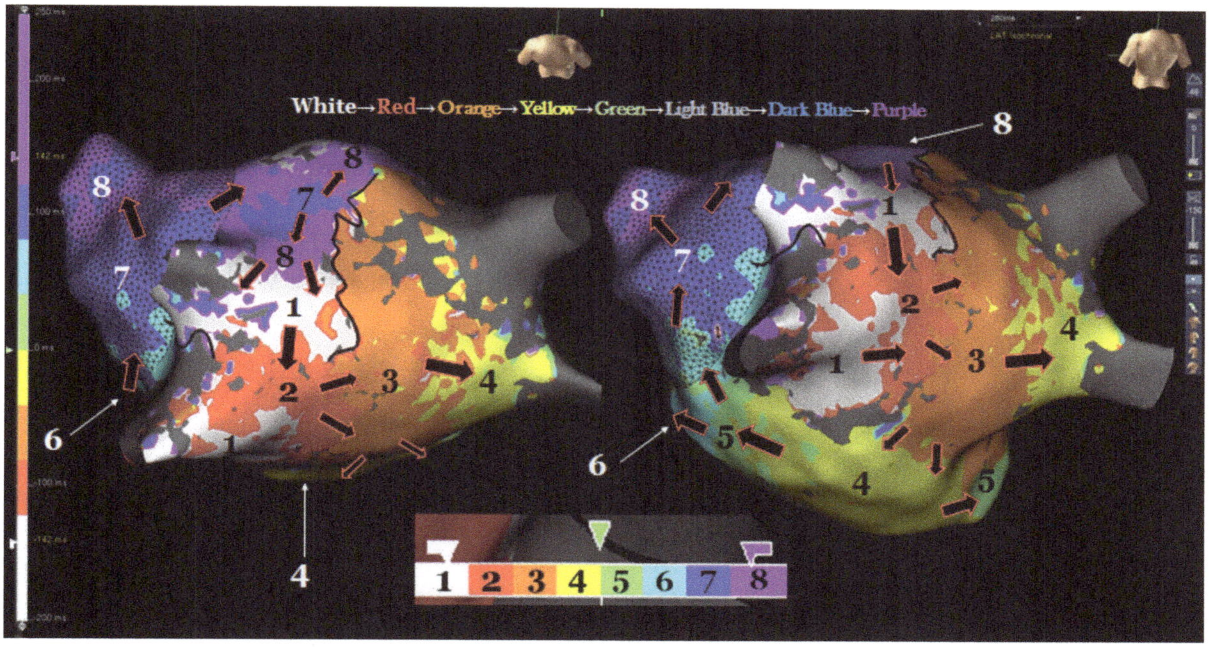

Figure 12.2 The left atrium seen from a superior view on the left and a posterolateral view on the right. The tachycardia progresses from White → Red → Orange → Yellow → Green → Light Blue → Dark Blue → Purple. The color scheme shows a roof-dependent flutter. Ablation lesions at the roof, between the **black lines** in the area between the **white region** (area 10) and the **red region** (area 2), terminated the tachycardia.

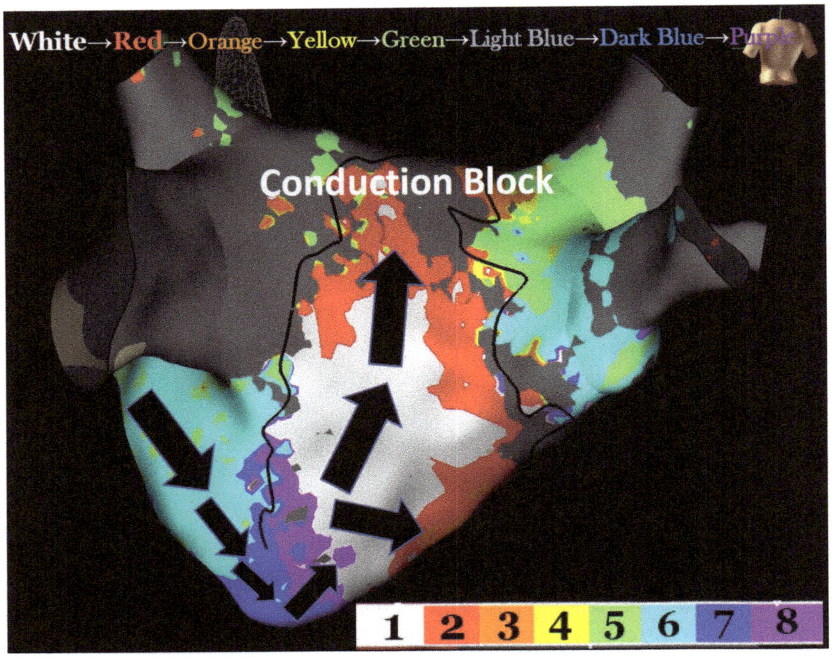

Figure 12.3 Posterior view of the LA. The tachycardia progresses from White → Red → Orange → Yellow → Green → Light Blue → Dark Blue → Purple. The color scheme shows an atypical flutter that runs between a previous ablation line (**black line**) and the mitral valve. The arrhythmia was terminated with 2 ablation lesions between the bottom of the prior ablation line and the mitral valve.

3. Voltage values are annotated automatically on the Precision system and stored for each Local Activation Time (LAT) point. The Low-V ID (LVID) was selected with the nominal setting of 1.0 mV. With this setting, an area of voltage lower than 1.0 mV will display as gray on the 3D map, which signifies scar. In brief, the LVID identifies low-voltage zones in activation maps. If a collected LAT point has a peak-to-peak (P-P) value lower than the specified LVID value, that point will display as gray and not be included in the color-coded timing scale. This helps to eliminate LAT points collected that were baseline noise on the electrogram. By increasing the LVID to a higher voltage value, more of the mapping data appears as gray or scar. Similarly, by decreasing the LVID, more of the mapping data appears as active tissue and is used in the activation mapping. The LVID is dynamically adjusted until only the largest voltage area in the previously identified critical slow conduction zone is shown. A narrow channel of higher voltage then becomes apparent in the slow conduction zone. After the target area was identified with HD-GVM, additional data points were obtained in this identified area, with a 3.5-mm irrigated tip contact sensing ablation catheter (TactiCath Catheter, Abbott). Points were only taken when contact force was greater than 10 g and less than 40 g. Collecting additional data points with the contact-sensing catheter further defined the area targeted for ablation. By using this method, we have been able to quickly and successfully terminate 92% of all atypical flutters.[19]

In situations when the CARTO mapping system is used, there are a number of similarities but a few notable differences.

1. Integration of ICE images into the electroanatomic map allows the interatrial fossa, esophagus, LA contours, and PV ostia to be pre-identified on the 3D map prior to transseptal puncture. Identifying these structures before entering the LA can facilitate atraumatic catheter manipulation when refining the 3D map in the LA.

2. Any non-Biosense Webster catheter, needle, or wire can be visualized on the mapping system. This specific feature allows the BRK needle, and the tip of a SafeSept Wire (Pressure Products, San Pedro, CA), to be visualized on 3D mapping when alligator clips are attached to the back of the BRK apparatus. This ability improves non-fluoroscopic transseptal puncture, as it integrates all imaging and electroanatomic data onto a single map.

3. The ConfiDense module allows for continuous collection of activation and anatomic points using either cycle length stability or a cycle length range. Once these points are collected, a Ripple map can display both voltage and activation maps simultaneously to aid with identification of a critical isthmus in aAFL.

Movement of the Catheters

Once inside the LA, the movement of the catheters can be monitored on ICE as well as the 3D anatomic mapping system. There are some unique movements necessary for a non-fluoroscopic procedure compared to traditional mapping. The first is obtaining an increased amount of data points inside the chamber of interest. Because our visualization of the chamber is mainly with the mapping system, we obtain a detailed map and usually acquire more points than usual. With the EnSite Precision mapping system, the operator usually obtains up to 75,000 data points per chamber. By obtaining a detailed map, one can identify all of the individual anatomic variants within the chamber. Using high-resolution mapping allows us to minimize extrapolations made by the software and improve map fidelity. Additionally, the authors decrease the internal projection, external projection, and fill thresholds values from their baseline value of 10 mm to 5 mm. This ensures that points taken are more accurate and are not far field potentials. After identifying the area of interest for ablation, additional data points are taken with the contact-sensing catheter. The benefit of the contact sensing is that it confirms that the data points are on the adjacent atrial myocardium and not far-field signals.

The second change is the visualization of the ablation catheter and sheath position. There are several methods to determine the position of the catheter and sheath individually and the relation to the sheath to the catheter. ICE visualization is the primary method of determining the location of the sheath and the ablation catheter. We usually try to keep ablation catheter distal electrodes a few millimeters outside the sheath. This provides better control of the ablation catheter during the case. The sheath and catheter positions can be determined by ICE.

Additionally, with the mapping system, the operator can identify the relationship of the ablation catheter and sheath. When the ablation catheter is completely outside the sheath, electrograms are visualized on both the proximal and distal poles. Additionally, the ablation catheter has a more traditional shape. As the catheter is pulled into the sheath, the proximal electrode is no longer sensing electrograms, and the impedance increases. This change in impedance can be seen on the mapping system screen as the catheter will artificially elongate on the proximal end while the distal end has a normal appearance.

As the catheter is further withdrawn into the sheath, the catheter elongates throughout its entire body (**Figure 12.4**). During the case, the authors routinely withdraw and advance the catheter to determine the relation of the sheath to the ablation catheter and to keep the ablation catheter proximal poles a few millimeters outside of the sheath. In the CARTO mapping system, when the proximal electrode is covered by the sheath, the distal electrode changes color which helps in sheath localization. Recently released mapping catheters from Abbott have a sheath filter for the most proximal poles of the mapping catheter. In addition, the Vizigo (Biosense Webster) steerable bidirectional sheath will soon be available commercially in North America. The Vizigo sheath is currently available in other markets. This sheath has 4 electrodes that can be visualized on the 3D anatomic map and can be used to determine the location of the sheath and catheters.

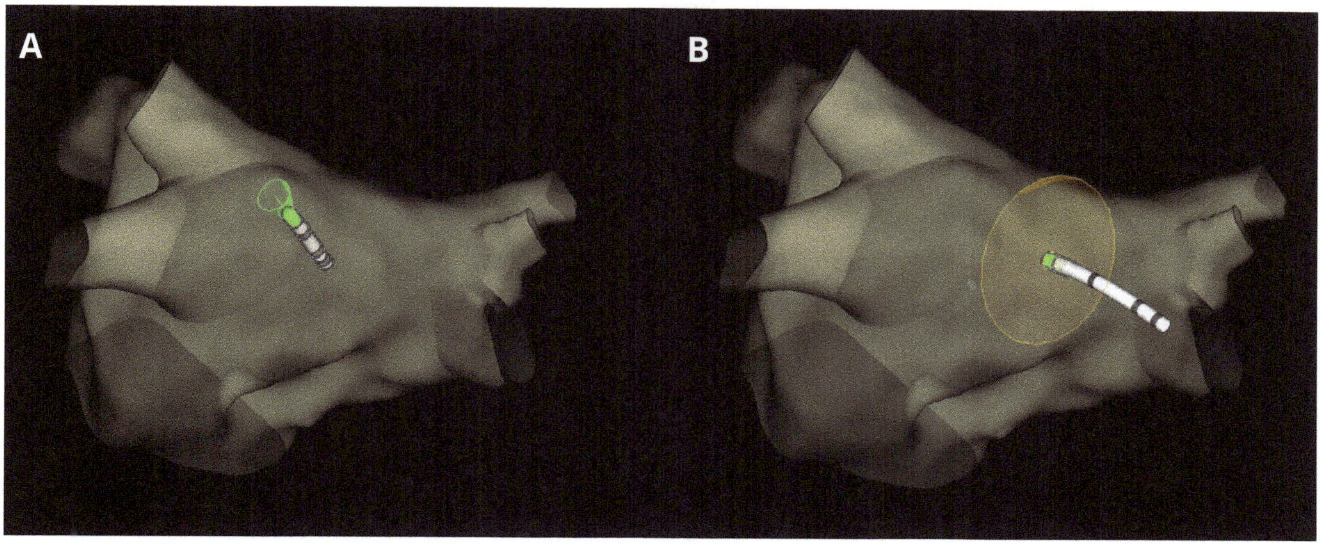

Figure 12.4 **A:** The ablation catheter fully outside the sheath. **B:** The ablation catheter partially inside the sheath. The distal end elongates as the impedance changes.

ICE Guidance and Special Considerations for Particular Flutters

The use of ICE as a supplement to the electroanatomic map and to guide catheter manipulation is a critical element of non-fluoroscopic ablation. ICE guidance helps visualize irregularities in the endocardial surface, such as ridges and pouches, which are not well visualized on electroanatomic maps. Such irregularities can make ablation challenging and often require catheter reorientation. ICE guidance can also ensure good catheter-to-tissue contact as a good supplement to contact force sensing. In the CARTO system, green tip overlay of the ablation catheter tip on the ICE image helps visualize tip–tissue interface.

Specifically, visualization of the coumadin ridge can be quite helpful in flutters involving the left atrial appendage and left superior pulmonary vein. Visualization of this ridge is accomplished by placing the ICE catheter in the home view from the mid RA and then rotating the catheter counter clockwise such that the left atrial appendage and left superior pulmonary vein are in view simultaneously with posterior flexion and rightward direction (**Figure 12.5**). Other helpful structures to visualize are the left atrial roof and posterior wall (**Figures 12.6** and **12.7**), which are critical in roof-dependent flutters and have important anatomic associations with the esophagus and ascending aorta. These structures can be visualized from the home view, first visualizing the left superior pulmonary vein and then rotating clockwise until the right superior pulmonary vein comes into view.

In addition, an esophageal temperature probe can also be placed via ICE localization. Using the posterior view of the LA, the esophagus is seen below the LA. As the temperature probe is advanced and withdrawn, the location of the probe can be determined on ICE.

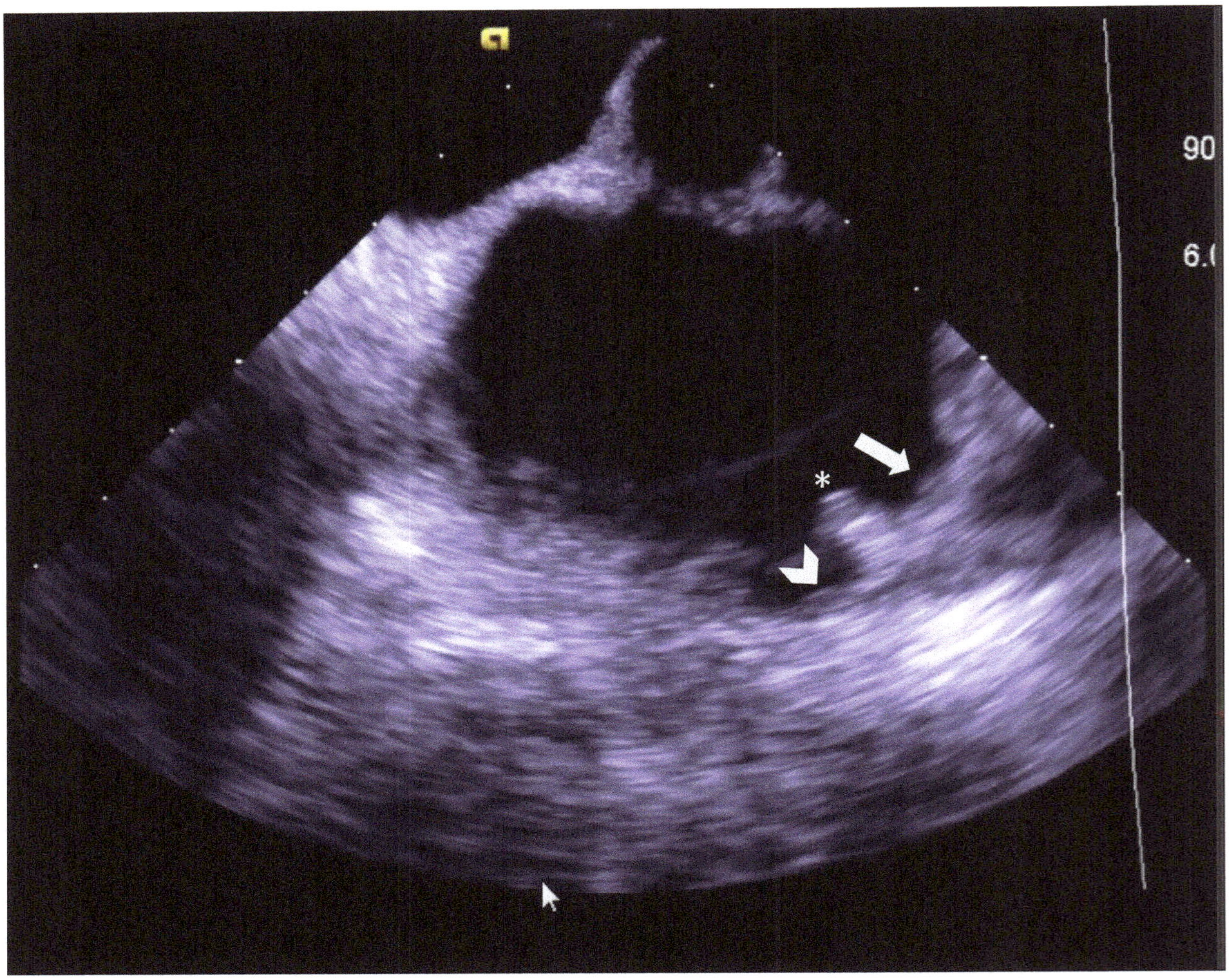

Figure 12.5 ICE visualization of the coumadin ridge (**asterisk**) and the LAA (**arrow**) and LSPV (**arrowhead**), which can be a critical location for atypical flutter circuits.

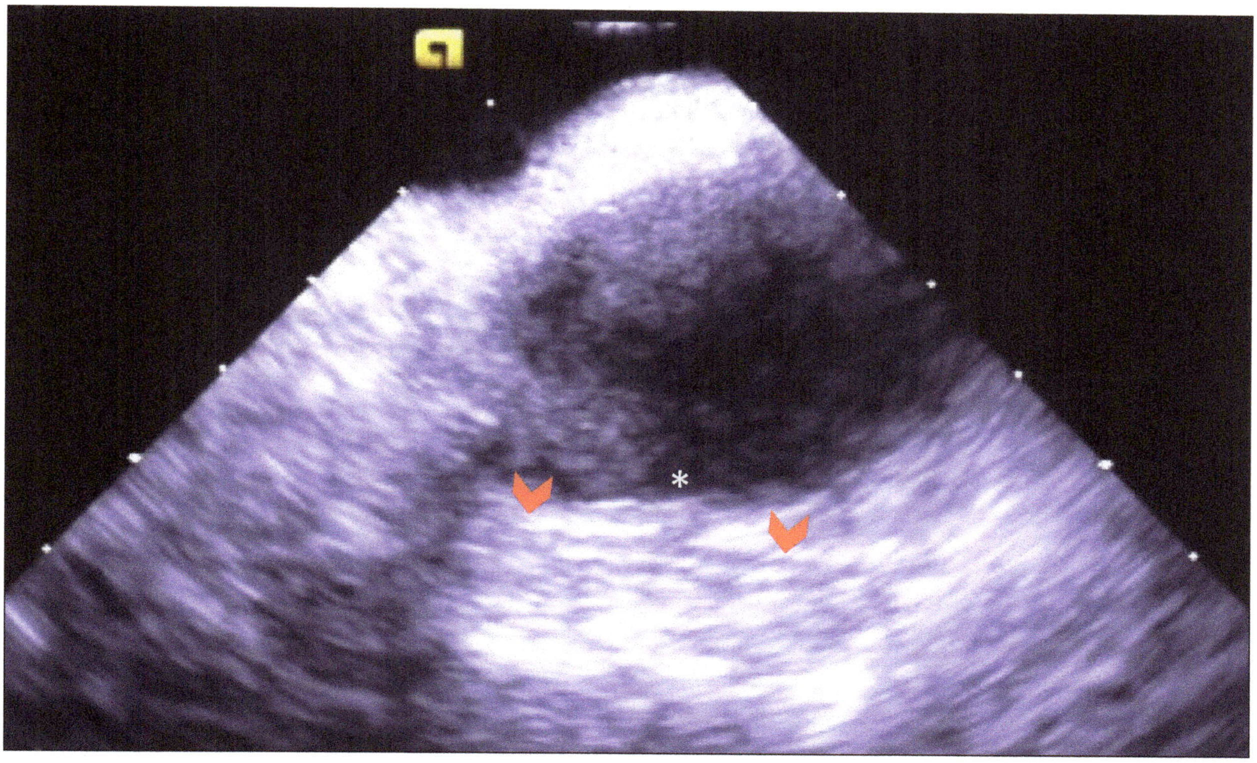

Figure 12.6 ICE visualization of the posterior wall (**asterisk**) highlighting its close relationship to the esophagus (**red arrowheads**).

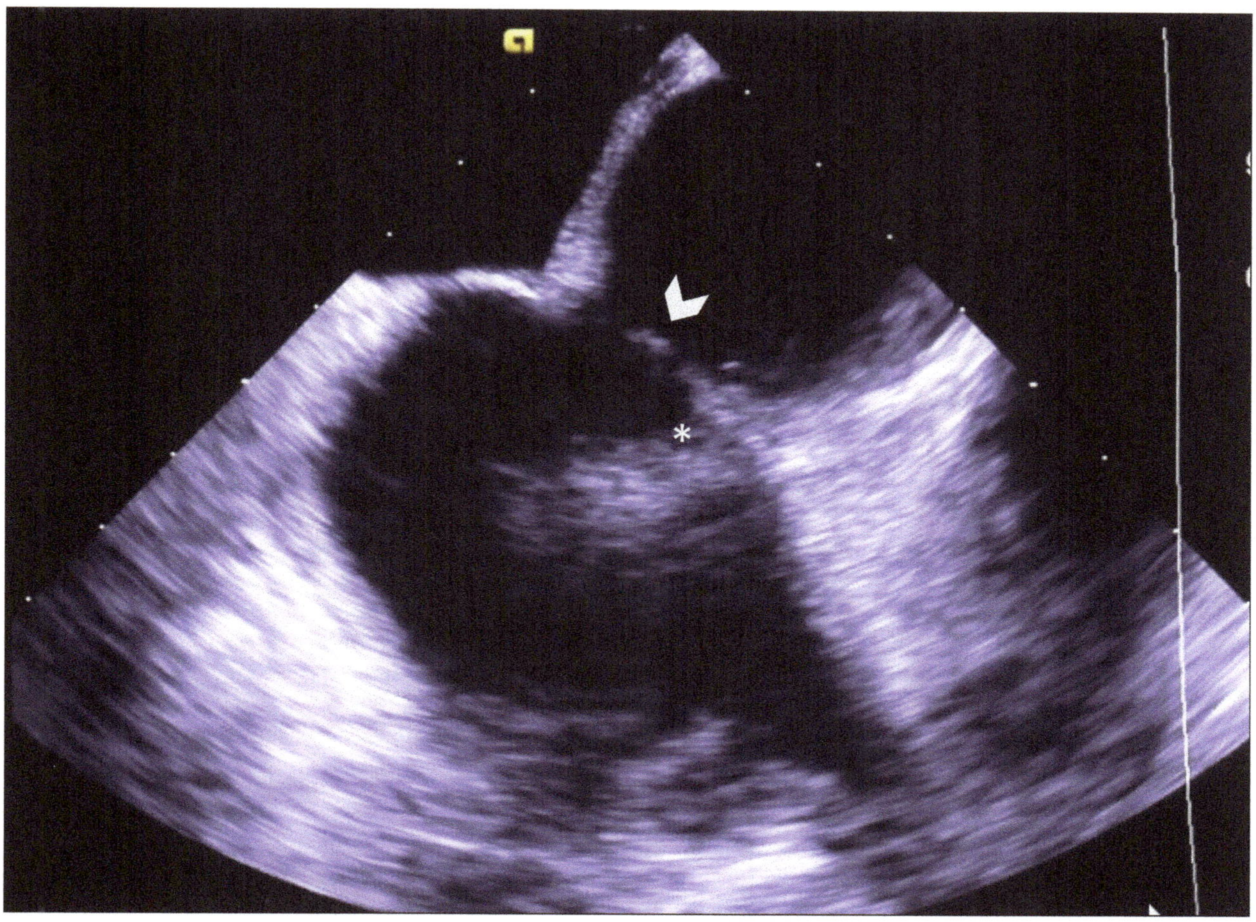

Figure 12.7 ICE visualization of the LA roof (**asterisk**) and its close relationship to the ascending aorta (**arrowhead**).

Complications

By using a non-fluoroscopic approach to ablation, the authors' overall complication rate with LA cases has remained unchanged at approximately 2%. Additionally, potential complications can be discovered earlier. Pericardial effusions are noted earlier with ICE as well as 3D mapping. ICE visualization of an early effusion has become our gold standard. After each step in the mapping and ablation process, we visualize the inferoposterior left ventricle, as this is where pericardial fluid will collect. In addition, with an effusion there will be a significant variation in the impedance and therefore, change in the appearance of the ablation catheter on the 3D mapping system. We have noticed these changes before a change in hemodynamics or the change in appearance of the lateral heart border on fluoroscopy.

Conclusion

Atypical atrial flutters are known to be challenging ablations. With the advent of more advanced mapping systems and increasing use of ICE, the procedure can be performed safely and successfully with procedural benefits to the patient and operators.

References

1. Heidbuchel H, Wittkampf FHM, Vano E, et al. Practical ways to reduce radiation dose for patients and staff during device implantations and electrophysiological procedures. *EP Europace.* 2014;16:946–964.
2. Haïssaguerre M, Jaïs P, Shah DC, et al. Spontaneous initiation of atrial fibrillation by ectopic beats originating in the pulmonary veins. *N Engl J Med.* 1998;339:659–666.
3. Haïssaguerre M, Shah DC, Jaïs P, et al. Electrophysiological breakthroughs from the left atrium to the pulmonary veins. *Circulation.* 2000;102:2463–2465.
4. Haïssaguerre M, Jaïs P, Shah DC, et al. Electrophysiological end point for catheter ablation of atrial fibrillation initiated from multiple pulmonary venous foci. *Circulation.* 2000;101:1409–417.
5. Pappone C, Rosanio S, Oreto G, et al. Circumferential radiofrequency ablation of pulmonary vein ostia. *Circulation.* 2000;102:2619–2628.
6. Oral H, Scharf C, Chugh A, et al. Catheter ablation for paroxysmal atrial fibrillation. *Circulation.* 2003;108: 2355–2360.
7. Haïssaguerre M, Hocini M, Sanders P, et al. Catheter ablation of long-lasting persistent atrial fibrillation: Clinical outcome and mechanisms of subsequent arrhythmias. *J Cardiovasc Electrophysiol.* 2005;16:1138–1147.
8. Patel AM, d'Avila A, Neuzil P, et al. Atrial tachycardia after ablation of persistent atrial fibrillation. *Circulation: Arrhythmia Electrophysiol.* 2008;1:14–22.
9. Kobza R, Hindricks G, Tanner H, et al. Late recurrent arrhythmias after ablation of atrial fibrillation: Incidence, mechanisms, and treatment. *Heart Rhythm.* 2004;1: 676–683.
10. Gerstenfeld EP, Callans DJ, Dixit S, et al. Mechanisms of organized left atrial tachycardias occurring after pulmonary vein isolation. *Circulation.* 2004;110:1351–1357.
11. Deisenhofer I, Estner H, Zrenner B, et al. Left atrial tachycardia after circumferential pulmonary vein ablation for atrial fibrillation: Incidence, electrophysiological characteristics, and results of radiofrequency ablation. *EP Europace.* 2006;8:573–582.
12. Veenhuyzen GD, Knecht S, O'Neill MD, et al. Atrial tachycardias encountered during and after catheter ablation for atrial fibrillation: Part I: Classification, incidence, management. *Pacing Clin Electrophysiol.* 2009;32:393–398.
13. Sawhney N, Anousheh R, Chen W, Feld GK. Circumferential pulmonary vein ablation with additional linear ablation results in an increased incidence of left atrial flutter compared with segmental pulmonary vein isolation as an initial approach to ablation of paroxysmal atrial fibrillation. *Circulation: Arrhythm Electrophysiol.* 2010;3:243–248.
14. Chugh A, Oral H, Lemola K, et al. Prevalence, mechanisms, and clinical significance of macroreentrant atrial tachycardia during and following left atrial ablation for atrial fibrillation. *Heart Rhythm.* 2005;2:464–471.
15. Wazni OM, Saliba W, Fahmy T et al. Atrial arrhythmias after surgical maze: Findings during catheter ablation. *J Am Coll Cardiol.* 2006;48:1405–1409.
16. Weerasooriya R, Jaïs P, Wright M, et al. Catheter ablation of atrial tachycardia following atrial fibrillation ablation. *J Cardiovasc Electrophysiol.* 2009;20:833–838.
17. Lerman BB, Markowitz SM, Liu CF, Thomas G, Ip JE, Cheung JW. Fluoroless catheter ablation of atrial fibrillation. *Heart Rhythm.* 2017;14:928–934.
18. Bulava A, Hanis J, Eisenberger M. Catheter ablation of atrial fibrillation using zero-fluoroscopy technique: A randomized trial. *Pacing Clin Electrophysiol.* 2015;38:797–806.
19. Eitel C, Hindricks G, Dagres N, Sommer P, Piorkowski C. EnSite Velocity™ cardiac mapping system: A new platform for 3D mapping of cardiac arrhythmias. *Expert Rev Med Devices.* 2010;7:185–192.
20. Bailin SJ, Korthas MA, Weers NJ, Hoffman CJ. Direct visualization of the slow pathway using voltage gradient mapping: A novel approach for successful ablation of atrioventricular nodal reentry tachycardia. *EP Europace.* 2011;13: 1188–1194.
21. Sundaram S, Choe W, Jordan R, et al. Catheter ablation of atypical atrial flutter: A novel 3D anatomic mapping approach to quickly localize and terminate atypical atrial flutter. *J Interv Card Electrophysiol.* 2017;49:307–318.
22. Choe W, Sundaram S, Jordan R, et al. A novel 3D anatomic mapping approach using multipoint high-density voltage gradient mapping to quickly localize and terminate typical atrial flutter. *J Interv Card Electrophysiol.* 2017;49: 319–326.

Video Legend

Video 12S Chapter summary and step-by-step procedures by Mansour Razminia. [3:55]

Section 3

Ablation of Atrial Fibrillation

13

How to Perform Radiofrequency Ablation of Atrial Fibrillation Using No Fluoroscopy

Robin Singh, MD; Paul C. Zei, MD, PhD

Background

Radiofrequency (RF) catheter ablation for atrial fibrillation (AF) has evolved significantly since the first description of targeting focal pulmonary vein (PV) triggers by Haïssaguerre and colleagues.[1] The field has witnessed an evolution and refinement of various RF techniques, including abandonment of a segmental, ostial approach[2] in favor of antral circumferential lesion sets,[3] in large part to minimize the risk of PV stenosis. Point-by-point contiguous lesions have given way to continuous "drag" lesion sets, resulting in shorter procedural times and increased durability of PV isolation (PVI).[4] A growing number of operators are adopting a short-duration, high-power (up to 50 W) RF ablation approach,[5] given dramatically shorter reported procedural times, and a theoretical benefit of creating effective lesions primarily through resistive heating, while minimizing conductive heating that may increase the risks of thermal injury to extra-cardiac structures. Lesion durability has also likely improved due to numerous technological innovations, including irrigated tip ablation catheters with contact force sensing, steerable sheaths, as well as real-time measures of ablation energy delivery.[6,7]

While PVI remains integral for both paroxysmal and persistent AF patients, the utility of additional ablation remains unclear given the results of STAR AF II[8] and other studies.[9] As a result, there remains considerable heterogeneity in approaches to persistent AF. The current approach of the authors is to target organized atrial arrhythmias following PVI with focal or linear ablation, but if AF persists, to perform external cardioversion with subsequent attempts to induce non-PV triggers with programmed atrial stimulation and/or administration of chronotropic agents such as IV isoproterenol. A voltage map in sinus rhythm may help localize abnormal, potentially proarrhythmic substrate that may be targeted for ablation (**Figure 13.1**). Posterior wall isolation[10] may be pursued in select patients presenting for repeat procedures, while targeting complex, fractionated electrograms (CFAE)[11] or mapping rotors,[12] and other additional ablation targets remains relatively controversial (e.g., Topera, Abbott, Abbott Park, IL).[13] Various complex mapping catheters, enabling the rapid acquisition of a large number of data points during electroanatomic mapping (EAM), have facilitated techniques for rapid and precise mapping of potential ablation targets and validating clinical end points (e.g., PentaRay, Biosense Webster, Irvine, CA; Rhythmia, Boston Scientific, Charlestown, MA; Advisor HD Grid Mapping Catheter, SE, Abbott). While discussing the merits of the aforementioned approaches is beyond the scope of this chapter, we aim to provide insights into the fundamental approaches to low/zero fluoroscopy mapping and ablation, which can be adapted to future techniques, with current zero-fluoroscopy techniques utilizing primarily EAM and intracardiac echocardiography (ICE).

Fluoroscopy Reduction Techniques for Catheter Ablation of Cardiac Arrhythmias. © 2019 Mansour Razminia, Paul C. Zei, eds.
Cardiotext Publishing, ISBN: 978-1-942909-30-9.

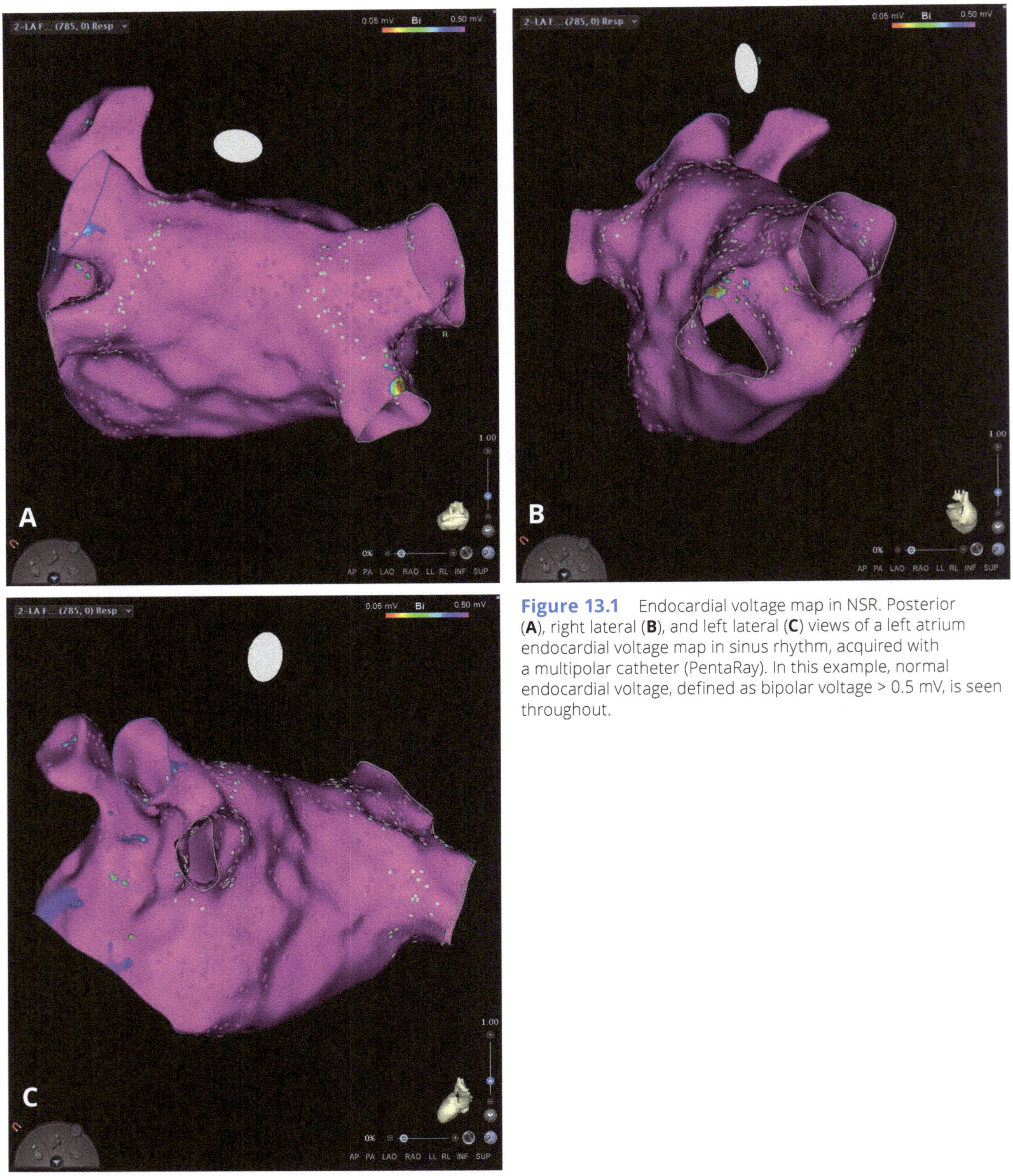

Figure 13.1 Endocardial voltage map in NSR. Posterior (**A**), right lateral (**B**), and left lateral (**C**) views of a left atrium endocardial voltage map in sinus rhythm, acquired with a multipolar catheter (PentaRay). In this example, normal endocardial voltage, defined as bipolar voltage > 0.5 mV, is seen throughout.

Procedure

Access and Catheter Placement

The absence of an intracardiac thrombus is typically confirmed with a preoperative TEE, although there is increasing utilization of ICE to interrogate the left atrial appendage (LAA) intraprocedurally.[14] Following induction of general anesthesia, bilateral femoral venous access is obtained utilizing a vascular ultrasound probe (Chapter 5), with placement of access sheaths for advancement of catheters. These include a multielectrode mapping catheter (e.g., PentaRay or Lasso, Biosense Webster; Advisor HD Grid Mapping Catheter, SE,

Abbott), an ablation catheter usually with contact force sensing (CF), (e.g., SmartTouch SF, Biosense Webster; TactiCath, Abbott), an ICE catheter (e.g., CARTOSOUND, Biosense Webster; ViewFlex, Abbott), and a multipolar reference catheter in the coronary sinus (CS). Following sheath placement, we typically administer serial boluses of intravenous heparin to maintain an activated clotting time (ACT) of >400 seconds, with periodic monitoring of ACT values generally every 15 minutes.

Safety Monitoring

To ensure safe and accurate manipulation of catheters within the heart, an adequate anatomic roadmap is essential. A combination of detailed EAM and ICE provides the optimal combination of detailed anatomy, physiologic correlation, and real-time visualization of catheters. Although relatively uncommon, the most significant procedural complications encountered during AF ablation include pericardial effusion with cardiac tamponade, PV stenosis, phrenic nerve injury, and risk of developing atrioesophageal fistula.

Frequent visualization of the catheters on ICE (**Figure 13.2**), use of contact-force sensing during ablation, periodic monitoring for nascent effusion, and accurate creation of an anatomic shell to guide catheter positioning are all essential to avoid perforation and/or cardiac tamponade. Frequent communication with the anesthesia team enables prompt evaluation of the pericardial space at the earliest signs of hemodynamic compromise. Since pericardial effusions tend to accumulate in a dependent fashion, familiarity with obtaining views of the posterior LA wall, posterior left ventricle, and the posterolateral right atrium (RA) is essential. Following ablation, a comprehensive evaluation to exclude pericardial effusion is requisite.

Accurate demarcation of the PV ostia is obtained prior to antral ablation to prevent PV stenosis, by constructing detailed anatomy using a multielectrode mapping catheter. Care should be taken to avoid excessive deformation of the chamber walls or accepting "internal points," both of which can distort true anatomy. Certain anatomic locations, especially the ridge separating the LAA from the left superior pulmonary vein (LSPV) as well as the left inferior pulmonary vein (LIPV), can be challenging. This ridge can be precisely defined by dragging the contact-force catheter along the ridge with adequate CF until the ablation catheter flips from either the LSPV to the LAA, or vice versa.

Pace mapping the course of the phrenic nerve in both the superior vena cava (SVC) and right superior pulmonary vein (RSPV) while creating anatomic tags to delineate its course is also useful. This may often reveal a location in close proximity to the intended wide area circumferential ablation (WACA) lesion set, typically along the anterior aspect of the RSPV. In such instances, reevaluation with pace mapping immediately prior to ablation provides additional reassurance that the phrenic nerve is avoided with ablation.

The various approaches to monitoring esophageal temperature are discussed elsewhere in this text (Chapter 8). The most widely adopted approach involves the manipulation of a single electrode esophageal temperature probe traditionally under fluoroscopy. We advocate a technique of attaching (suturing) a quadripolar mapping catheter (e.g., Josephson, Abbott) to the temperature probe with the distal electrode offset approximately 1 cm proximal to the thermistor, allowing visualization of the unit on the mapping system (**Figure 13.3**). There is evidence that the metallic electrodes may create a current sink during RF that can preferentially direct RF energy towards the esophagus,[15] which may be avoided by such an offset fixation. The temperature probe, visualized on the mapping system, is then moved along the esophageal lumen such that the thermistor opposes the ablation site. Tracking and adjusting the electrode position can also be performed via visualization of the electrode tip within the esophagus on ICE. As is the case for "conventional" fluoroscopic visualization, the location of the temperature probe only provides a linear, one-dimensional representation of the esophageal lumen. It should be kept in mind that the remainder of the underrepresented esophagus may be located a significant distance laterally from the visualized probe location. Therefore, any posterior wall ablation should be performed with that in mind.

Mapping and Anatomy Creation

Following the advancement of the ICE catheter to the RA (Chapter 2), a mapping or ablation catheter is similarly advanced to the RA with visualization on the mapping system and ICE. The mapping/ablation catheter is then utilized to create an EAM of the RA that allows for adequate definition of the SVC, tricuspid valve (TV), His bundle, and proximal CS, with visualization of the latter allowing subsequent placement of a CS reference catheter without fluoroscopy. High-output pacing, generally along the posterior-lateral SVC, is performed to identify the course of the phrenic nerve. Transseptal access without fluoroscopy is obtained (Chapter 6); the authors utilize a "drag" approach whereby the transseptal unit (sheath/dilator/needle) is advanced over a wire to the SVC and pulled down into the interatrial septum utilizing ICE visualization. We typically deploy a RF-enabled needle (Baylis NRG, Baylis Medical, Montreal, Canada), with double transseptal access for placement of a long, nonsteerable SL1 sheath as well as a long, steerable sheath (Vizigo, Biosense Webster) in the LA.

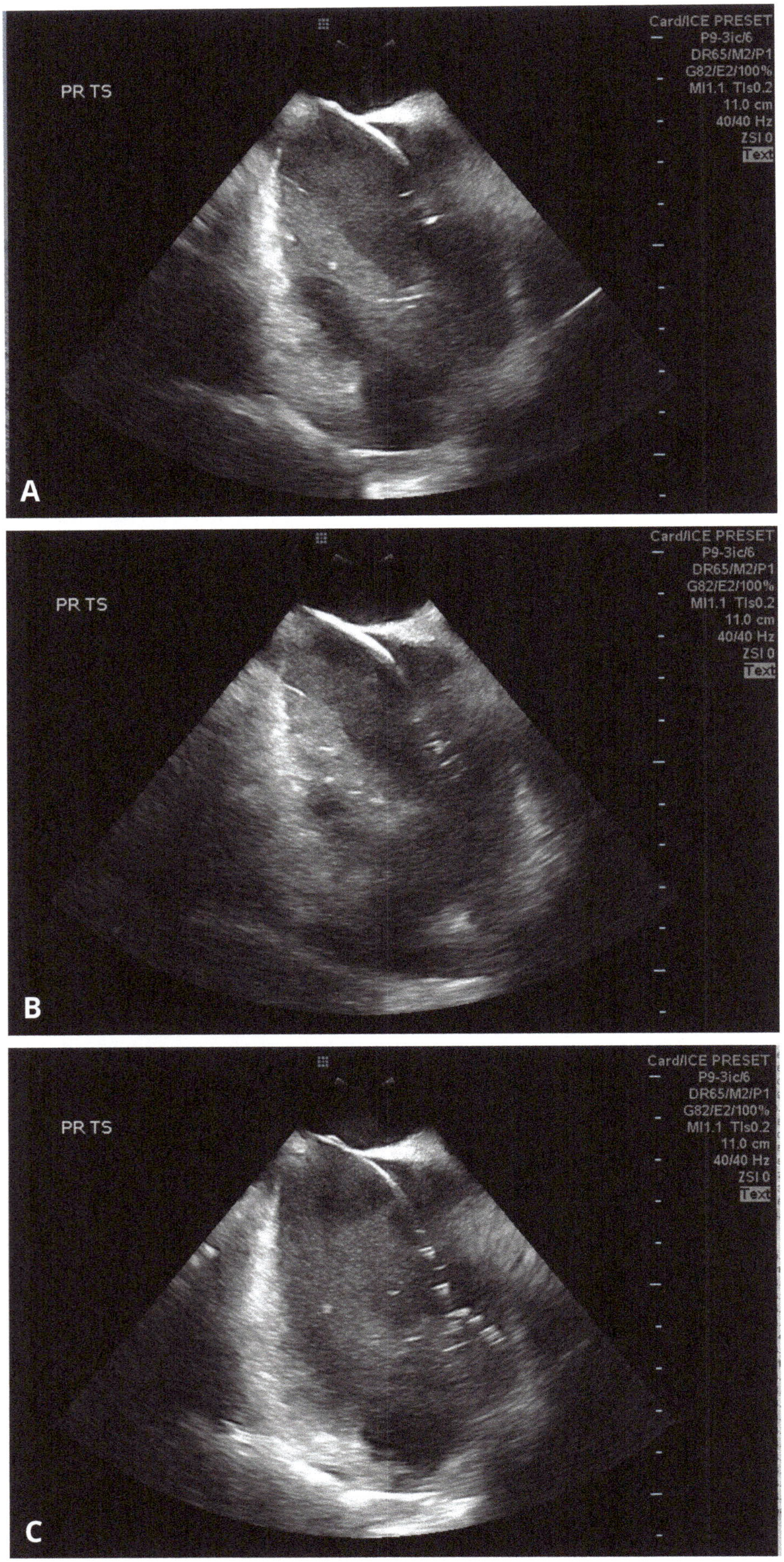

Figure 13.2 Visualization of catheters on ICE (long transseptal sheath). In this image, the ICE probe is directed towards the left atrium, toward the left superior pulmonary vein and posterior wall. A PentaRay mapping catheter is directed towards the left superior pulmonary vein (LSPV), with progressive still images of the advancement of the PentaRay out of the transseptal sheaths (**A–C**). Please see **Video 13.1** for additional images.

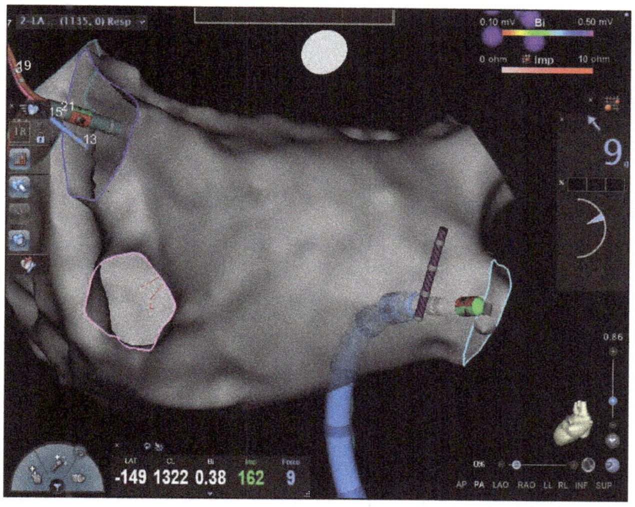

Figure 13.3 Visualization of the esophageal probe location on CARTO. A PA view of a left atrial endocardial map, with visualization of a quadripolar (Josephson, Abbott) mapping catheter attached to the esophageal temperature probe within the esophageal lumen. Note that the quad catheter is typically attached at a fixed offset from the tip of the temperature probe to prevent the possibility of RF/heat transfer to the quad electrodes (see text). In this example, the esophageal temperature probe (and esophagus) are located adjacent to the right inferior pulmonary vein.

Ablation

The ablation and high-density mapping catheters are advanced via the steerable and fixed curve long sheaths, respectively, to the LA via ICE (**Figure 13.4**). A dense (typically >2000 points) EAM is created of the LA, identifying all the PVs, the LAA, and the mitral valve (MV) annulus. RF energy is then delivered to create a continuous WACA lesion set around each pair of ipsilateral PVs. Specific catheter movements may be accomplished through direct catheter steering mechanisms or with augmentation with the long steerable sheath. Most sheaths currently are not directly visualized in the mapping system; thus, catheter curve, direction, and extension within the LA must be visualized through ICE. Utilizing a sheath that can be visualized within the mapping system (Vizigo, Biosense Webster) can facilitate this process (**Figure 13.5**). As mentioned, the authors typically utilize a hybrid drag approach with continuous RF delivery, maintaining the catheter at each ablation location for a prescribed time based on a combination of variables including power, anatomic location, catheter stability, impedance decrease, and electrogram amplitude diminishment.

At the time of this writing, the evolution of several novel RF delivery strategies is ongoing, with the potential for these various techniques to be incorporated into standard AF RF ablation in the future. Real-time measures of RF energy delivery that may predict lesion formation include ablation index (AI), which incorporates contact force, power, and time of RF,[6] force-time integral (FTI), which simply integrates contact force over time,[7] may have benefit. Delivery of short duration (4–5 seconds), high power (50W) lesions in order to shorten lesion formation time and minimize lesion depth is also gaining acceptance.[5] Automated algorithms to mark RF ablation sites have also been developed.[16] It is quite likely that such approaches can be easily incorporated into a reduced/zero fluoroscopy workflow.

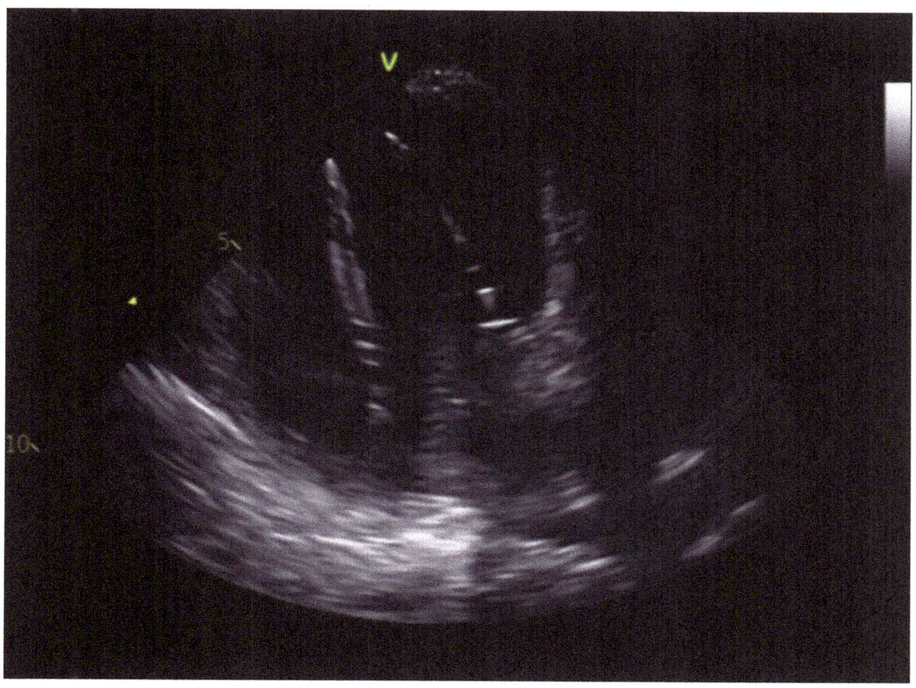

Figure 13.4 ICE visualization of PentaRay and SmartTouch introduced in LA. An ICE image of the left atrium demonstrates both a PentaRay and ablation catheter in the left atrium, directed towards the LSPV and posterior wall, respectively. Please see **Video 13.2** for additional information.

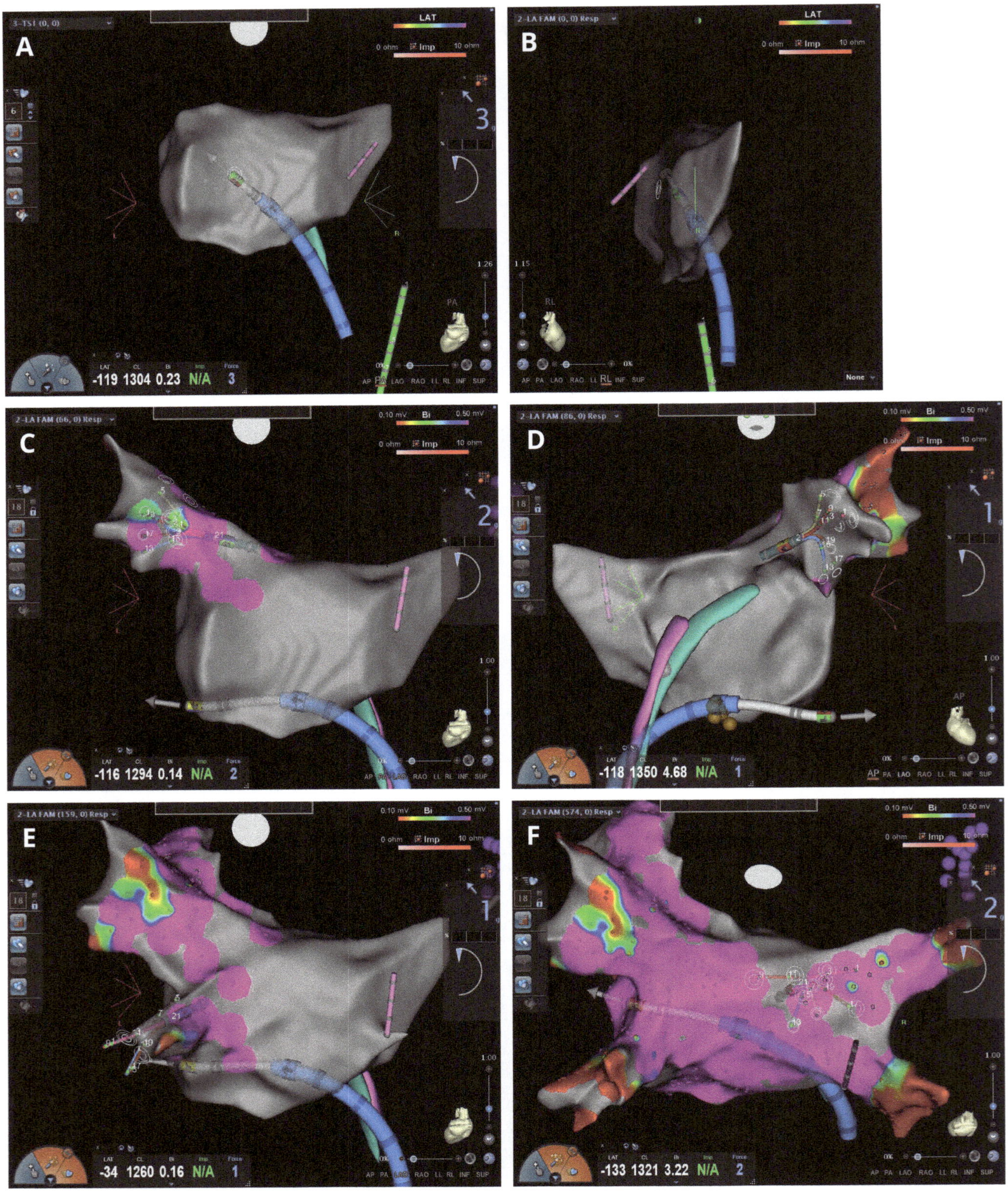

Figure 13.5 Steerable sheath (Vizigo) visualization on CARTO. Still images of endocardial mapping with a multipolar (PentaRay) catheter, with the ablation catheter visualized within the left atrium, passed through a steerable sheath visualized on the mapping system. This allows reliable manipulation of the steerable sheath (and ablation catheter) primarily via the mapping system. Note that Figures 13.5A–F show progressive mapping creation of an endocardial left atrial map using a multipolar mapping catheter (PentaRay) and ablation catheter (Smartouch STSF), with assistance of a steerable sheath (Vizigo) that can be visualized on the mapping system.

Validation

In accordance with the 2017 HRS expert consensus statement on AF ablation,[17] the authors advocate utilizing more than one modality to validate complete PV electrical isolation. This may include some subset of these techniques: confirmation of entrance block as well as exit block with and without pacing, voltage mapping in sinus rhythm to demonstrate "electrically silent" PVs, and drug perturbation with agents such as IV adenosine or isoproterenol to evaluate for dormant conduction. Specifically, the operator may advance the PentaRay mapping catheter sequentially into each of the PVs, with confirmation of both entrance block as well as performance of sequential pacing utilizing all distal bipoles to demonstrate exit block. IV adenosine is administered 20 minutes following initial PVI to unmask any dormant conduction.[18] A repeat electroanatomic map of the LA including endocardial voltage in NSR is also obtained to provide additional validation.[19]

Additional Ablation

In patients with paroxysmal AF, current data support PVI as the cornerstone of the ablation procedure.[20] Various additional ablation lesion sets have been endorsed over the years, but currently there is no consensus on an ideal approach. The most common barrier to posterior LA wall isolation[21] is inadequate ablation due to esophageal temperature elevation. High-density mapping postablation may assist in confirmation of PW isolation. If linear ablation is performed, in addition to traditional pacing maneuvers to confirm electrical block, we remap the endocardial voltage in the chamber of interest following ablation, assessing for areas of low voltage consistent with block and/or lack of conduction into the zone of interest (**Figure 13.6**). Activation mapping, performed in sinus or paced rhythm, may be an additional confirmation of block. If non-PV trigger ablation is contemplated,[22] multielectrode catheters can assist in accurate and more rapid localization of ablation targets. If mapping complex signals such as fractionated electrograms (CFAEs)[11] and rotors,[12] additional mapping catheters may be employed, including "basket" catheters.[23] Since real-time EAM visualization of these catheters is not currently reliable, ICE remains an integral modality for catheter manipulation.

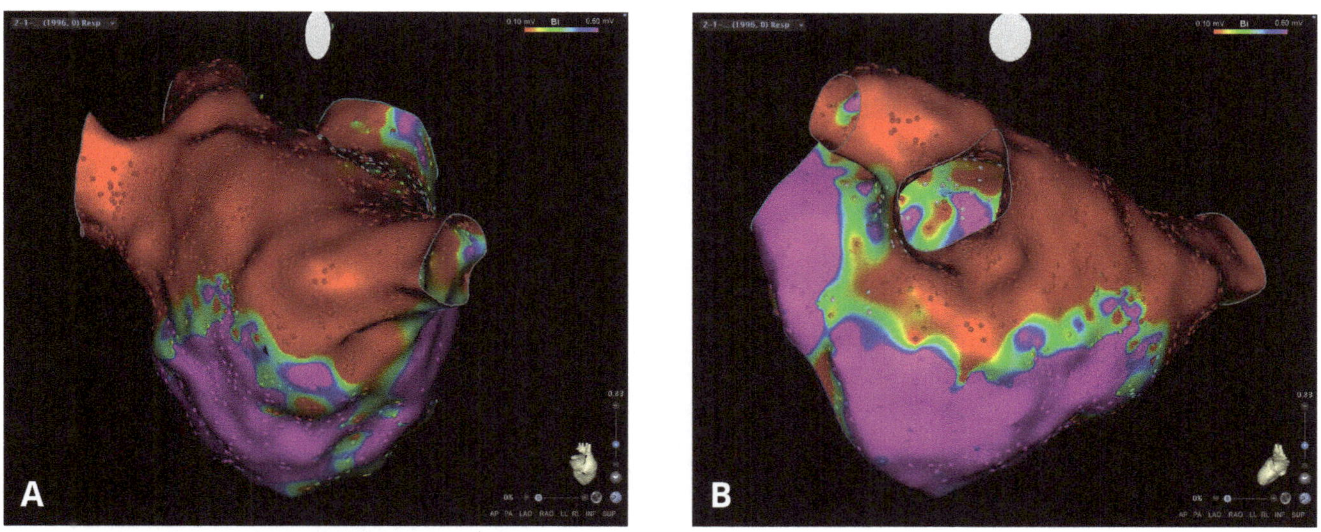

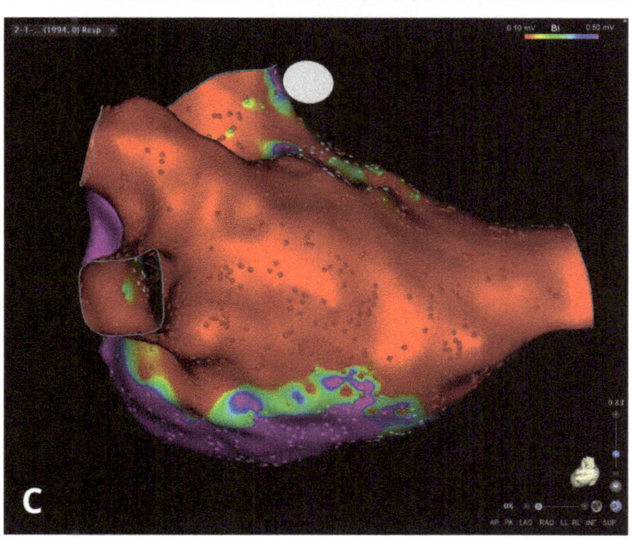

Figure 13.6 LA posterior wall isolation. Right lateral (**A**), PA (**B**), and left lateral (**C**) views of a left atrium after posterior wall ablation to achieve PW electrical isolation. The displayed voltage map demonstrates low voltage, consistent with electrical isolation of the posterior wall. Note that in this patient a common right pulmonary vein (rare) variant is present, and there is evidence of low voltage/abnormal substrate in part of the left atrial appendage.

Future Directions

Novel approaches to identifying ablation targets utilizing cardiac MR (DECAAF II)[24] as well as biomarkers evaluating intra-atrial dyssynchrony to predict ablation success[25] are currently being evaluated. Data from the RADIANCE study demonstrating effective PV isolation utilizing an irrigated, multielectrode RF balloon (Biosense Webster) were presented in 2017.[26] The HeartLight laser balloon catheter (CardioFocus, Marlborough, MA), approved by the FDA in 2016, allows for direct tissue visualization potentially obviating the need for EAM, as well as the ability to titrate delivery of power.[27] Other non-thermal ablation techniques, such as electroporation resulting in cell membrane permeabilization and subsequent apoptosis in contrast to cell necrosis induced by traditional RF application, have drawn significant research interest.[28] These examples serve to highlight the exciting potential for continued growth and development within the field of AF ablation. Ultimately, regardless of the novel approaches developed in the future, existing as well as new tools likely can be seamlessly incorporated into a reduced/zero fluoroscopy workflow.

References

1. Jaïs P, Haïssaguerre M, Shah DC, et al. A focal source of atrial fibrillation treated by discrete radiofrequency ablation. *Circulation.* 1997 Feb 4; 95(3):572–576.
2. Oral H, Knight BP, Ozaydin M, et al. Segmental ostial ablation to isolate the pulmonary veins during atrial fibrillation: Feasibility and mechanistic insights. *Circulation.* 2002 Sep 3;106(10):1256–1262.
3. Mansour M, Ruskin J, Keane D. Efficacy and safety of segmental ostial versus circumferential extra-ostial pulmonary vein isolation for atrial fibrillation. *J Cardiovasc Electrophysiol.* 2004 May;15(5):532–537.
4. Yokokawa M, Bhandari AK, Tada H, et al. Comparison of the point-by-point versus catheter dragging technique for curative radiofrequency ablation of atrial fibrillation. *Pacing Clin Electrophysiol.*2011 Jan;34(1):15–22.
5. Winkle R, Moskovitz R, Mead R, et al. Atrial fibrillation ablation using very short duration 50 W ablations and contact force sensing catheters. *J Interv Card Electrophysiol.* 2018 Jun;52(1):1–8.
6. Hussein A, Das M, Chaturvedi V, et al. Prospective use of ablation index targets improves clinical outcomes following ablation for atrial fibrillation. *J Cardiovasc Electrophysiol.* 2017;28:1037–1047.
7. Fabien S, Decebal G, Youssef M, Marouane M, Sok-Sithikun B, Nadir S. Contact force and force-time integral in atrial radiofrequency ablation predict transmurality of lesions. *EP Europace.* 2014 May;16(5):660–667.
8. Verma A, Jiang C, Betts T, et al. Approaches to catheter ablation for persistent atrial fibrillation. *N Engl J Med.* 2015 May;372:1812–1822.
9. Ejima K, Arai K, Suzuki T, et al. Long-term outcome and preprocedural predictors of atrial tachyarrhythmia recurrence following pulmonary vein antrum isolation-based catheter ablation in patients with non-paroxysmal atrial fibrillation. *J Cardiol.* 2014 July;64(1):57–63.
10. Tahir K, Mounsey JP, Hummel J. Posterior wall isolation in atrial fibrillation. *J Innov Card Rhythm Manag.* 2018;9:3186–3194.
11. Caldwell J, Redfearn D. Ablation of complex fractionated atrial electrograms in catheter ablation for AF; Where have we been and where are we going? *Curr Cardiol Rev.* 2012;8(4):347–353.
12. Krummen DE, Swarup V, Narayan SM. The role of rotors in atrial fibrillation. *J Thoracic Di.* 2015;7(2):142–151.
13. Nedios S, Sommer P, Bollmann A, Hindricks G. Advanced mapping systems to guide atrial fibrillation ablation: Electrical information that matters. *J Atr Fibrillation.* 2016; 8(6):1337.
14. Baran J, Stec S, Pilichowska-Paszkiet E, et al. Intracardiac echocardiography for detection of thrombus in the left atrial appendage: Comparison with transesophageal echocardiography in patients undergoing ablation for atrial fibrillation: The Action-ICE I study. *Circulation: Arrhythm Electrophysiol.* 2013 Nov;6:1074–1081.
15. Perez J, D'Avila A, Aryana A, Berjano E. Electrical and thermal effects of esophageal temperature probes on radiofrequency catheter ablation of atrial fibrillation: Results from a computational modeling study. *J Cardiovasc Electrophysiol.* 2015;26:556–564.
16. Anter E, Tschabrunn CM, Contreras-Valdes FM, Buxton AE, Josephson ME. Radiofrequency ablation annotation algorithm reduces the incidence of linear gaps and reconnection after pulmonary vein isolation. *Heart Rhythm.* 2014 May;11(5):783–790.
17. Calkins H, Hindricks G, Cappato R, et al. 2017 HRS/EHRA/ECAS/APHRS/SOLAECE expert consensus statement on catheter and surgical ablation of atrial fibrillation. *Heart Rhythm.* 2017 Oct;14(10):e275–e444.
18. Macle L, Khairy P, Weerasooriya R, et al. Adenosine-guided pulmonary vein isolation for the treatment of paroxysmal atrial fibrillation: an international, multicentre, randomised superiority trial. *Lancet.* 2015;386(9994):672–679.
19. Masuda M, Fujita M, Iida O, et al. Comparison of left atrial voltage between sinus rhythm and atrial fibrillation in association with electrogram waveform. *Pacing Clin Electrophysiol.* 2017 May;40(5):559–567.
20. Santangeli P, Lin D. Catheter ablation of paroxysmal atrial fibrillation: Have we achieved cure with pulmonary vein isolation? *Methodist Debakey Cardiovasc J.* 2015;11(2):71–75.
21. Tahir K, Mounsey JP, Hummel J. Posterior wall isolation in atrial fibrillation. *J Innov Card Rhythm Manag.* 2018;9:3186–3194.
22. Hayashi K, Yoshimori A, Nagashima M et al. Importance of nonpulmonary vein foci in catheter ablation for paroxysmal atrial fibrillation. *Heart Rhythm.* 2015 Sept;12(9):1918–1924.
23. Hummel J. Atrial mapping with basket catheters. *JACC Clin Electrophysiol.* 2016 Feb;2(1):66–68.

24. Marrouche NF. Efficacy of DE-MRI-Guided Ablation vs. Conventional Catheter Ablation of Atrial Fibrillation (DECAAF II). Clinical Trial NCT02529319 (https://clinicaltrials.gov/ct2/show/NCT02529319). Accessed August 6, 2018.
25. Ciuffo L, Susumu T, Esra Gucuk I, et al. Intra-atrial dyssynchrony during sinus rhythm predicts recurrence after the first catheter ablation for atrial fibrillation. *JACC Cardiovasc Imaging.* 2018 Jan 17. pii: S1936-878X(17)31151-8. doi: 10.1016/j.jcmg.2017.11.028 [Epub ahead of print]
26. Fornell D. Multi-electrode RF balloon efficient for acute pulmonary vein isolation. *Diagnostic Intervent Cardiol.* 2017. https://www.dicardiology.com/article/multi-electrode-rf-balloon-efficient-acute-pulmonary-vein-isolation. Accessed August 6, 2018.
27. CardioFocus laser endoscopic ablation system cleared in Japan. *Diagnostic Intervent Cardiol.* 2017. https://www.dicardiology.com/content/cardiofocus-laser-endoscopic-ablation-system-cleared-japan. Accessed August 6, 2018.
28. Wojtaszczyk A, Caluori G, Pesi M, Melajova K, Starek Z. Irreversible electroporation ablation for atrial fibrillation. *J Cardiovasc Electrophysiol.* 2018 Apr;29(4):643–651.

Video Legends

Video 13.1 ICE images of the left atrium showing a PentaRay and ablation catheter in the chamber, demonstrating the ability to visualize catheters in the left atrium in real time during mapping and ablation. [00:05]

Video 13.2 ICE images of the left atrium showing a PentaRay exiting the transseptal sheath into the left atrium, demonstrating the ability to track catheter movement and relationship to the left atrium continuously in real time. [00:42]

14

How to Perform Cryoballoon Ablation of Atrial Fibrillation Using No Fluoroscopy

Hany Demo, MD; Oliver D'Silva, MD; Mansour Razminia, MD

Introduction

Cryoballoon ablation (CBA) offers a single-delivery approach to pulmonary vein isolation (PVI) that is an alternative to the traditional point-to-point radiofrequency ablation (RFA) methodology.

The conventional-method CBA of atrial fibrillation (AF) involves the use of fluoroscopy for visual guidance, with fluoroscopy times averaging 20 to 60 minutes.[1-3]

The commonplace use of 3-dimensional (3D) electroanatomic mapping (EAM) systems along with intracardiac echocardiography (ICE) allows the operator to eliminate fluoroscopy during cryoballoon ablation procedures.[4]

Preprocedural Preparation

In the authors' lab, preprocedural computed tomography (CT) or cardiac magnetic resonance imaging (CMR) are not routinely performed. A preprocedural transesophageal echocardiogram (TEE) is obtained should there be any risk of left atrial (LA) thrombus. The procedure is typically performed on uninterrupted anticoagulation with warfarin or direct oral anticoagulants (DOAC).

Procedure

Vascular Access and Creation of Right Atrial Geometry

Percutaneous femoral venous access is obtained by the modified Seldinger technique guided by vascular ultrasound. One 14-Fr sheath (Input PS, Medtronic, Minneapolis, MN) is placed in the right femoral vein; one 10-Fr long sheath (Super Arrow-Flex introducer, Teleflex, Morrisville, NC) and another 7-Fr sheath (Input PS, Medtronic) are placed in the left femoral vein. A 9-Fr ICE catheter (ViewFlex, Abbott, Abbott Park, IL) is inserted through the 10-Fr long sheath in the left femoral vein and advanced to the inferior vena cava (IVC) while maintaining an echo-free space at the tip of the transducer (**Figure 14.1**). The ICE catheter is then advanced to the right atrium (RA). The ICE catheter is maneuvered into the right ventricle to evaluate for any pericardial effusion (**Figure 14.2**). Baseline images are stored.

Fluoroscopy Reduction Techniques for Catheter Ablation of Cardiac Arrhythmias. © 2019 Mansour Razminia, Paul C. Zei, eds.
Cardiotext Publishing, ISBN: 978-1-942909-30-9.

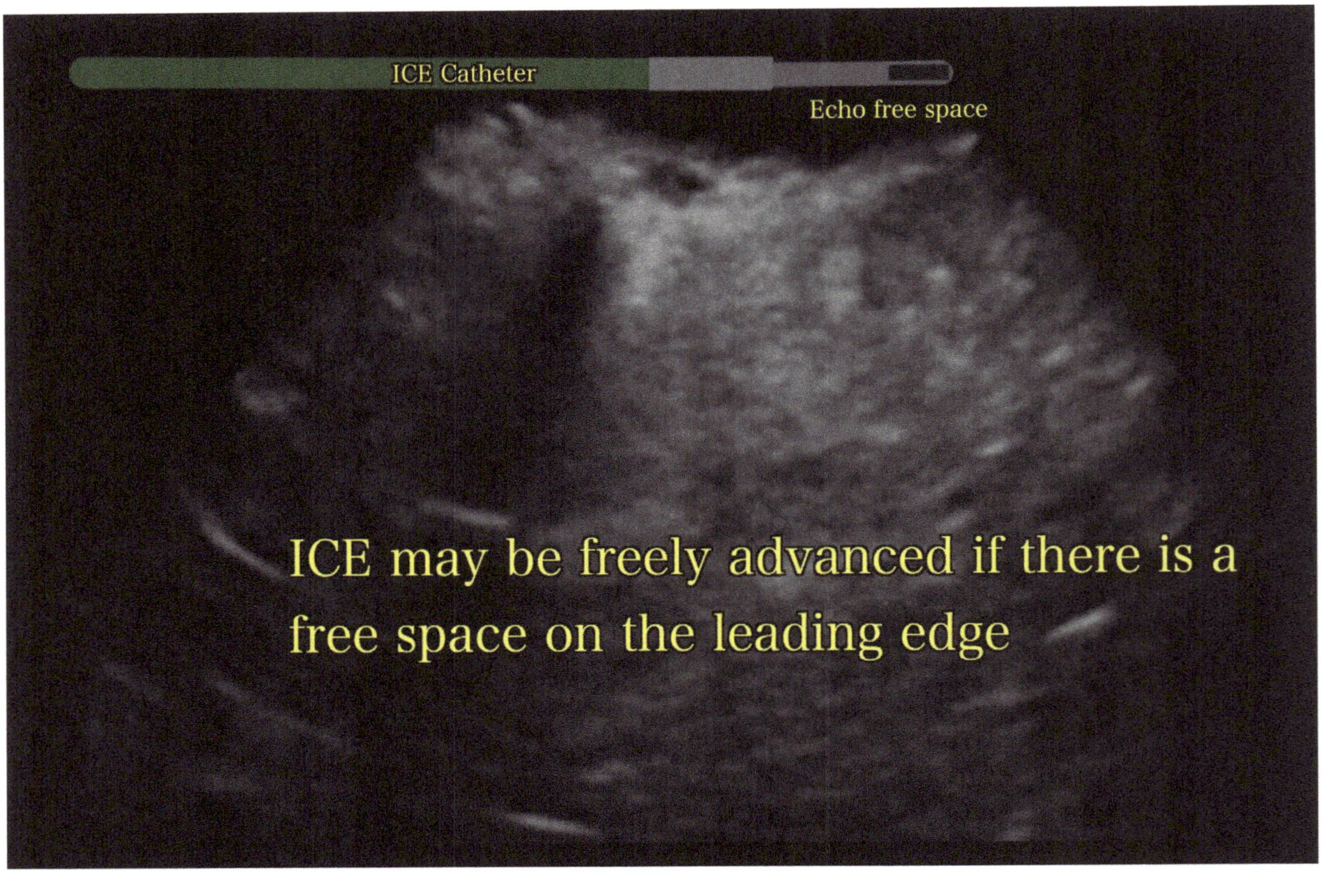

Figure 14.1 Maintaining an echo-free space at the tip of the transducer is essential during ICE advancement.

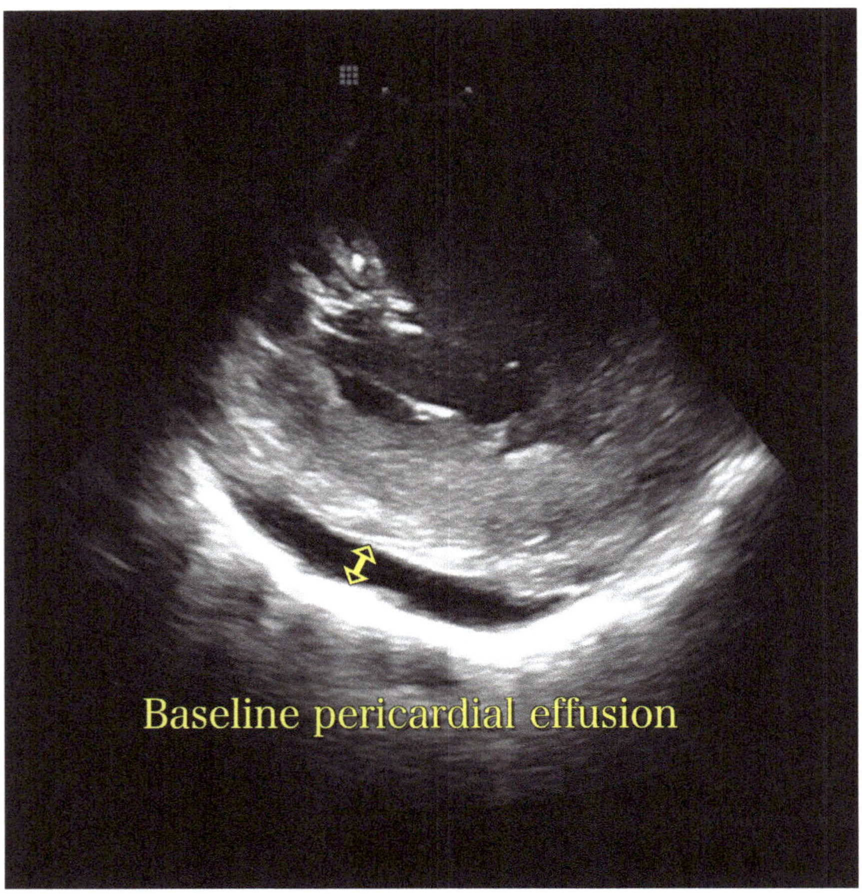

Figure 14.2 ICE catheter in the right ventricle showing baseline pericardial effusion prior to ablation.

EnSite is currently the only feasible mapping system that will allow EAM creation and diagnostic catheter visualization without a proprietary ablation/mapping catheter. In addition, beyond mapping systems, cryoballoon ablation requires significant utilization of ICE to adequately visualize the ablation catheter throughout the procedure. The 6-Fr decapolar catheter (Inquiry, Ten Ten Diagnostic Catheter, Abbott) is inserted into the left femoral vein and advanced to the IVC under the guidance of the EAM system (EnSite Velocity, Abbott). Geometry of the IVC is collected as the decapolar catheter is advanced to the IVC. The appearance of electrograms on the distal bipoles of the decapolar catheter indicates when the catheter tip has reached the border of the inferior RA and IVC (**Figure 14.3**). The decapolar catheter is then advanced into the RA and into the superior vena cava (SVC). The RA-SVC junction is marked by a loss of electrogram signals on the distal poles of the decapolar catheter as the catheter enters the SVC (**Figure 14.4**). Geometry of the SVC is collected on the EAM system. The decapolar catheter is then withdrawn into the RA. Under ICE and EAM guidance, 3D geometries of the RA and coronary sinus (CS) are collected.

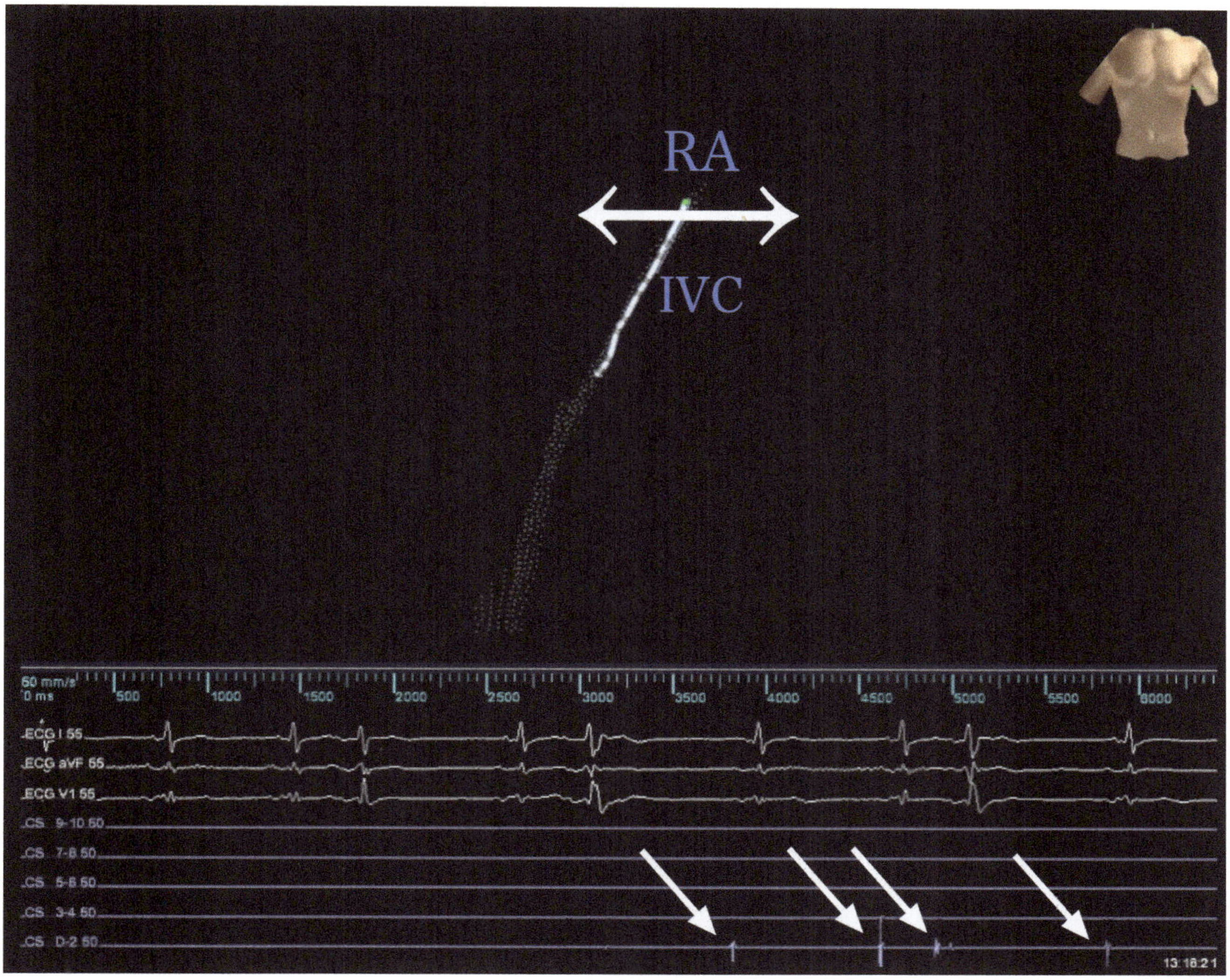

Figure 14.3 The appearance of electrograms on distal bipoles of the decapolar catheter (**red arrows**) indicates the catheter tip has reached junction of IVC and RA. RA: right atrium; IVC: inferior vena cava.

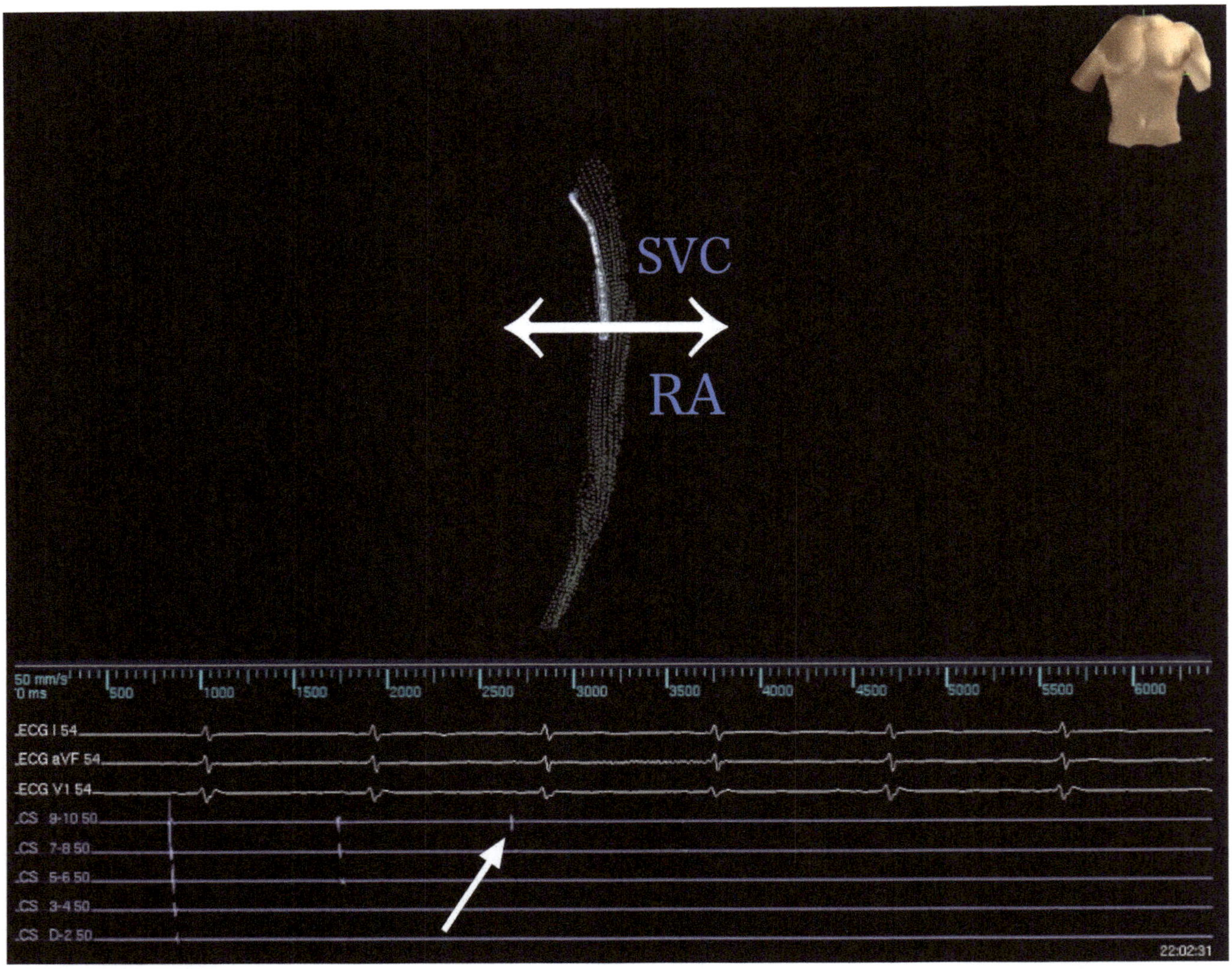

Figure 14.4 The RA-SVC junction is marked by loss of electrogram signals on the distal poles of the decapolar catheter as the catheter enters the SVC. RA: right atrium; SVC: superior vena cava.

Transseptal Puncture

A weight-based heparin bolus is administered prior to the transseptal puncture. The activated clotting time (ACT) is monitored throughout the procedure and intravenous heparin boluses are administered to target an ACT of 350 to 400 seconds.

From the home view on ICE, clockwise rotation is added to visualize the interatrial septum and the left atrium. Then, a posterior tilt is added, and minimal counterclockwise rotation is applied to visualize the SVC (**Figure 14.5**). Next, through the 14-Fr sheath, a 180-cm 0.032-in J-wire (fixed-core J-tip guidewire, Medtronic) is advanced inside the SVC under direct visualization of the ICE. The transseptal sheath–dilator assembly (SL-0, Abbott) is inserted through the 14-Fr sheath and advanced over the wire into the SVC (**Figure 14.6**). The wire is then withdrawn from the body. The transseptal needle (NRG RF Transseptal needle, Baylis Medical, Montreal, Canada) is placed in the sheath-dilator assembly. The sheath–dilator assembly is withdrawn minimally to expose the blunt tip of the RF Transseptal needle. The transseptal assembly is withdrawn into the RA, while tracked on the EAM system (**Figure 14.7**) and on ICE, until tenting of the interatrial septum is seen on ICE (**Figure 14.8**). In contrast to RF transseptal access, which requires left pulmonary vein visualization on ICE while performing transseptal puncture, a relatively anterior and inferior transseptal puncture is preferred for cryoballoon ablation. This can be achieved by visualizing the transseptal needle tip on the inferior part of the septum after the ICE catheter is rotated slightly counterclockwise relative to the location of the two left-sided pulmonary veins as we start visualizing the LAA (**Figure 14.9**). Hemodynamic pressure monitoring is used to confirm entry into the LA along with direct ICE visualization.

If a standard transseptal needle, rather than an RF transseptal needle, is used, the operator would rely solely on ICE to track the sheath–dilator assembly position, without exposing the needle tip, as it is withdrawn from the SVC down to the interatrial septum.

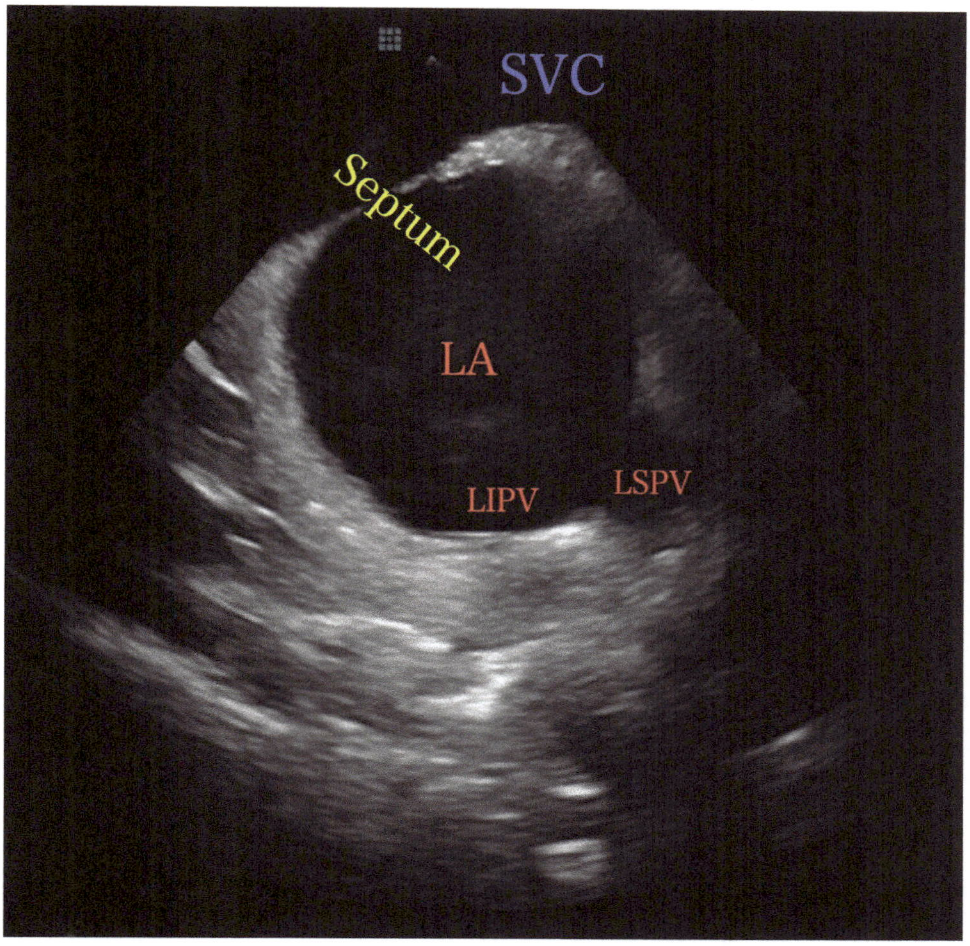

Figure 14.5 From the home view on ICE, clockwise rotation is added to visualize the interatrial septum and the left atrium. Then a posterior tilt is added, and minimal counterclockwise rotation is applied to visualize the SVC. SVC: superior vena cava; LSPV: left superior pulmonary vein; LIPV: left inferior pulmonary vein.

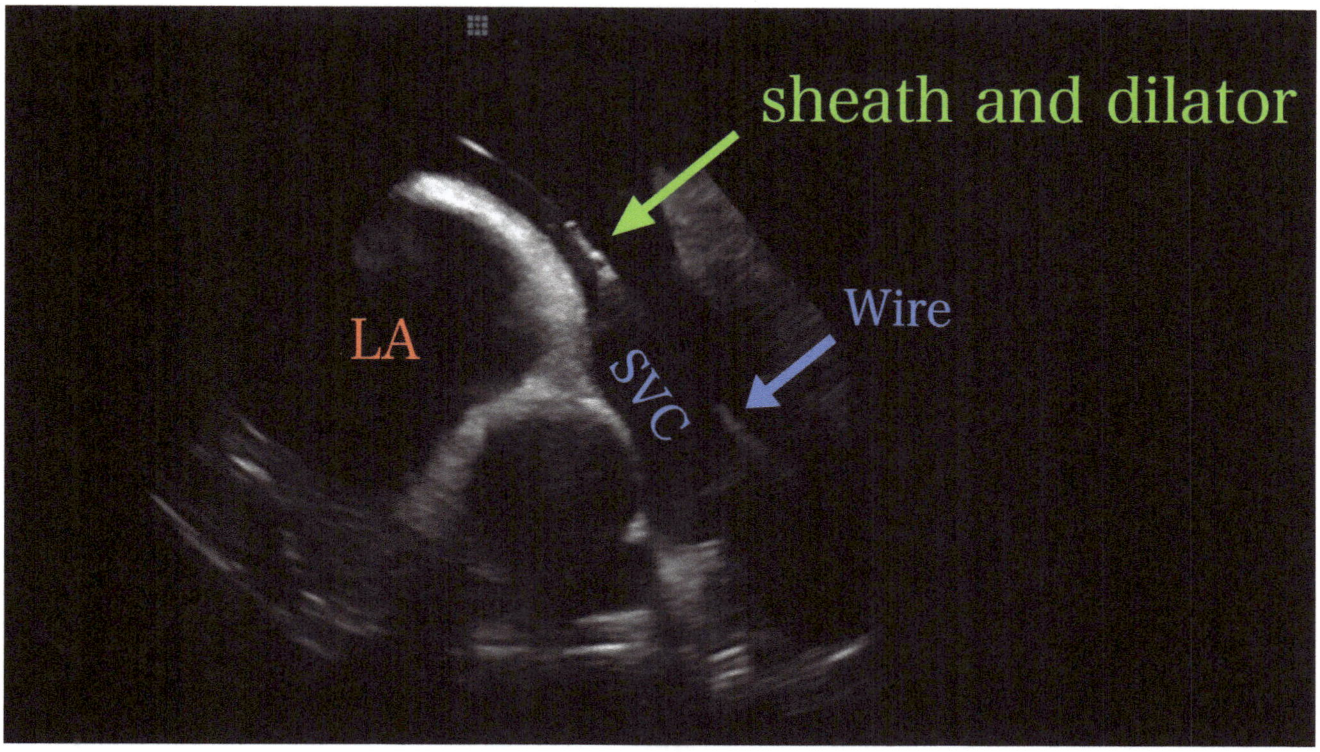

Figure 14.6 The transseptal sheath–dilator assembly is advanced over the wire into the SVC. LA: left atrium; SVC: superior vena cava.

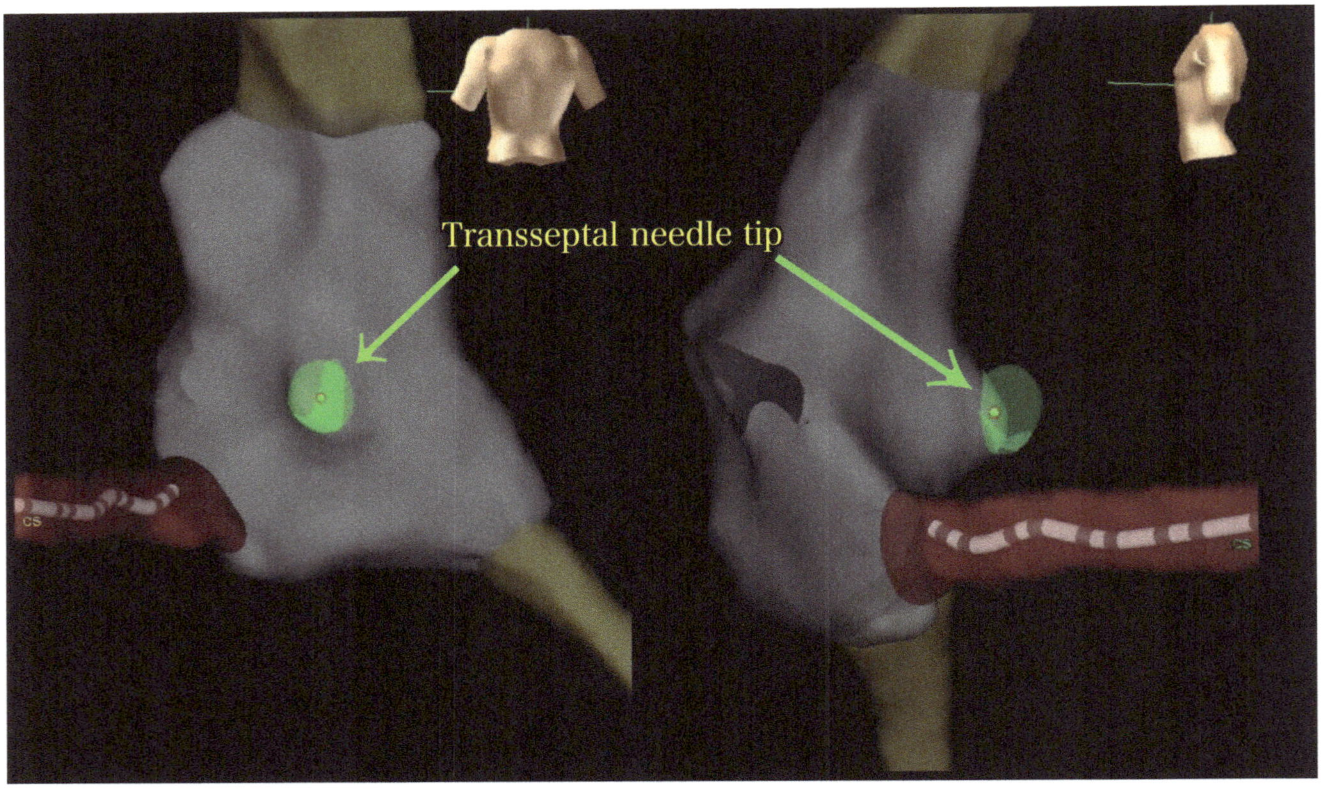

Figure 14.7 The blunt tip of the RF transseptal needle as shown on EAM system prior to performing the transseptal puncture.

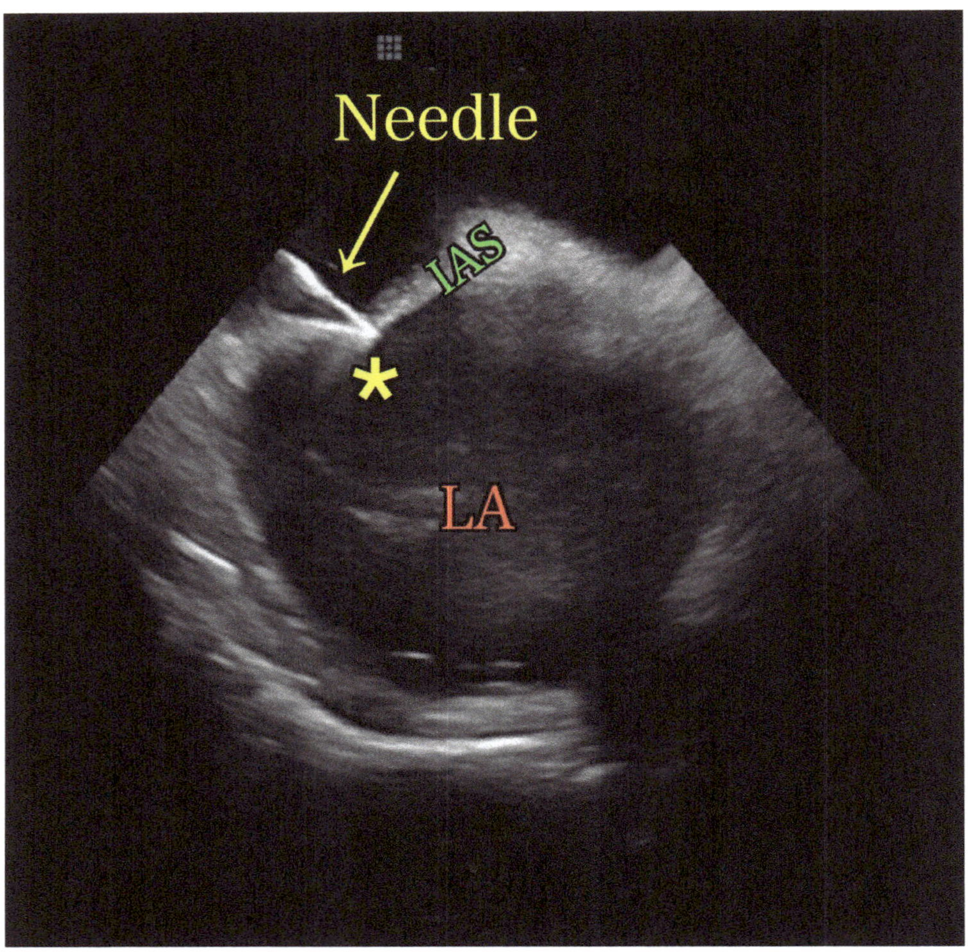

Figure 14.8 Tenting of the interatrial septum (*) caused by the transseptal needle as seen on ICE. LA: left atrium; IAS: interatrial septum.

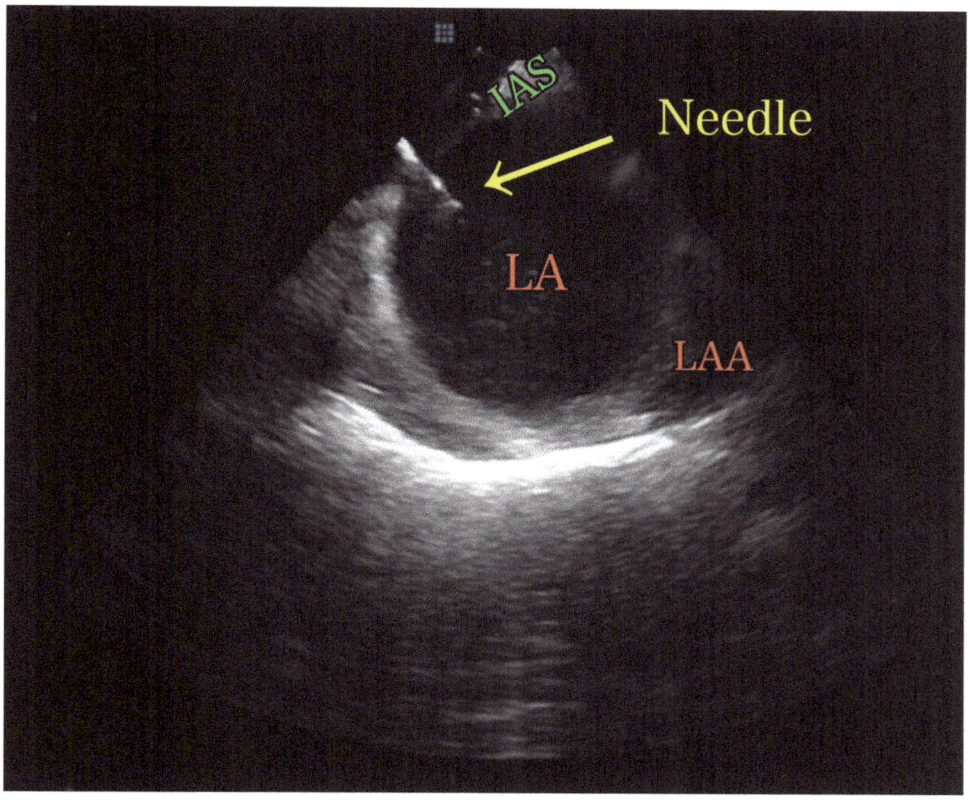

Figure 14.9 A relatively anterior and inferior transseptal puncture is preferred for cryoballoon ablation. As the left atrial appendage come in view, it indicates an anterior site of entry. LA: left atrium; LAA: left atrial appendage; IAS: interatrial septum.

Sheath Exchange

In preparation for CBA, the J-wire is advanced through the transseptal sheath into the left superior PV (LSPV), the location of which is confirmed under ICE (**Figure 14.10**). While maintaining the J-wire in the LSPV, the SL-0 sheath is withdrawn from the body along with the short 14 F access sheath and exchanged for a 15-Fr steerable sheath (FlexCath Advance, Medtronic). The 10.5-Fr, 28-mm cryoballoon (Arctic Front Advance, Medtronic) and a 10-pole circular mapping catheter (Achieve, Medtronic) are placed through the FlexCath into the LA. The 6-Fr decapolar catheter is inserted through the 7-Fr sheath in the left femoral vein and advanced under EAM guidance to the SVC in order to stimulate the phrenic nerve during CBA of right-sided PVs.

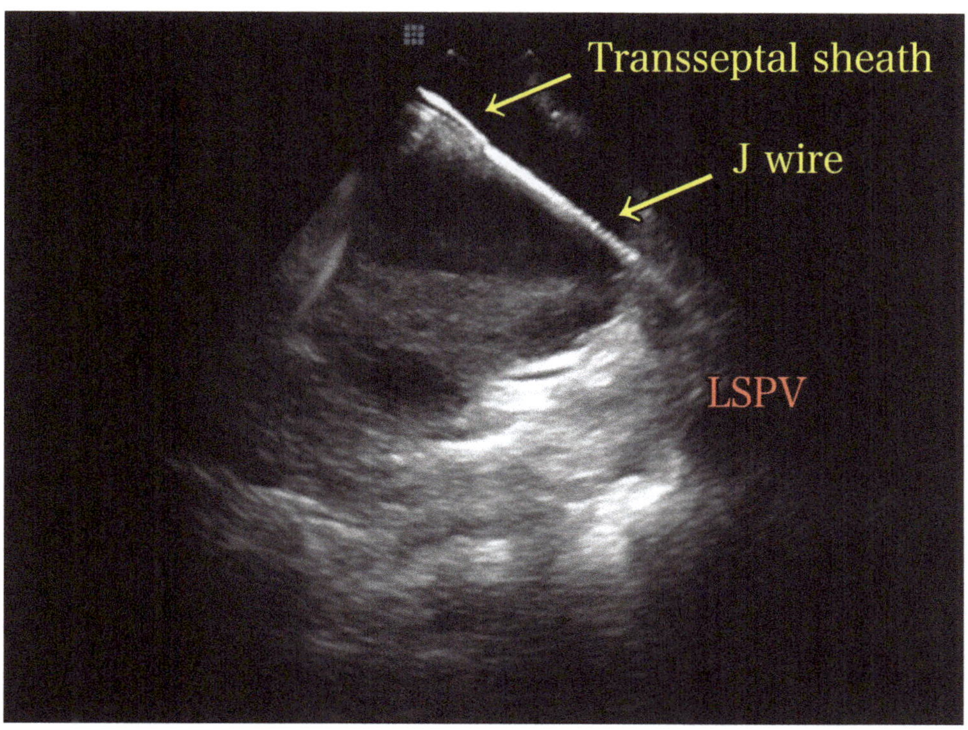

Figure 14.10 The J-wire is advanced through the transseptal sheath into the left superior pulmonary vein. LSPV: left superior pulmonary vein.

Tip 1: Facilitating Sheath Exchange Across a Difficult Septum

If the FlexCath sheath could not be advanced into the LA due to the sheath-dilator step-up, we recommend the pull-push technique. The FlexCath sheath and dilator are minimally withdrawn to the RA while maintaining the J-wire in the LSPV. The decapolar catheter is withdrawn from the SVC down to the RA such that the tip of the decapolar catheter can be seen adjacent to the J-wire as it traverses from RA to LA (**Figure 14.11**). Maintaining this view, the decapolar catheter is advanced directly along the side of the J-wire, through the same hole, into the left atrium. The FlexCath and dilator are readvanced over the wire until septum tenting is observed. At this point, the decapolar catheter is simultaneously withdrawn while advancing the FlexCath, resulting in successful entry of the FlexCath into the LA (**Figure 14.12**).

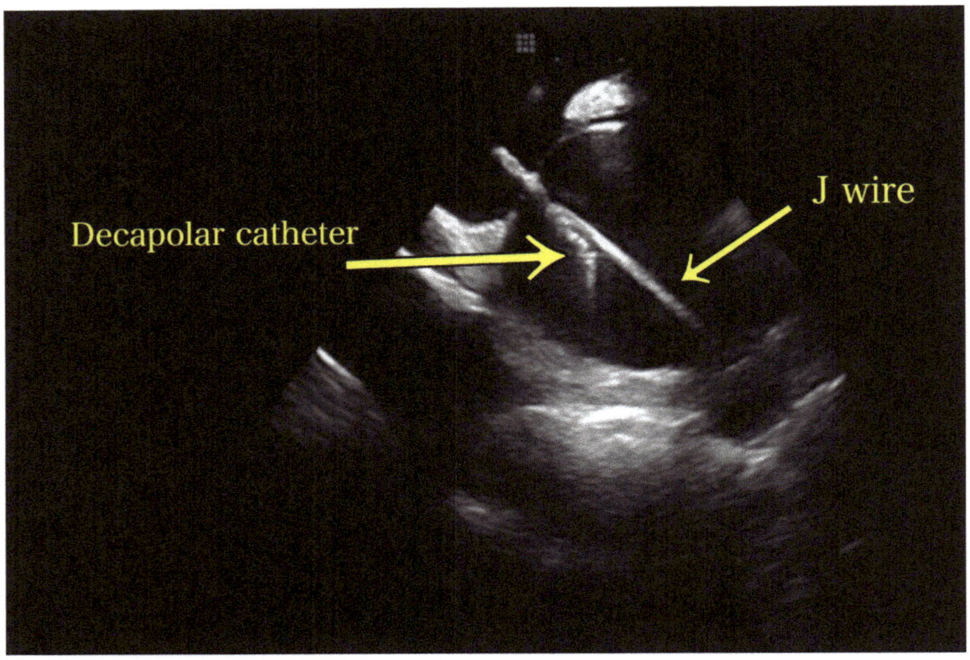

Figure 14.11 Decapolar catheter is advanced alongside the J-wire through the transseptal puncture.

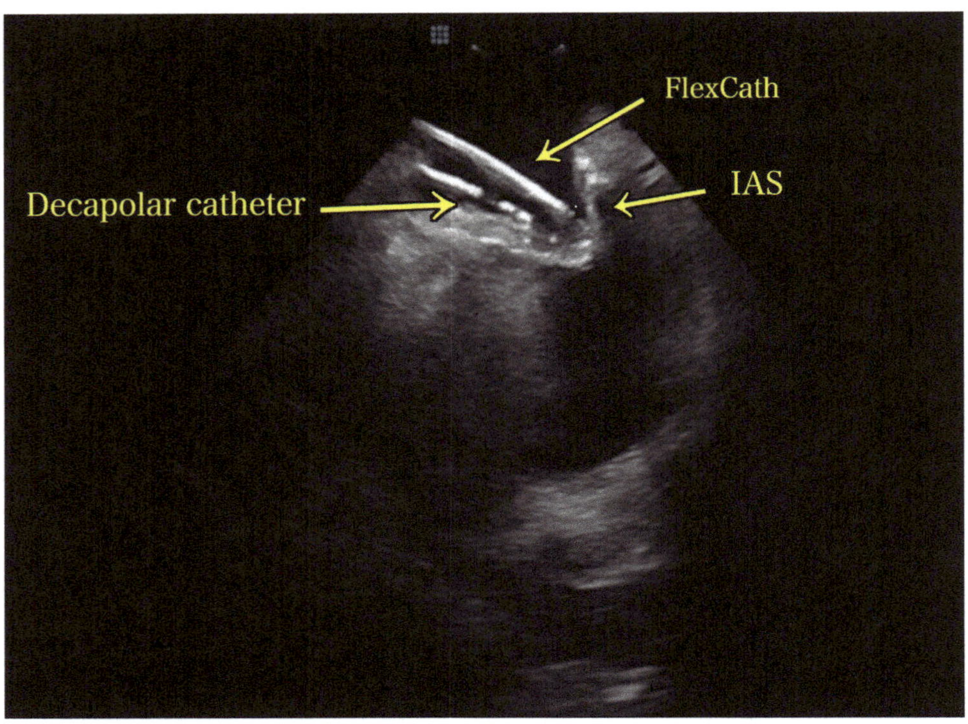

Figure 14.12 Push-Pull Technique. The FlexCath and dilator are advanced over the wire until septum tenting is observed. At this point, the decapolar catheter is simultaneously withdrawn while advancing the FlexCath dilator assembly, resulting in successful entry of the FlexCath into the LA. IAS: interatrial septum.

Tip 2: Placing the ICE Catheter in the LA for Improved Visualization

For superior visualization of the PVs, the ICE catheter can be advanced into the LA. The ICE catheter will be introduced through the same transseptal puncture. After successful transseptal exchange, the J-wire is left in the LSPV. Then, the FlexCath–dilator assembly is pulled back in to the RA, maintaining the J-wire in the LSPV. Then, while applying an anterior curve to the ICE catheter, the entry point of the J-wire through the transseptal puncture is visualized on ICE. (**Figure 14.13**). The ICE is advanced parallel to the J-wire through the same transseptal puncture. The FlexCath–dilator assembly is then readvanced into the LA. The dilator and wire are removed. Once ICE is in the LA, adding a posterior tilt will facilitate visualization of the left pulmonary veins and clockwise rotation would facilitate visualization of the right pulmonary veins.

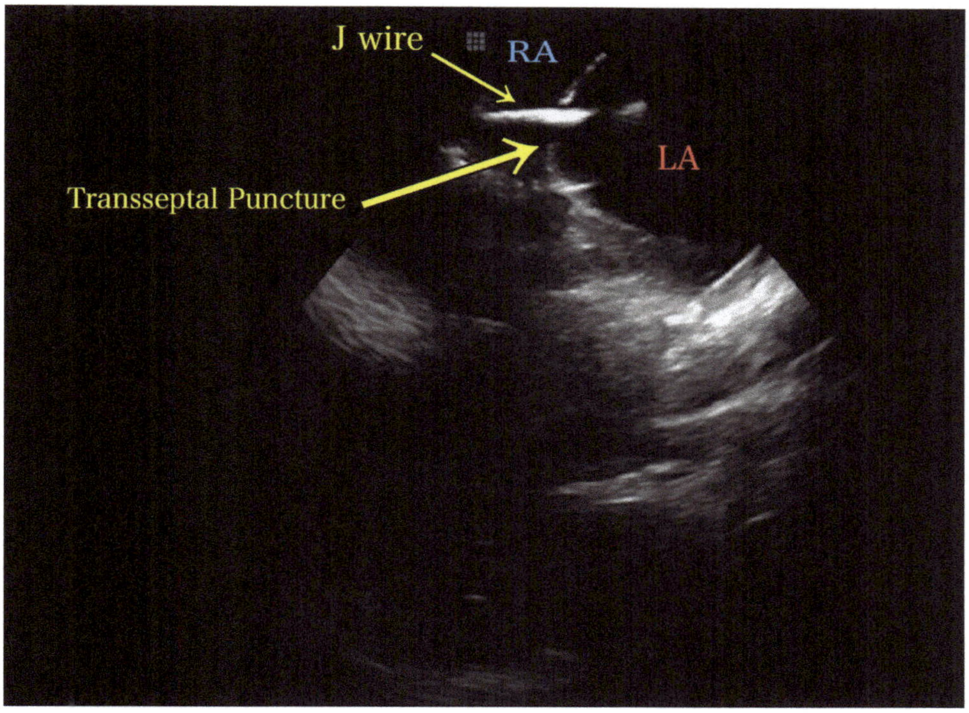

Figure 14.13 By applying anterior curve to the ICE catheter, the entry point of the J-wire through the transseptal puncture is visualized on ICE. The ICE is advanced parallel to the J-wire through the same transseptal puncture into the left atrium. LA: left atrium; RA: right atrium.

Cryoballoon Ablation

The ostia of the PVs, as visualized by ICE, are delineated on the EnSite system using the Achieve catheter. A 3D geometry of the pulmonary veins (PVs) and LA on the EnSite system is created as the operator sequentially isolates the PVs.

The Achieve catheter is advanced into the LSPV. The balloon is inflated and moved to the antrum of the vein. ICE is utilized to confirm the alignment of the transseptal sheath and the balloon prior to cryo application (**Figure 14.14**). Achievement of a pulmonary capillary wedge pressure waveform on hemodynamic pressure monitoring signifies complete occlusion of the vein (**Figure 14.15**). A lack of color-flow Doppler within the targeted PV serves as an additional indicator of adequate PV occlusion. A thorough search for leaks on color-flow Doppler should be performed by applying small degrees of clockwise and counterclockwise rotation to evaluate for leaks posteriorly and anteriorly. It is also imperative to ensure that the sheath, balloon, and vein are coaxial in the same view. If the balloon appears to be coaxial to the vein but the sheath is not clearly seen in this view, then slight clockwise or counterclockwise rotation may be applied to the ICE to determine the relative location of the sheath; from there, a counter maneuver is applied to the sheath to achieve coaxiality. For example, if the ICE catheter is rotated slightly clockwise to find the sheath relative to the balloon and vein, then the sheath should be rotated slightly counterclockwise to bring it coaxial to the balloon and vein. Finally, to ensure a relatively antral location of the balloon during ablation, the majority of the equator of the balloon should be seen on ICE like a "golf ball on tee" (**Figure 14.16**).[5]

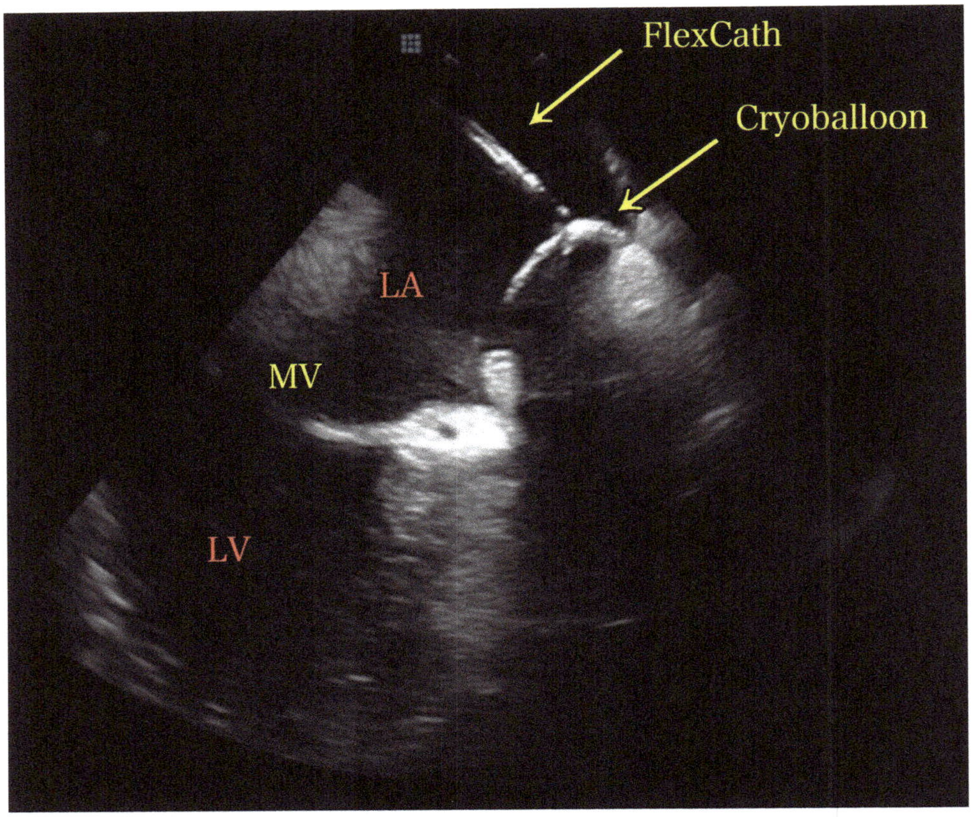

Figure 14.14 Alignment of the transseptal sheath and the balloon is confirmed on ICE prior to cryo application. LV: left ventricle; LA: left atrium; MV: mitral valve.

Cryotherapy is then applied. The goal temperature is –40°C to –50°C. Each application lasts up to 180 seconds, with the goal of achieving PV conduction block within the first 60 seconds.[6] In general, we apply 2 applications per vein.

In order to maneuver from the left-sided pulmonary veins over to the right-sided pulmonary veins, the deflated balloon is withdrawn into the sheath, leaving the Achieve catheter outside of the sheath, which can be seen on ICE and on the EAM system. If the ICE catheter is inside the LA, then it can be rotated clockwise to visualize the RIPV longitudinally. In order to achieve the same view if the ICE catheter is in the RA, the ICE should be minimally withdrawn, and a left steer applied prior to rotating the catheter clockwise.

The sheath is then maximally deflected and rotated 180 degrees clockwise. At this point, the Achieve catheter should be seen close to or within the ostium (os) of the RIPV. The Achieve catheter should be maneuvered well into the RIPV as clearly seen on the longitudinal ICE view. A loss of voltage and usually a tubular geometric shape can be seen on the EnSite system as the Achieve catheter is advanced into the vein.

Prior to CBA for the right-sided PVs, the 6-Fr decapolar catheter is used to pace the SVC at high output to monitor the integrity of the phrenic nerve during cryo applications. Diaphragmatic capture is monitored through compound motor action potentials (CMAP)[7,8] and by manual tactile monitoring of right-sided diaphragmatic stimulation. If the CMAP amplitude diminishes or a palpable loss of diaphragmatic contraction is noted, cryotherapy is immediately discontinued.

After isolation of each pulmonary vein, the Achieve catheter is used to confirm entrance and exit block. Based on operator preference, intravenous adenosine may then be administered after treatment of each vein to confirm sustained electrical isolation.

At the conclusion of the procedure, the transseptal assembly is withdrawn from the LA to the RA and intravenous protamine is administered. All catheters are removed.

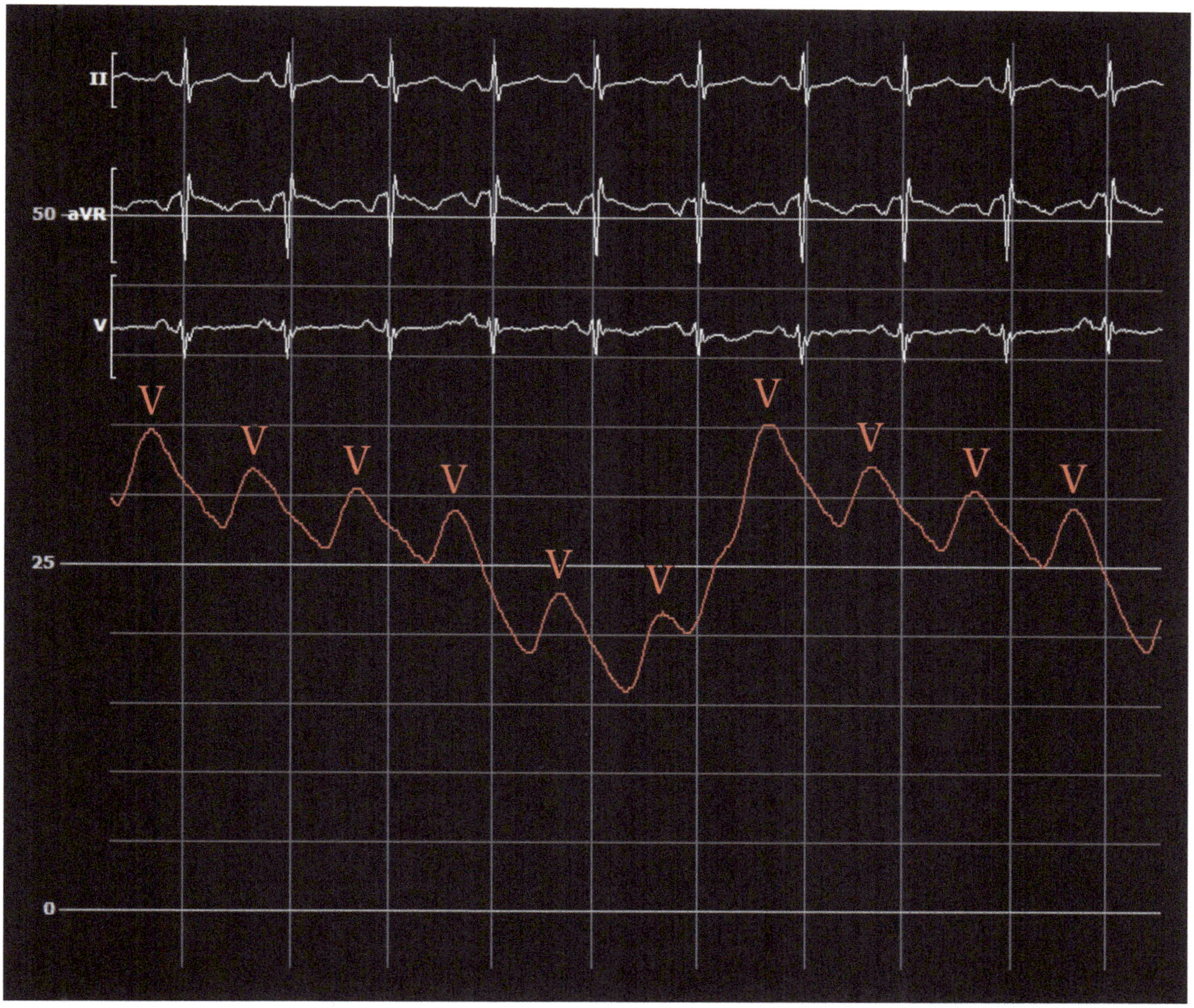

Figure 14.15 Pulmonary capillary wedge pressure waveform on hemodynamic pressure monitoring signifies complete occlusion of the vein.

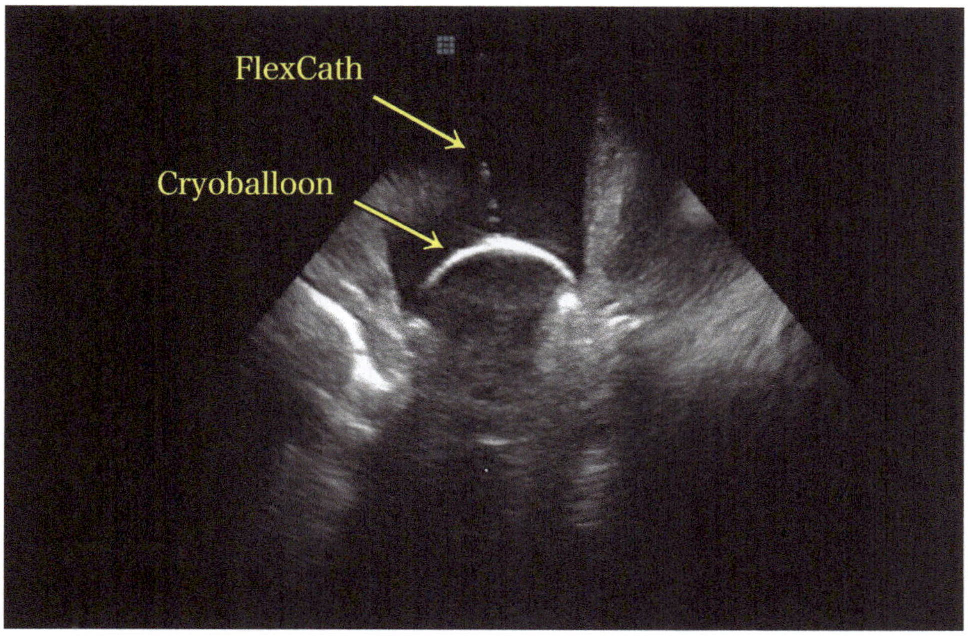

Figure 14.16 A relatively antral location of the balloon during ablation is preferred, where the majority of the equator of the balloon should be seen on ICE like a "golf ball on tee" as shown on this example of right inferior pulmonary vein (RIPV) isolation.

Advantages and Limitations

As with other non-fluoroscopic ablation procedures, non-fluoroscopic CBA offers the advantages of avoiding delivery of harmful radiation to the patient, EP lab staff, and physicians. The avoidance of wearing heavy lead garments can result in reduced orthopedic injuries and disabilities for EP lab staff and physicians. Also, pregnant EP lab staff members and members of the anesthesia team can safely assist in the fluoroscopy-free cryoballoon procedure.

As the non-fluoroscopic cryoballoon ablation technique does not use any contrast to confirm pulmonary vein occlusion, the risks of contrast-induced renal injury and allergic reactions are completely avoided.

The extensive reliance on ICE in the non-fluoroscopic technique often results in a better understanding of anatomic variations and obstacles such as the left common PV and/or right middle PV, or an unusual take off of an accessory PV (**Figure 14.17**). In fact, the use of ICE immediately identified a case of cor triatriatum sinister and facilitated successful ablation (**Figure 14.18**). Proficient use of ICE may eliminate the need for routine preprocedural imaging including CT and CMR for purposes of identifying anatomic variations.

A potential disadvantage of non-fluoroscopic cryoballoon ablation is the cost associated with ICE and the EAM system. However, in many labs, these technologies are routinely used during cryoballoon ablation procedures. Finally, if routine preprocedural CT and CMR are not performed, then significant cost-savings may be achieved. Long-term cost effectiveness may involve potentially overlooked factors such as avoidance of employee disability due to orthopedic injury.

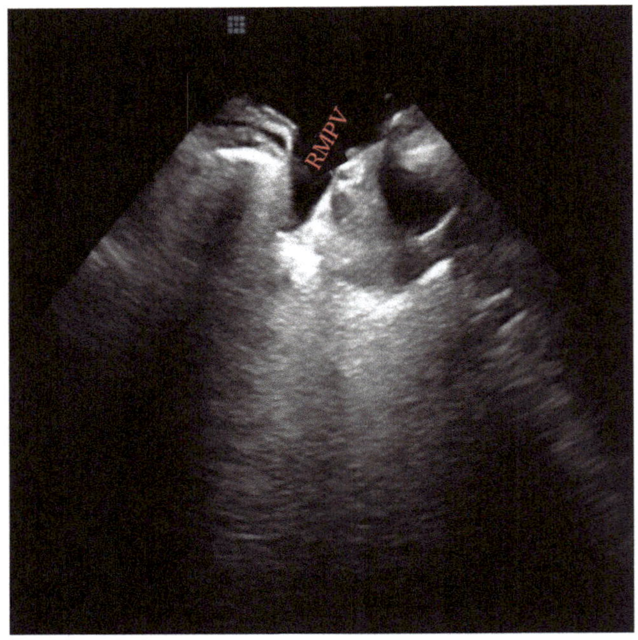

Figure 14.17 Right middle pulmonary vein noted on ICE.

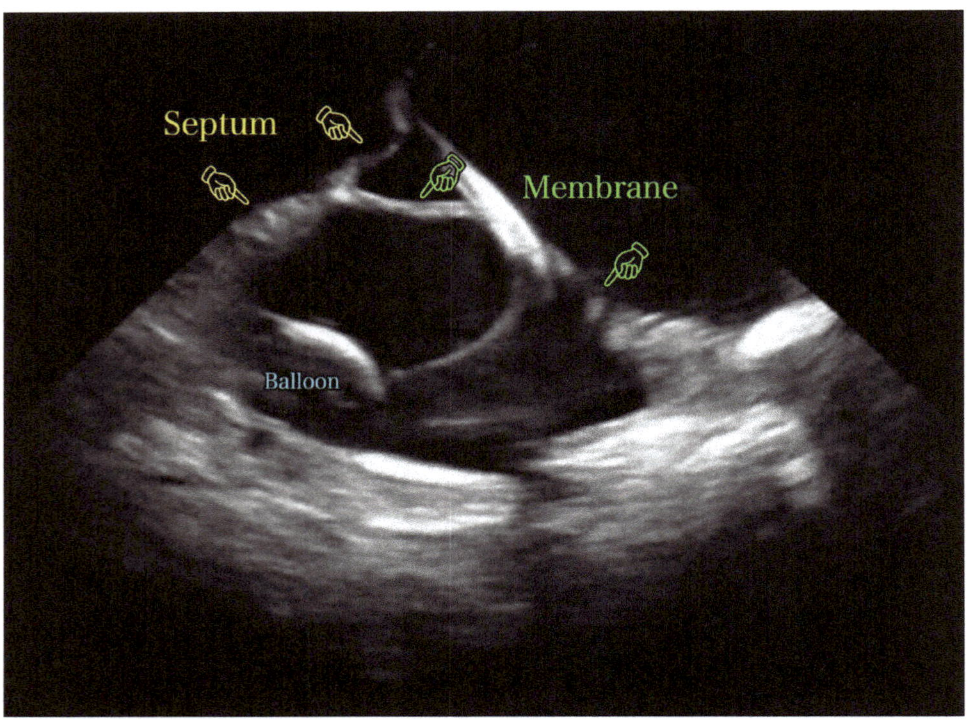

Figure 14.18 Cryoballoon ablation of right inferior pulmonary vein in a patient with cor triatriatum sinister.

Conclusion

Radiation risk to patients and EP staff during catheter ablation procedures is considerable and efforts should be made to try to eliminate unnecessary exposure whenever possible. The non-fluoroscopic cryoballoon ablation technique can be performed routinely via the use of ICE and the 3D mapping system. This technique offers several advantages over traditional fluoroscopy-based cryoballoon ablation including facile identification of anatomic variants, the avoidance of contrast, avoidance of radiation risks to patient and EP staff members, and the potential for decreased orthopedic injuries for EP lab staff.

References

1. Packer DL, Kowal RC, Wheelan KR, et al. Cryoballoon ablation of pulmonary veins for paroxysmal atrial fibrillation: First results of the North American Arctic Front (STOP AF) pivotal trial. *J Am Coll Cardiol.* 2013;61(16):1713–1723.
2. Mugnai G, Chierchia G, de Asmundis C, et al. Comparison of pulmonary vein isolation using cryoballoon versus conventional radiofrequency for paroxysmal atrial fibrillation. *Am J Cardiol.* 2014;113(9):1509–1513.
3. Bohó A, Mišíková S, Spurný P, et al. Complications of circumferential pulmonary vein isolation using the cryoballoon technique: Incidence and predictors. *Int J Cardiol.* 2014;171(2):217–223.
4. Razminia M, Demo H, Arrieta-Garcia C, D'Silva OJ, Wang T, Kehoe R. Non-fluoroscopic ablation of atrial fibrillation using cryoballoon. *J Atr Fibrillation.* 2014;7(1):1093.
5. Su W, Kowal R, Kowalski M, et al. Best practice guide for cryoballoon ablation in atrial fibrillation: The compilation experience of more than 3000 procedures. *Heart Rhythm.* 12(7):1658–1666.
6. Aryana A, Kenigsberg DN, Kowalski M, et al. Verification of a novel atrial fibrillation cryoablation dosing algorithm guided by time-to-pulmonary vein isolation: Results from the Cryo-DOSING Study (Cryoballoon-ablation DOSING Based on the Assessment of Time-to-Effect and Pulmonary Vein Isolation Guidance). *Heart Rhythm.* 2017;13(12):2306–2313.
7. Franceschi F, Dubuc M, Guerra PG, et al. Diaphragmatic electromyography during cryoballoon ablation: a novel concept in the prevention of phrenic nerve palsy. *Heart Rhythm.* 2011;8(6):885–891.
8. Lakhani M, Saiful F, Parikh V, Goyal N, Bekheit S, Kowalski M. Recordings of diaphragmatic electromyograms during cryoballoon ablation for atrial fibrillation accurately predict phrenic nerve injury. *Heart Rhythm.* 2014;11(3):369–374.

Video Legend

Video 14S Chapter summary and step-by-step procedures by Mansour Razminia. [33:42]

Section 4

Ablation of Ventricular Arrhythmias

15

How to Perform Premature Ventricular Complex Ablation Originating from the Right Ventricle and Right Ventricular Outflow Tract Using No Fluoroscopy

Christopher I. Jones, MD; Roderick Tung, MD

Introduction

The right ventricular outflow tract (RVOT) is the most common site of origin for idiopathic premature ventricular complexes (PVCs) and ventricular tachycardia (VT) in patients without underlying structural heart disease.[1,2] The majority of outflow tract VTs are focal and adenosine-sensitive, induced by cyclic adenosine monophosphate-mediated delayed afterdepolarizations. These triggered activity mechanisms differ from scar-mediated reentry in patients with structural heart disease.[6] The appreciation of PVC-mediated cardiomyopathy in setting of high-burden ectopy (>20%) and PVC-triggered polymorphic VT has expanded the indications for PVC ablation in the right ventricle (RV).[3-5]

Ablation of VT has traditionally been performed with fluoroscopic guidance, which provides visualization of the cardiac silhouette with inferred cardiac chamber location and direct visualization of catheter manipulation within the heart. While substrate-based ablation strategies are predicated upon a voltage-based substrate map, electroanatomic mapping (EAM) has become the mainstay for activation mapping and pace mapping for idiopathic PVCs arising from the RV and RVOT. The use of fluoroscopy is associated with orthopedic-related complications, operator fatigue, and latent health risks related to radiation exposure. To reduce the burden of these attendant risks from fluoroscopy, minimal- to zero-fluoroscopy techniques have been developed over the past decade with the aid of intracardiac echocardiography (ICE) and greater reliance on EAM systems. This chapter will focus on our non-fluoroscopic approach to RVOT ventricular arrhythmias (VAs), which highlights the anatomic course from the inferior approach to critical regions that are typical sites of origin.

Anatomic Considerations and ECG Localization

The RVOT is the tubular region of heart connecting the right ventricle to the pulmonary artery. Anatomically, the RVOT wraps anteriorly and leftward around the left ventricular outflow tract (LVOT) and aortic root with the pulmonary valve positioned superior to the level of the aortic valve. The RVOT is defined superiorly by the pulmonic valve and inferiorly by the RV inflow tract and the superior tricuspid valvular annulus, which includes both the His and proximal right bundle branch (**Figure 15.1**). The RVOT free wall serves as the lateral border, and the medial border of the RVOT is synonymous with the septal wall. The septal RVOT contains the most basal interventricular septum prior to the curving anterior and superior to the LVOT after the septomarginal trabeculation.[6] The posteroseptal RVOT is the most common site for idiopathic VA origin and is immediately adjacent and anterior to the right coronary cusp (RCC) (**Figure 15.2**). The junction of the RCC and left coronary cusp (LCC) is adjacent to the pulmonic valve, whereas sites in the pulmonary cusps above the valve are leftward and superior to the left main coronary artery.

Fluoroscopy Reduction Techniques for Catheter Ablation of Cardiac Arrhythmias. © 2019 Mansour Razminia, Paul C. Zei, eds.
Cardiotext Publishing, ISBN: 978-1-942909-30-9.

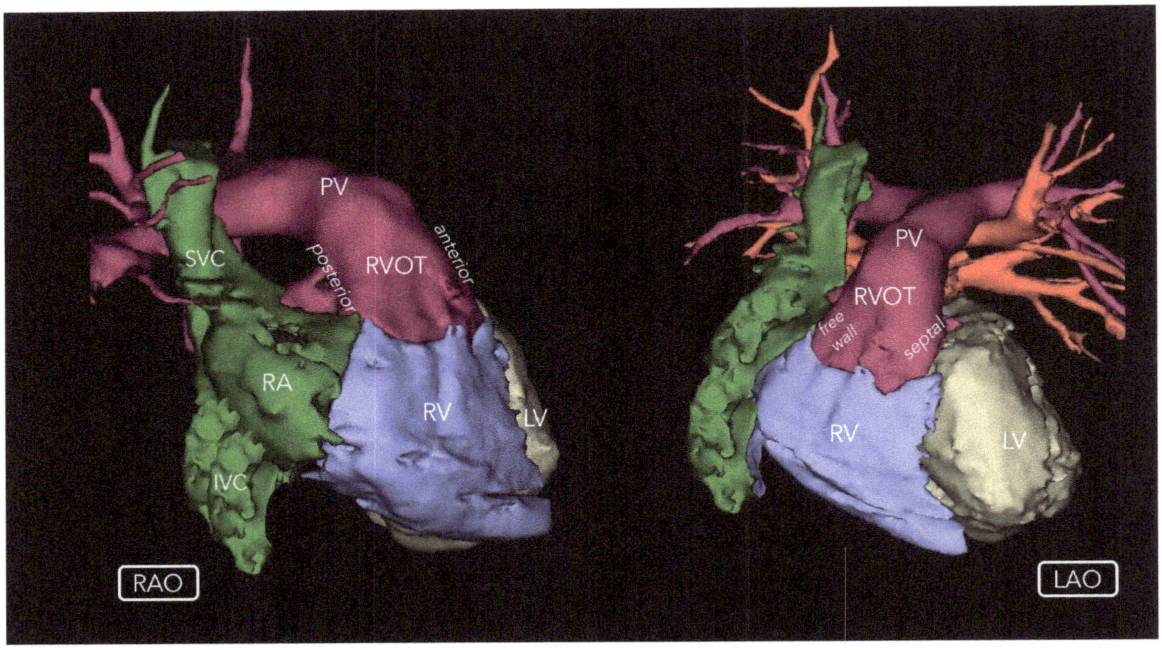

Figure 15.1 Anatomy of the RVOT from a reconstruction of a computed tomography scan. The RV is shown in **blue** and the RVOT is depicted in **magenta**. Right anterior oblique (RAO) view shows the anterior and posterior regions of the RVOT. Left anterior oblique (LAO) view shows the free wall and the septal side that is adjacent to the left ventricle. The RVOT runs superior and leftward toward the pulmonic valve (PV). RA: right atrium; SVC: superior vena cava; IVC: inferior vena cava.

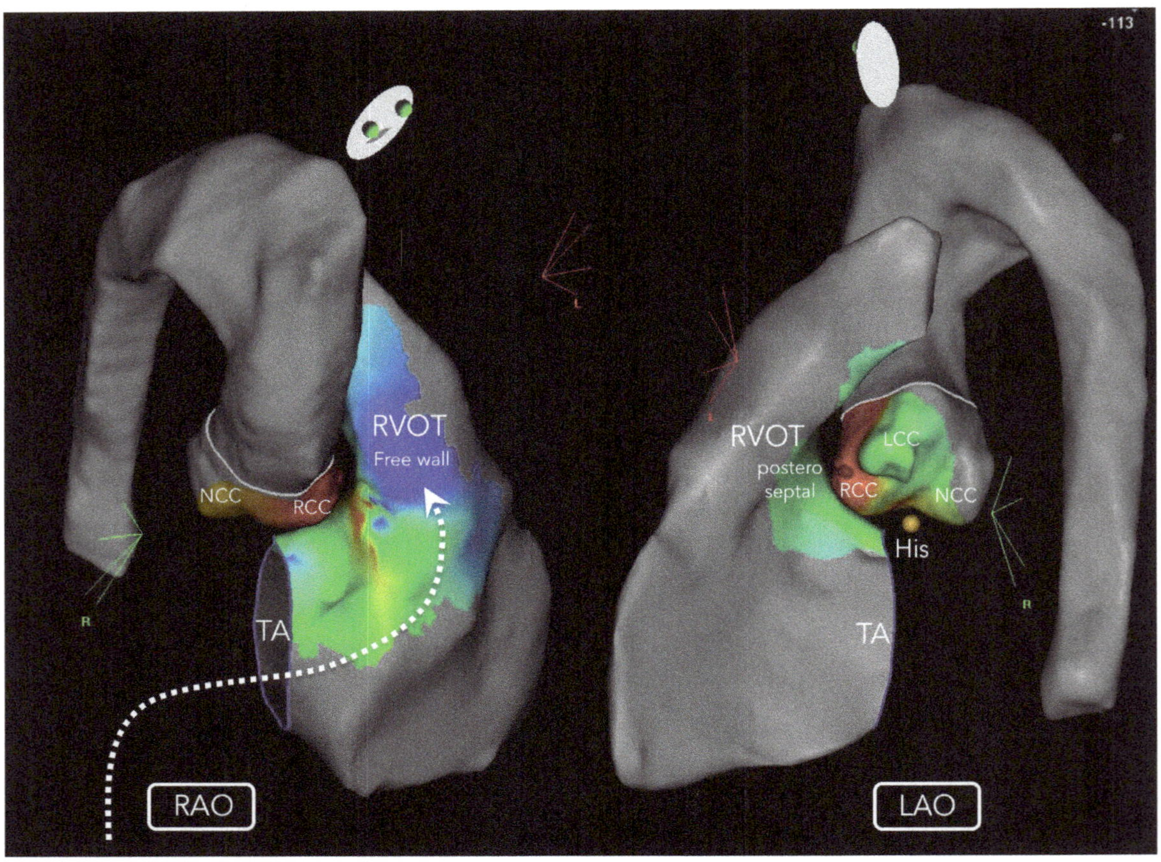

Figure 15.2 The relationship between the aortic root and RVOT is shown, with the RVOT wrapped leftward and superiorly around the aorta. The RCC abuts the posterior RVOT, and arrhythmias mapped earliest in the posteroseptal RVOT may represent early breakout from a RCC site of origin. Note that the RCC is immediately posterior to the RVOT in the RAO view. Manipulation of the mapping catheter on EAM requires a reverse S-shaped route (**arrow**). The junction of the non-coronary cusp (NCC) and RCC contains the penetrating portion of the bundle of His.

One of the typical ECG features of VT originating from the RVOT is left bundle branch block (LBBB) inferior axis morphology with late precordial transition zone after V_3.[7] A later transition after V_4 suggests a more anterior source, which may be arising from the free wall. Arrhythmias originating from the anterior RVOT will exhibit a right-axis deviation with an isoelectric or QS pattern in lead I, whereas a posterior RVOT site of origin typically features a prominent R pattern in lead I. VT originating from the septal RVOT exhibits a narrower monophasic R wave inferiorly, and arrhythmias originating from the lateral free wall of the RVOT exhibit a broader, notched QRS complex inferiorly.[8]

PVCs arising from the pulmonary cusps above the valve exhibit negative lead I and tall inferior lead amplitude.[9] PVCs may originate from the myocardial muscle sleeves, which extend from the RVOT in a manner similar to the way the left atrial muscle sleeves extend into the pulmonary veins.[10] When targeting VT localized to the superior aspects of the RVOT, mapping within and above the pulmonary cusps is important, as myocardial sleeves extending above the pulmonary valve may be identified by local prepotentials. ICE is extremely useful to delineating the valve plane. A tight "candy cane" curl may be useful to map within the pulmonary cusps to achieve contact by undeflection.[11]

Intracavitary structures that are known sources of PVCs include the moderator band and papillary muscles. The moderator band, which has been implicated as a trigger for polymorphic ventricular tachycardia (PMVT) or fibrillation (PMVF) contains the right bundle and runs from the septomarginal band cranially with insertion adjacent to the anterior papillary muscle. The septal papillary muscle arises from the postero-caudal limb of the septomarginal band and is the least prominent of the 3 papillary muscles. Septal papillary muscles are characterized by a LBBB inferior axis and early precordial transition. The posterior papillary muscle frequently has 2 parts and is attached to the inferior RV. PVCs arising from the anterior and posterior papillary muscles typically show a superior axis with late precordial transition after V_4.[12] Moderator band sites of origin are similar to PVCs arising from the anterior papillary muscle.[13]

Finally, PVCs less commonly may also arise from the tricuspid annulus, free wall, and apex of the RV.[14] The approach to tricuspid annulus PVCs requires a steerable sheath to optimize catheter contact and stability with a large curve to reach the underside of the tricuspid leaflets. A reverse S-curve can be helpful for mapping superior tricuspid annular sites.

Preprocedural Planning

In preparation for VT ablation, antiarrhythmic medications are typically discontinued for at least 3 half-lives and the patient is brought to the electrophysiology (EP) laboratory in a nonsedated, fasting state. Prior to initiation of sedation, the awake patient is monitored with ECG electrodes. The EAM patches are applied in the standard positions on the chest and back. Impedance-based systems (EnSite, Abbott, Abbott Park, IL) allow for tracking of any diagnostic catheter advanced from the femoral veins, whereas geometry needs to be created with sensor-enable catheters in order to visualize the chamber of interest with mapping systems that utilize magnetic and impedance localization.

While general anesthesia and sedation are known to suppress both spontaneous and programmed induction of VT, the balance between patient comfort and potential suppression of PVCs must be maintained.

Prior to initiation of sedation, the patient is monitored for ectopy to establish a template of the clinical morphology. If no spontaneous VT occurs, we typically administer isoproterenol at low dose (2 mcg/min), then high dose 10–20 mcg/min), followed by washout with adjunctive calcium and phenylephrine/epinephrine. General anesthesia is typically avoided when focal mechanisms are suspected.

Preprocedural imaging is performed when signs or symptoms (epsilon wave, QRS, fractionation, T-wave inversions, or RV dysfunction) of arrhythmogenic RV cardiomyopathy are suggested or present. MRI can be useful to rule out regions of focal dyskinesia or delayed enhancement. Notched inferior lead patterns that suggest free wall or lateral tricuspid annulus involvement are more common in arrhythmogenic right ventricular cardiomyopathy (ARVC) than in idiopathic RVOT cases.

Procedural Approach

Right and left femoral venous access is obtained, and a coronary sinus catheter may be used as an internal reference, along with a phased-array intracardiac echocardiography (ICE) catheter, and mapping catheter. Non-fluoroscopic advancement of the ICE catheter is performed by maintaining an echolucent space along the superior border of the ICE display at 1 o'clock to 3 o'clock on the window. If the operator feels any resistance, the catheter is withdrawn and redirected.

Rightward and posterior tilt are then performed upon entry into the right atrium from the view of the fossa ovalis. This view allows visualization of the SVC-RA junction. A 180-cm, 0.032-in J-wire is then advanced through the 8.5-Fr femoral sheath and advanced to the SVC-RA junction. A steerable (Agilis) or fixed sheath (SR0 or SL0) is then advanced to provide more support for mapping in the RVOT. If a magnetic sensor-based system such as CARTO (Biosense Webster, Irvine, CA) or Rhythmia (Boston Scientific, Marlborough, MA) is used, a diagnostic catheter cannot be visualized unless the ablation catheter is first used to create geometry or matrix in the desired region. As a result, preselection of an ablation catheter must be made, taking into account options of contact force, irrigation, and catheter curve, all prior to detailed mapping of the potential ablation target.

Atrial electrograms are seen as soon as the catheter crosses the junction between the inferior vena cava (IVC) and the RA. The mapping catheter is then pulled back down to the IVC-RA junction until electrograms used to create a full geometry of the IVC are no longer present. The mapping catheter is then advanced superiorly with posterior tilt until a loss of atrial electrograms is seen, indicating entry into the SVC, and the geometry is further delineated in this region to outline the RA-SVC junction. Care must be exercised to advance into the SVC with a slight posterior angulation from the IVC as to not enter the RA appendage, which could lead to perforation. The catheter is then used to create RA geometry by anterior flexion toward to the tricuspid annulus, where 1:1 AV ratio can be annotated to delineate the valve plane. With undeflection and septal clockwise torque, the His bundle is mapped and tagged as a reference point. The home view on ICE is critical to assess the relationship between the RV inflow and His bundle location, which is seen adjacent to the junction of the NCC and RCC (**Figure 15.3**).

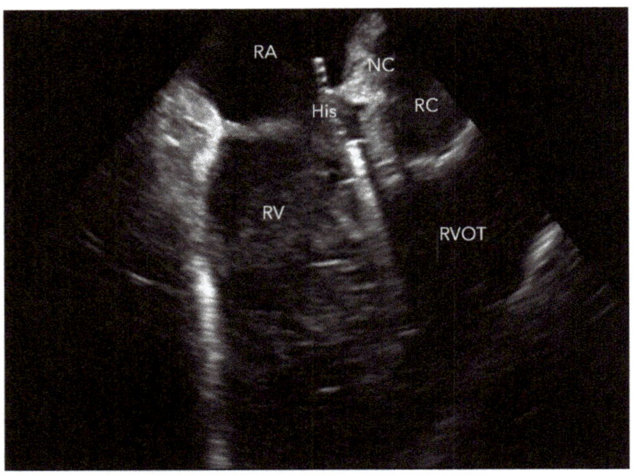

Figure 15.3 Intracardiac echocardiography "home" view showing the RA, triscuspid valve, with multielectrode catheter across the annulus to record a His bundle at the junction of the non-coronary and right coronary cusp. The RV and RVOT are easily visualized in this view to guide catheter positioning and ensure stability.

The coronary sinus catheter can be placed with EAM guidance in both RAO and LAO position to direct inferoposterior and leftward, respectively. The catheter can also be placed with the use of only ICE. The catheter is positioned at the His reference point under ICE, then deflected inferiorly toward 6 o'clock (tricuspid annulus) and torqued clockwise, where ICE can visualize the funnel shape of the CS ostium (os) on ICE with the same clockwise torque. With advancement of the catheter with clockwise rotation and undeflection, the typical near-field atrial and far-field ventricular components are seen. Additional clockwise torque on ICE allows for visualization of the catheter inferior to the left atrium running in the AV groove.

For mapping of the RV inflow and RVOT, the real-time EAM views are maintained in RAO and LAO projection and under ICE visualization, the sheath is deflected inferiorly to allow the mapping catheter to be advanced through the tricuspid valve annulus and into the RV cavity. Ventricular electrograms are visualized to confirm entry into the RV. The geometry is created similarly as in the RA, all of which can be visualized on ICE. It is important to avoid bumping the His (previously annotated and tagged on EAM) and right bundle during mapping, and if existing left bundle branch block is present, a backup quadripolar RV catheter for pacing can be considered. The authors typically avoid mapping the entire apex of the RV to avoid risk of perforation, unless critical for the targeted arrhythmia and contact force is observed when advancing the most anterior and superior portion of the RVOT to avoid perforation.

The mapping or ablation catheter is flexed inferiorly and then clocked upward to advance from the RV towards the RVOT (**Figure 15.4**). If a bidirectional catheter is used, the catheter can be advanced past the His and deflected upward with posterior deflection to create a reverse S trajectory to enter the RVOT. The mapping catheter is advanced superiorly until there is loss of the ventricular signal, which signifies the plane of the pulmonic valve. The plane of the pulmonic valve can be approximated with several points to define the annulus. The mapping catheter is then flexed posteriorly in the RAO view to contact and map the posterior portion of the RVOT. To move anteriorly, the catheter is undeflected slowly. Extreme caution should be exercised with antegrade movements while defining the anterior RVOT, which is the most superior portion of the geometry in RAO. The use of contact-force sensing may improve safety, with a warning set at >20 g of force to avoid perforation of the anterior RVOT, the thinnest portion of the RVOT.

After the posterior and anterior portion of the RVOT have been defined, the septal (leftward) and lateral (rightward free wall) aspects are then mapped. Counterclockwise torque of the reverse S curve will navigate the catheter leftward toward the septal side, and clockwise torque allows for mapping of the free wall. Once the geometry is complete, we then perform activation mapping if there is adequate VA burden, or pace mapping if there is insufficiently ambient ectopy. Isoproterenol is administered if no spontaneous ectopy is seen.

ICE is invaluable when mapping intracavitary structures to ascertain contact and complete sampling of each side of the papillary muscle or moderator band. Integrated ultrasound (CARTOSOUND, Biosense Webster) is useful, as an indicator is present to localize the catheter within the ultrasound field. Because stability can be challenging, ICE visualization may also assess lesion formation during radiofrequency (RF) delivery. Differentiation between the anterior papillary muscle and moderator is difficult as they are frequently connected. The identification of Purkinje potentials is an additional sign of adequate contact with an intracavitary structure.

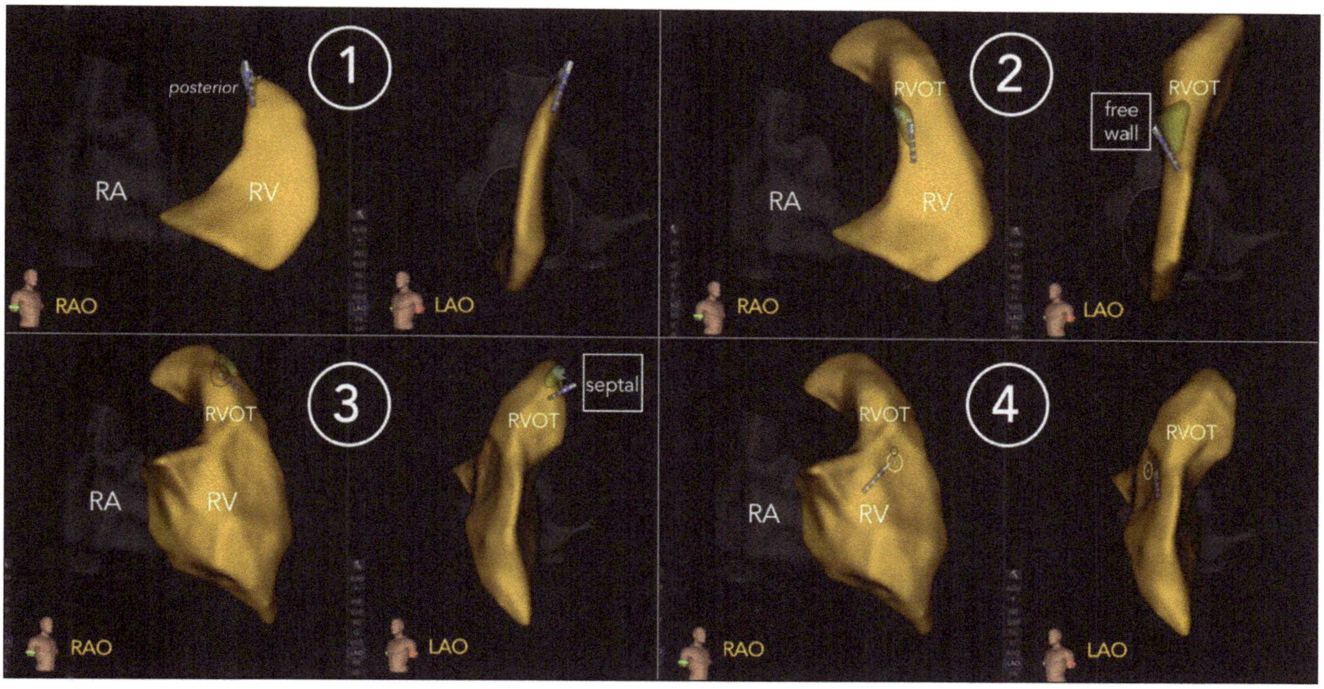

Figure 15.4 Four sequential views using a non-fluoroscopic technique (Rhythmia, Boston Scientific) with impedance and magnetic tracking. **Step 1:** RAO and LAO views are shown to create RV and RVOT geometry with attention to curve the catheter posteriorly to avoid perforation of the anterior RVOT in RAO view. The leftward orientation of the RVOT is seen in LAO as the catheter is advanced superiorly. **Step 2:** The free wall is mapped with clockwise rotation of the catheter. **Step 3:** The septal aspects of the RVOT are mapped with counterclockwise rotation of the catheter. **Step 4:** The entire geometry is completed without the need for fluoroscopy and mapping of the arrhythmia can commence by either pace mapping or activation mapping.

Activation Mapping and Ablation of VT

The goal of activation mapping is to localize the region with the earliest onset of RVOT endocardial activation by measuring from the earliest endocardial RVOT bipolar electrogram to the earliest QRS onset on the 12-lead ECG. As the geometry has been created during sinus rhythm, a non-fluoroscopic technique during PVCs can be performed safely within the confines of the electroanatomic shell. It is well known, however, that the geometry and location of the catheter can shift by 2–4 mm during a PVC, so it is important to create a separate activation map. When the site of earliest activation is localized, we increase the mapping density to insure concentric isochrones of progressively delayed endocardial activation around the site of earliest endocardial activation, creating a "bullseye." If the earliest site of activation is broad, mapping of an adjacent site (i.e., RCC and LVOT) is advised. Bipolar electrograms at the earliest site of activation have local high-frequency components with rapid slew rates and 10–45 ms pre QRS. Unipolar electrograms should show a rapid QS deflection indicating activation away from the recording tip. While prepotentials may be seen earlier than –30, it is uncommon to see complex fractionated electrograms and mid-diastolic late potentials typically seen in scar-mediated reentry.[1]

If the earliest site of activation cannot be discerned by activation mapping, pace mapping is then performed to approximate the exit morphology. Pace mapping is performed at the lowest output in attempt to improve specificity of local capture. Pace mapping scores have been developed that can quickly provide a percentage of similarity. Scores of >90% are preferred, but manual operator overread is recommended. A pace map can even be performed to create a region that has highest match, where the percentage of match can be manually converted to a timing (90% match is –90). With this approach, a worse pace map of 80% will appear –80 and farther away from the site of closest approximation. The resultant map appears to simulate an activation map with concentric display.

We typically perform ablation with an irrigated catheter in the RVOT to minimize temperature limitation on power delivery. A negative monophasic QS unipolar signal with rapid deflection from baseline on the distal electrode is confirmed on the ablation catheter in addition to the earliest bipolar prepotential. Alone, a QS unipolar signal in VT is not specific for identifying the best location for successful VT ablation as the area producing the QS complex can be larger than the site of earliest activation itself, up to 1 cm or wider in diameter. However, QS unipolar signal adds benefit when recorded from sites pre-QRS, as locations distal to the earliest site of activation would not be pre-QRS.[10]

RF energy is delivered at a maximum power output of 30-40 W, with 13–30 cc irrigation and a temperature limit of 42°C. Ideally, the operator will eliminate VA with focal origin on the first RF application because subsequent lesions may be limited by edema. The RF application duration is set to 60 seconds, and suppression is typically seen within 20 seconds unless an intramural source is suspected. In these cases, late suppression may be seen at 30–40 seconds. If suppression is seen, we typically ablate for 120 seconds at the site of elimination. Additional lesions above, below, left, and right can be performed to provide further consolidation around the successful site to decrease the chance of later recurrence. During delivery of RF, the operator must pay close attention to maintain appropriate catheter position, contact force, impedance, and power output to ensure safe and effective energy delivery. Rapid impedance drops >15 ohms have been associated with steam pops.

After presumed successful RF applications, we typically repeat the exact same induction protocol that was successful in triggering the CA. Endpoints following completion of RF include no spontaneous or inducible VT with and without isoproterenol. Sometimes the site of ablation may even be electrically unexcitable, although this is more common when ablating within scar. A 30-minute waiting period should be observed as well.[8,9]

At the conclusion of the procedure the ablation catheter is withdrawn into the sheath, which is indicated on EAM. Using the EAM and ICE, the straightened Agilis sheath and ablation catheter should be removed from the heart. The ICE catheter be positioned in the home view, flexed, and advanced into the RV, then clocked to exclude pericardial effusion.

Conclusion

While fluoroscopy-guided ablation has previously been the standard approach for complex ablation procedures, non-fluoroscopic procedures can be safely performed in clinical practice when mapping ablation arrhythmias arising from the RV and RVOT.[15] Knowledge of regional anatomy, EAM system guidance, and routine use of ICE allow for assessment of catheter location without fluoroscopy. ICE is invaluable when targeting intracavitary structures such as papillary muscles and the moderator band and the use of contact force is important for both safety and efficacy during mapping and ablation.

References

1. Lerman BB, Stein KM, Markowitz SM. Idiopathic right ventricular outflow tract tachycardia: A clinical approach. *Pacing Clin Electrophysiol.* 1996;19:2120–137.
2. Lerman BB, Stein KM, Markowitz SM, Mittal S, Slotwiner DJ. Right ventricular outflow tract tachycardia: an update. *Card Electrophysiol Rev.* 2002;6:668–671.
3. Yarlagadda RK, Iwai S, Stein KM, et al. Reversal of cardiomyopathy in patients with repetitive monomorphic ventricular ectopy originating from the right ventricular outflow tract. *Circulation.* 2005;112:1092–1097.
4. Haïssaguerre M, Extramiana F, Hocini M, et al. Mapping and ablation of ventricular fibrillation associated with long-QT and Brugada syndromes. *Circulation.* 2003;108:925–928.
5. Haïssaguerre M, Shah DC, Jaïs P, et al. Role of Purkinje conducting system in triggering of idiopathic ventricular fibrillation. *Lancet.* 2002;359:677–678.
6. Asirvatham SJ. Correlative anatomy for the invasive electrophysiologist: Outflow tract and supravalvar arrhythmia. *J Cardiovasc Electrophysiol.* 2009;20:955–968.
7. Movsowitz C, Schwartzman D, Callans DJ, et al. Idiopathic right ventricular outflow tract tachycardia: Narrowing the anatomic location for successful ablation. *Am Heart J.* 1996;131:930–936.
8. Dixit S, Gerstenfeld EP, Callans DJ, Marchlinski FE. Electrocardiographic patterns of superior right ventricular outflow tract tachycardias: Distinguishing septal and free-wall sites of origin. *J Cardiovasc Electrophysiol.* 2003;14:1–7.
9. Ebrille E, Chandra VM, Syed F, et al. Distinguishing ventricular arrhythmia originating from the right coronary cusp, peripulmonic valve area, and the right ventricular outflow tract: Utility of lead I. *J Cardiovasc Electrophysiol.* 2014;25:404–410.
10. Iwai S, Cantillon DJ, Kim RJ, et al. Right and left ventricular outflow tract tachycardias: Evidence for a common electrophysiologic mechanism. *J Cardiovasc Electrophysiol.* 2006;17:1052–1058.
11. Liao Z, Zhan X, Wu S, et al. Idiopathic ventricular arrhythmias originating from the pulmonary sinus cusp: Prevalence, electrocardiographic/electrophysiological characteristics, and catheter ablation. *J Am Coll Cardiol.* 2015;66:2633–2644.
12. Crawford T, Mueller G, Good E, et al. Ventricular arrhythmias originating from papillary muscles in the right ventricle. *Heart Rhythm.* 2010;7:725–730.
13. Sadek MM, Benhayon D, Sureddi R, et al. Idiopathic ventricular arrhythmias originating from the moderator band: Electrocardiographic characteristics and treatment by catheter ablation. *Heart Rhythm.* 2015;12:67–75.
14. Van Herendael H, Garcia F, Lin D, et al. Idiopathic right ventricular arrhythmias not arising from the outflow tract: Prevalence, electrocardiographic characteristics, and outcome of catheter ablation. *Heart Rhythm.* 2011;8:511–518.
15. Sadek MM, Ramirez FD, Nery PB, et al. Completely non-fluoroscopic catheter ablation of left atrial arrhythmias and ventricular tachycardia. *J Cardiovasc Electrophysiol.* 2019;30(1):78–88.

Video Legend

Video 15S Chapter summary and step-by-step procedures by Mansour Razminia. [6:28]

16

How to Perform Ablation in the Coronary Cusps Using No Fluoroscopy

José Mauricio Sánchez, MD

Background

Ablation of idiopathic premature ventricular complexes (PVCs) or idiopathic ventricular arrhythmias has become increasingly common.[1] Left ventricular outflow tract (LVOT) origin of ventricular foci of such clinical entities has become recognized as much more common than previously thought.[2] Additionally, mapping for possible ventricular arrhythmias from the outflow tract may require mapping both in the right ventricular outflow tract (RVOT) as well as the LVOT. The coronary cusps have emerged as an area of frequent origin of idiopathic PVCs. Ablation is frequently used to treat patients who are symptomatic from idiopathic ventricular arrhythmias, have resultant left ventricular dysfunction, or are high risk for development of left ventricular dysfunction.[3] This can also be performed safely within the coronary cusps. These arrhythmias can also be targeted in the coronary cusps with a fluoroscopy-free work flow to allow for accurate mapping that is safe and effective while avoiding unnecessary radiation to the operator and patient.

Technique

Setup and Access

Mapping and ablation within the coronary cusps and LVOT rely principally on recognition that the LVOT may play a role in origin of the ventricular arrhythmia. While details of determining when to consider examination of the LVOT will not be covered here, it is important to map the LVOT as well as the distal coronary sinus (CS) toward the LV summit if the PVC morphology suggests that this may be an origin of the arrhythmia.

Prior to gaining access into the arterial system, the author prefers to access the venous system and create a shell or geometry of the right atrium (RA) for catheter placement with the operator's 3D mapping system of choice. Sufficient venous access should be acquired for placement of a quadrapolar His catheter, a decapolar CS catheter, and a quadrapolar catheter in the right ventricular apex. Use of an 8-Fr sheath is preferred after gaining access to the right or left femoral artery by modified Seldinger technique. A 3.5-mm irrigated ablation catheter can then be visualized on mapping system of choice. Both the EnSite (Abbott, Abbott Park, IL) and CARTO3 (Biosense Webster, Irvine, CA) can be used. The EnSite system allows the catheter to be visualized by the mapping system through the entire process of advancing from the sheath tip retrograde toward the aorta. The CARTO3 system will only recognize the ablation catheter once it has advanced sufficiently into the abdomen near the patches and magnet system. In either case, great care should be taken when advancing the catheter. Any resistance should prompt immediate cessation of advancement and reevaluation of the process. The ablation catheter usually is able to

Fluoroscopy Reduction Techniques for Catheter Ablation of Cardiac Arrhythmias. © 2019 Mansour Razminia, Paul C. Zei, eds.
Cardiotext Publishing, ISBN: 978-1-942909-30-9.

be advanced without issue in a retrograde fashion. The exception to this rule is in patients with significant arterial or venous tortuosity. In these cases, a long sheath can be very helpful to navigate past these difficult areas. The availability of contact force-sensing ablation catheters may improve the safety of catheter advancement through the vascular tree without fluoroscopy.

A phased-array intracardiac echo (ICE) can be utilized from the vantage point of the femoral veins or iliac vein and inferior vena cava to visualize advancement of the ablation catheter within the arterial system (see **Video 16.1**). Once the ablation catheter is advanced, the ICE catheter can be advanced at the same time in order to maintain visualization of the catheter (see **Video 16.2** and **Video 16.3**). Once the catheter is at the level of the aortic arch, the operator must deflect the ablation catheter toward the right shoulder in order to descend in retrograde fashion into the ascending aorta. The ICE catheter can be placed into the SVC and directed toward the ascending aorta and follow the ablation catheter back down toward the cusps. The ablation catheter should be easily visualized with the ICE catheter (see **Video 16.4**). The ICE catheter can then be brought back into the RA for the home view (see **Figure 16.1**). The home view demonstrates the RA, RV, aortic cusps, and ascending aorta. These structures should be clearly visualized before proceeding with further manipulation in order for the operator to get a sense of the anatomy.

Mapping

Extensive mapping should be performed to generate a detailed 3D electroanatomic map of the LVOT and aortic cusps. Both the electrogram and location on map will help determine structure. All coronary cusps should be mapped. The non-coronary cusp (NCC) should be the most posterior cusp in 3D space with atrial electrogram signals seen due to its anatomical location above the intratrial septum. The right coronary cusp (RCC) will be anterior to this. Great care must be taken to document the presence of a His signal at or below the RCC. In the home ICE view from the RA vantage point, the cusps and aorta can be viewed in the long axis. In this view, the NCC will be the cusp that is on top. Rotation of the phased-array ICE catheter counter clockwise or rightward will bring the NCC and RCC into view (see **Video 16.5**). The right coronary artery can also be visualized here (**Figure 16.2**). The LCC will be located to the left of the RCC. Clockwise rotation of the ICE catheter will bring the LCC into view (see **Figure 16. 3** and **Video 16.6**). It is important to keep the tip of the ablation catheter toward the junction of the cusp and sinuses of Valsalva. The higher in the sinuses one moves, the greater the chance of damage to the coronary arteries. The left main coronary artery (LMCA) can usually be visualized in this long-axis view (see **Figure 16.4**). Additionally, color Doppler may be helpful on ICE to determine the location of ostium (os) of the major coronary arteries in order to avoid injury to these structures (see **Figure 16.5**; see **Video 16.7**). The short axis of the coronary cusps can also be visualized from the right ventricle. The ICE catheter can be deflected down in order to advance into the RV. The ICE catheter can then be rotated counterclockwise until the cusps come into view (**Figure 16.6**). The LMCA can be visualized here again (**Figure 16.7**). Again, color Doppler can be added for improved visualization (**Figure 16.8**). Visualization of the cusps can be achieved from the left atrium if necessary, either through a patent foramen ovale or via transseptal puncture into the LA. If the coronary artery cannot be visualized and the location of the earliest potential is higher in the cusp, coronary angiography may be needed to ensure ablation is safe. This is likely infrequent with excellent ICE images but may prove necessary with poorer imaging.

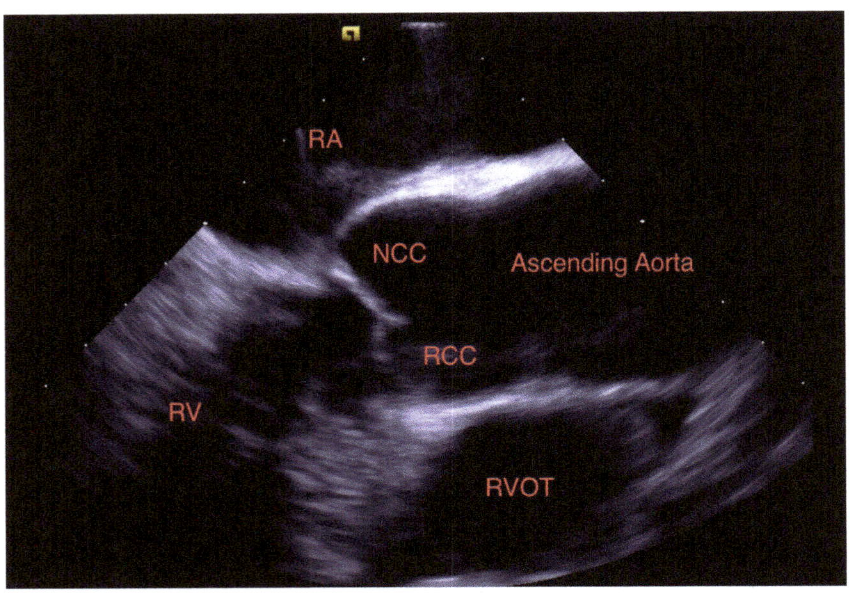

Figure 16.1 ICE home view of the RA, RV, and aortic cusps.

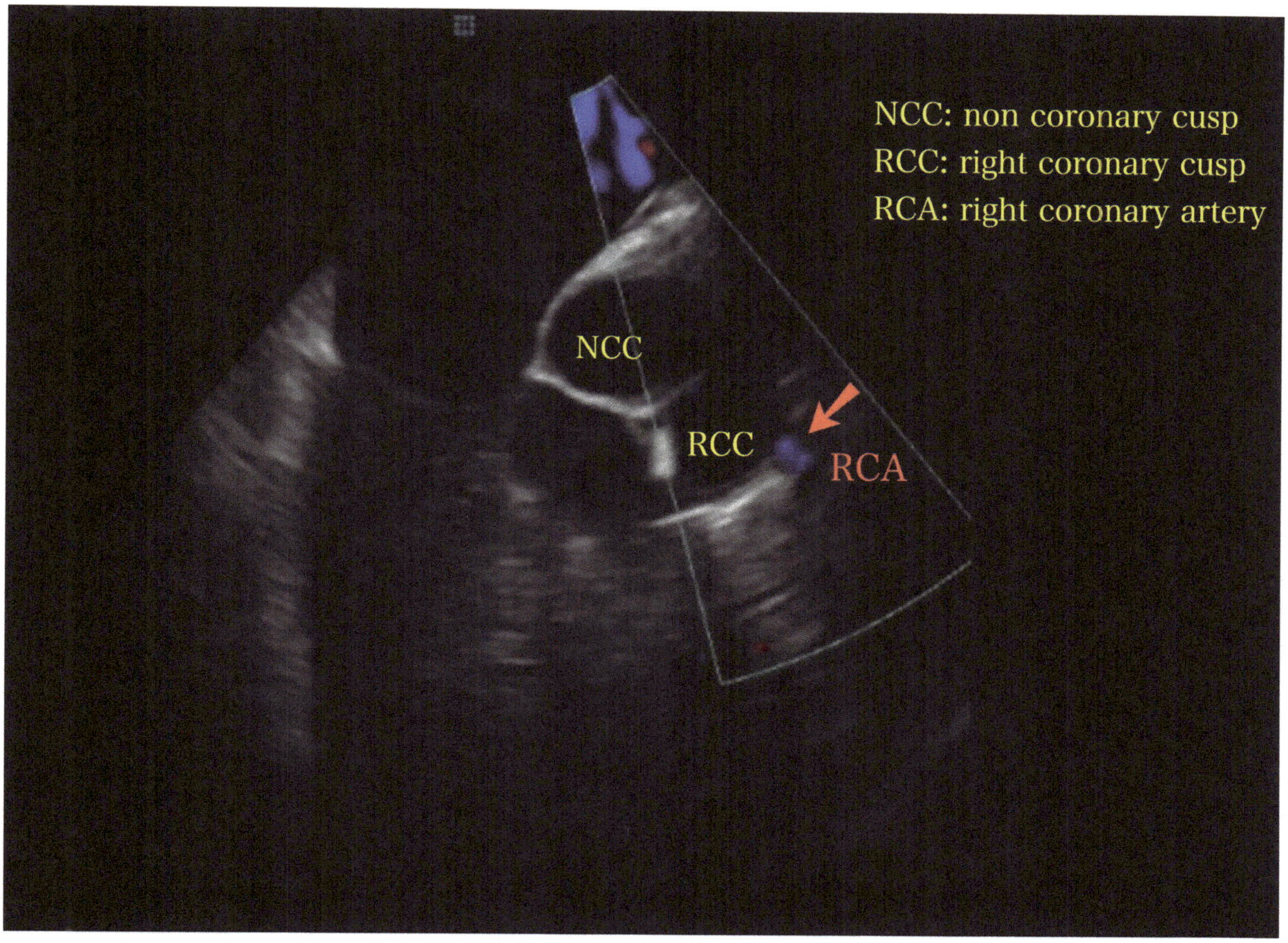

Figure 16.2 ICE view of the right coronary cusp and right coronary artery.

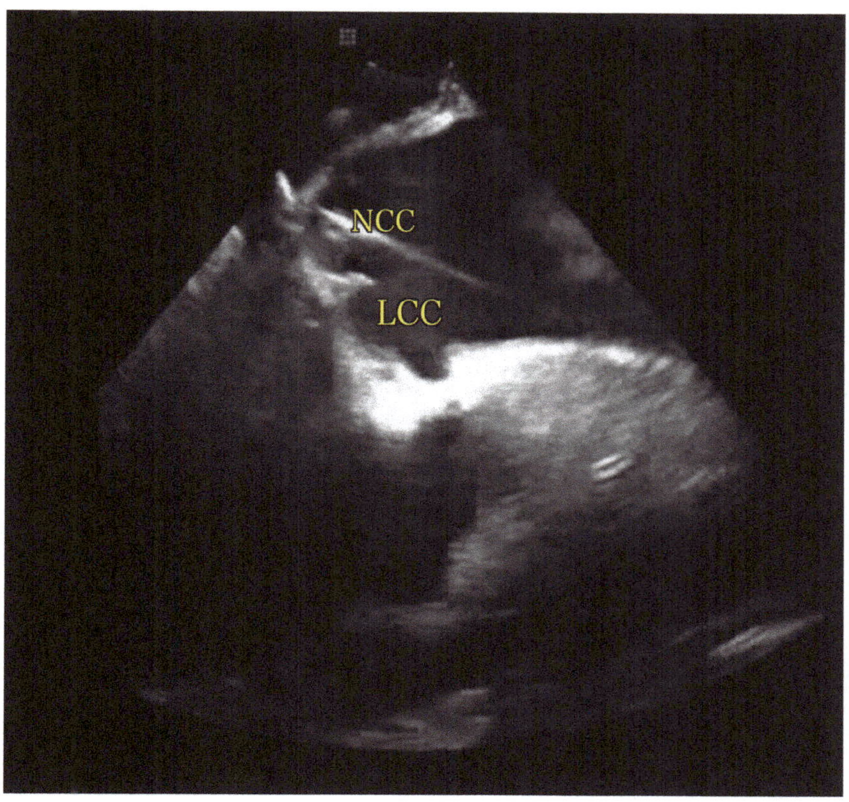

Figure 16.3 ICE view of the left coronary cusp.

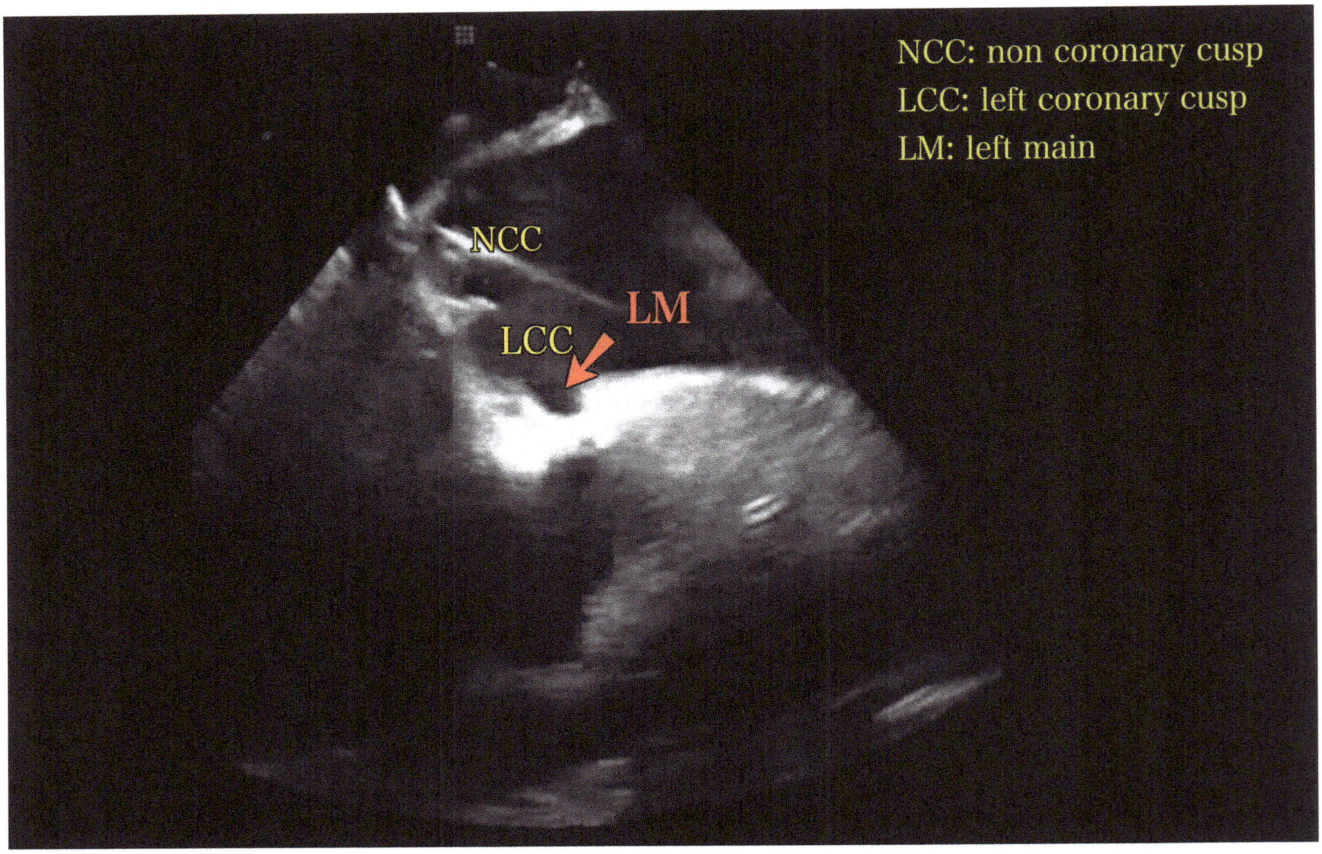

Figure 16.4 Long-axis ICE view of the left main coronary artery.

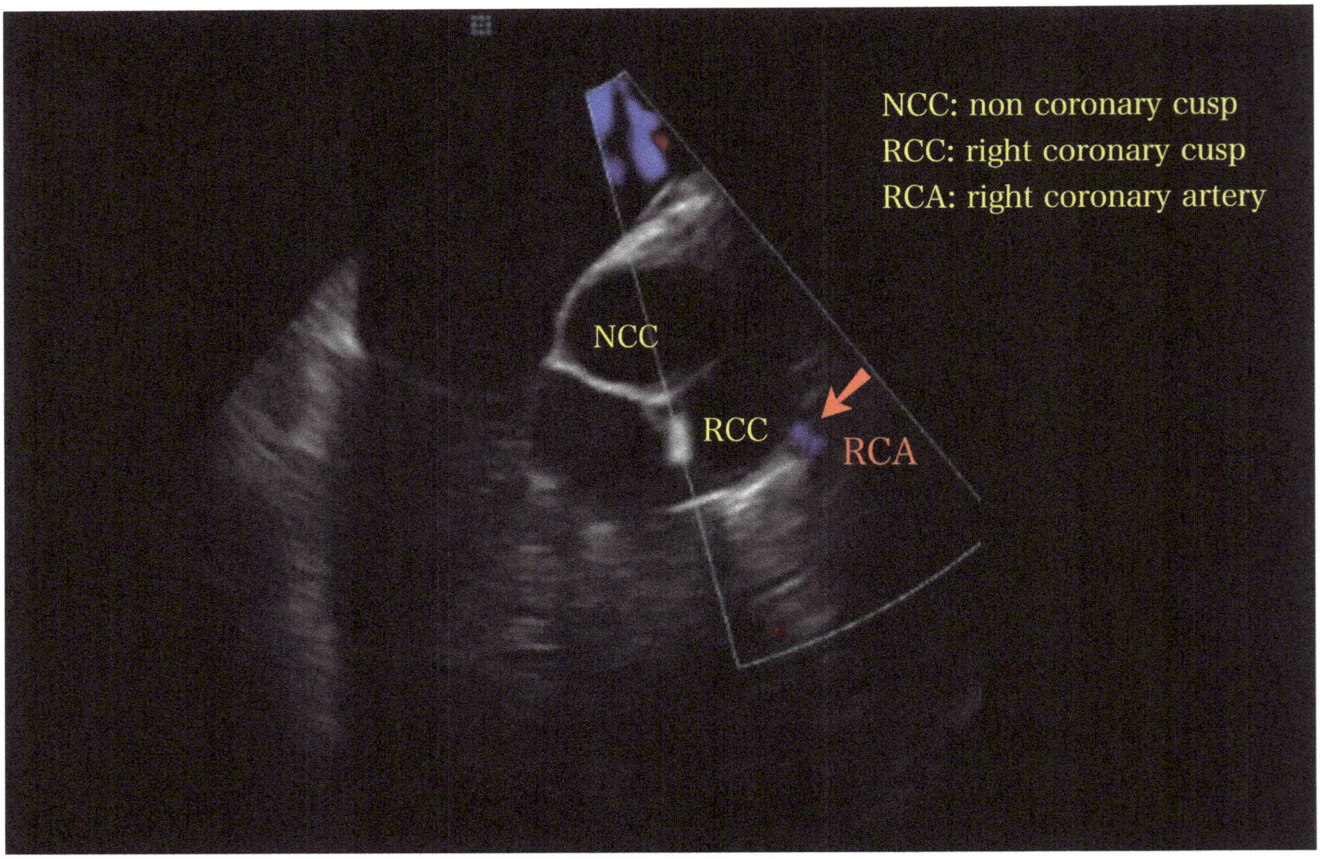

Figure 16.5 ICE image with color Doppler demonstrating arterial flow.

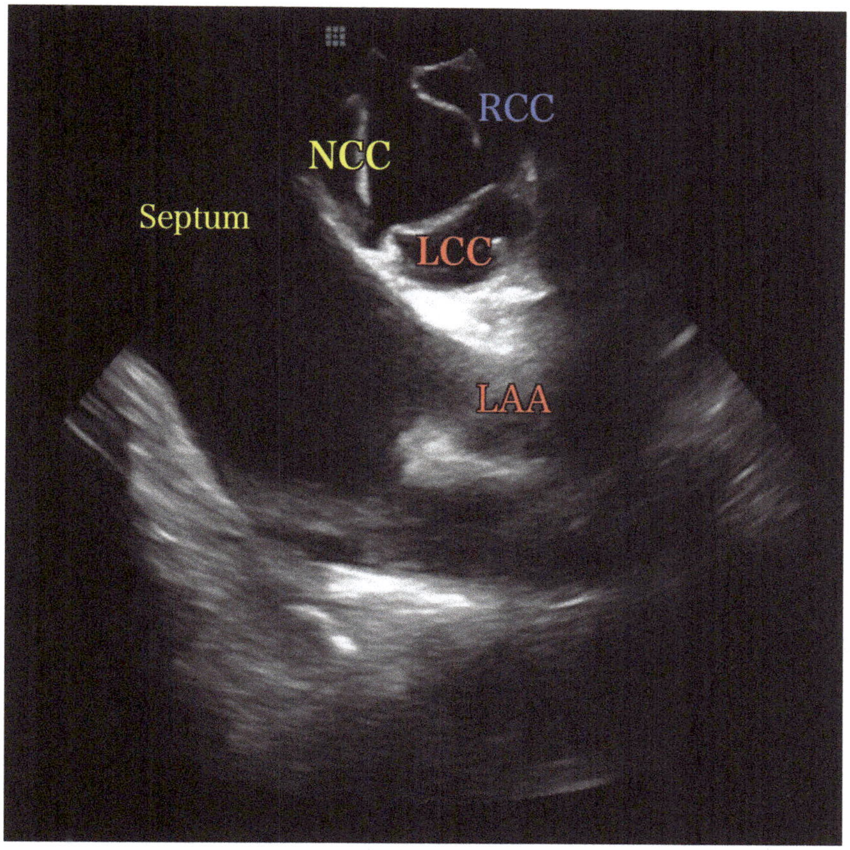

Figure 16.6 The short axis of the coronary cusps visualized from the right ventricle.

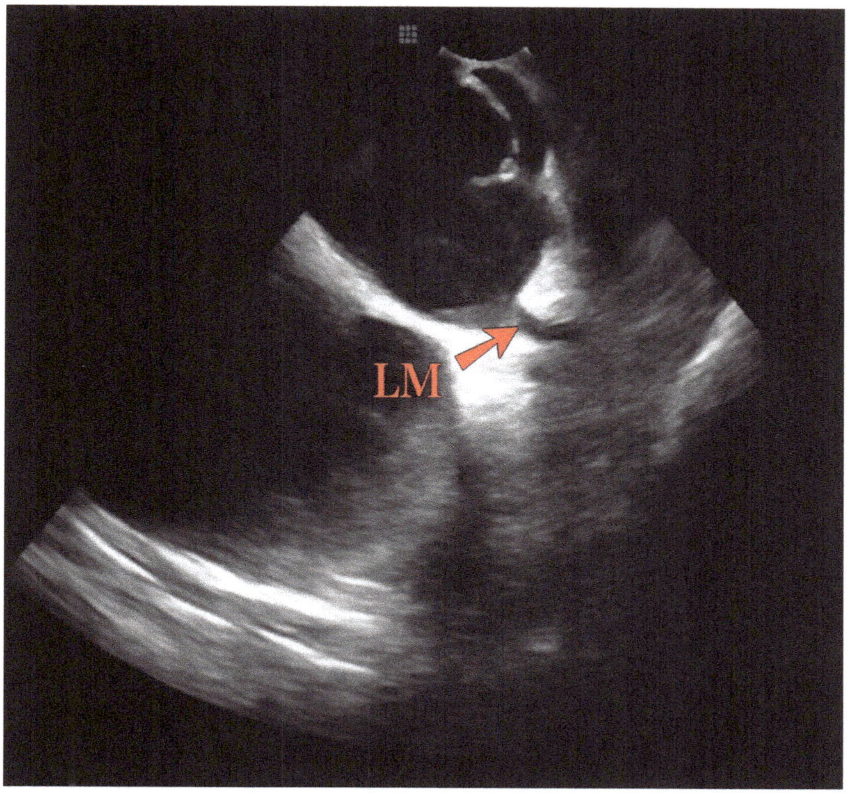

Figure 16.7 Short-axis ICE view of the left main and left coronary cusp.

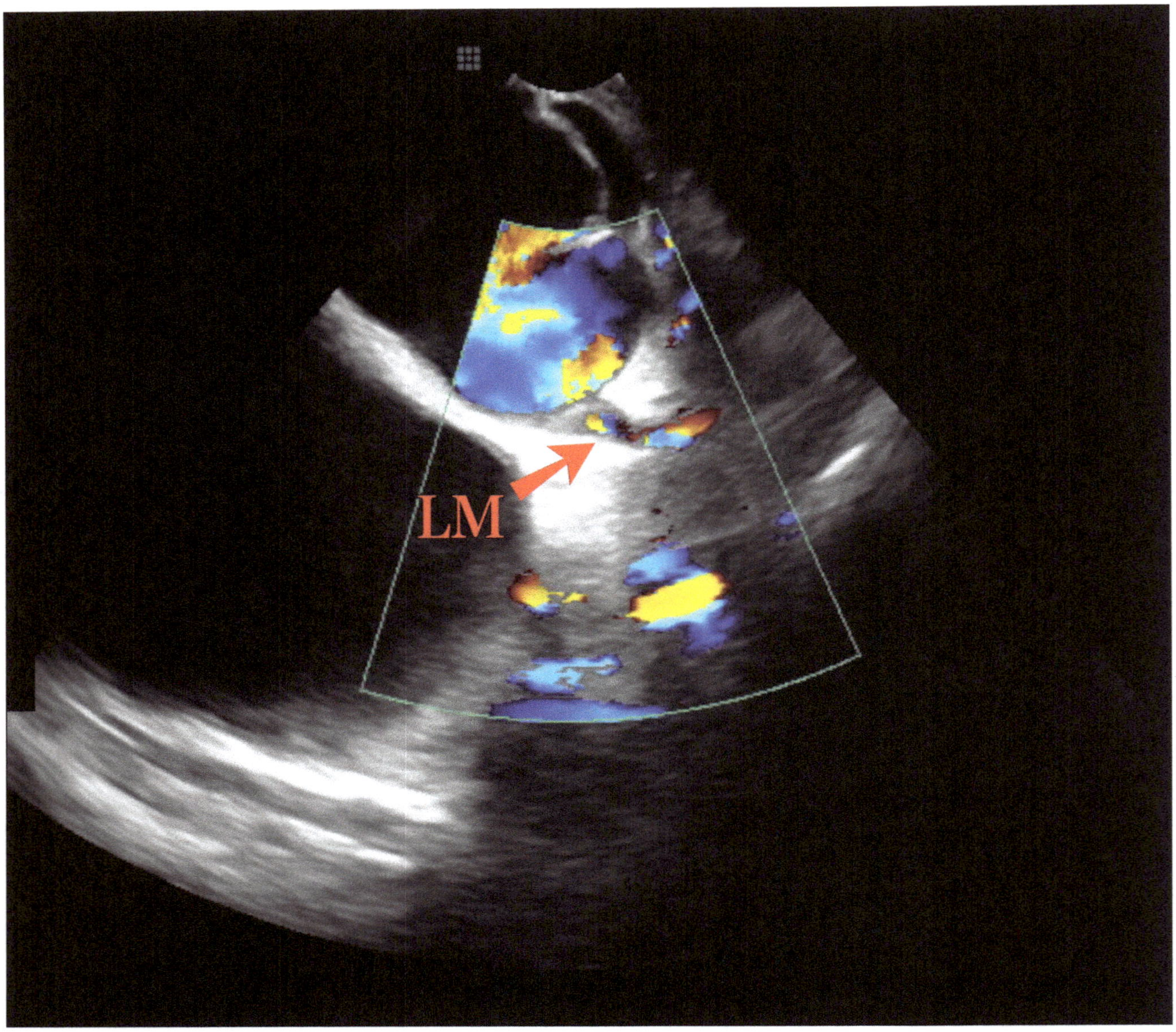

Figure 16.8 Color Doppler in short-axis ICE view of coronary cusps from RV to define coronary arteries.

Challenges

I have found that vascular tortuosity remains the most frequent challenge to non-fluoroscopic ablation in almost any setting. Patience is required as well as humility. This is true especially during the learning curve of fluoroscopy-free procedures. If occasional use of fluoroscopy is needed during the learning curve, this is not a failure but rather a learning opportunity. Long sheaths placed over long wires can help avoid difficulty in this regard for both ICE catheters as well as other steerable catheters. Response to tactile resistance is important to cultivate. A gentle and responsive demeanor can help avoid issues. Once catheters are placed within the heart, visualization with ICE and 3D mapping systems provides a plethora of real time electroanatomic and echocardiographic data that should be used in a complementary fashion. The operator is challenged to utilize both equally to confirm location and adequate positioning.

Conclusion

Fluoroscopy-free ablation within the coronary cusps is safe and effective. Excellent ICE imaging and familiarity with anatomy is key for success. Patience and integration of ICE and 3D mapping systems remains success.

References

1. Morady F, Kadish AH, DiCarlo L, et al. Long-term results of catheter ablation of idiopathic right ventricular tachycardia. *Circulation*.1990;82:2093–2099.
2. Coggins DL, Lee RJ, Sweeney J, et al. Radiofrequency catheter ablation as a cure for idiopathic tachycardia of both left and right ventricular origin. *J Am Coll Cardiol.* 1994;23:1333–1341.
3. Pedersen CT, Kay GN, Kalman J, et al. EHRA/HRS/APHRS expert consensus on ventricular arrhythmias. *Heart Rhythm.* 2014;11:e166–e196.

Video Legends

Video 16.1 Phased-array ICE used view and aid in ablation catheter navigating up the femoral artery and into the iliac and aorta retrograde through the arterial system. [00:03]

Video 16.2 ICE advanced within the venous system to visualize the ablation catheter. [00:03]

Video 16.3 ICE advanced within the venous system to visualize the ablation catheter. [00:03]

Video 16.4 The ICE catheter is placed into the SVC and directed toward the ascending aorta and follows the ablation catheter back down toward the cusps. [00:03]

Video 16.5 Rotation of the phased-array ICE catheter counter clockwise or rightward will bring the NCC and RCC into view. [00:02]

Video 16.6 The left coronary cusp will be located to the left of the RCC. Clockwise rotation of the ICE catheter will bring the LCC into view. [00:03]

Video 16.7 Color Doppler on ICE can be used to determine the location of ostium of the major coronary arteries in order to avoid injury to these structures. [00:03]

Video 16S Chapter summary and step-by-step procedures by Mansour Razminia. [5:29]

17

How to Perform Ablation of Premature Ventricular Complexes Originating from the Left Ventricular Outflow Tract Using No Fluoroscopy

Nicholas J. Costa, MD; Jim W. Cheung, MD

Introduction

The left ventricular outflow tract (LVOT) and its surrounding structures are a major source of both idiopathic and scar-mediated ventricular arrhythmias (VAs). It is estimated that nearly one-third of all VAs and 70% of left VAs occurring in structurally normal hearts originate from the LVOT.[1] Catheter ablation has been a mainstay of therapy for these arrhythmias, with success rates reaching over 90%. Typically, these procedures are performed under fluoroscopic guidance to position catheters for mapping and ablation, which expose both patients and staff to significant doses of radiation. One study estimated an average of 36 minutes of fluoroscopy exposure time during a typical ventricular tachycardia ablation, resulting in a dose area product of nearly 14,000 cGy/cm^2, which is associated with an estimated lifetime attributable cancer risk of 0.28% to an exposed patient.[2] Furthermore, operating staff usually wear lead aprons to reduce radiation exposure, which places stress on the spine and can lead to back injury and disability. Nearly 50% of cardiologists and radiologists wearing radiation protection during procedures reported back pain, in comparison to the estimated 28% of Americans who have chronic back pain.[3]

In the modern electrophysiology (EP) laboratory, a growing number of tools are available to enable ablation procedures to be performed without the aid of fluoroscopy. These techniques were initially used for right-sided ablation procedures but are now becoming common in left-sided procedures such as pulmonary vein isolation and ablation of VAs. Moreover, adoption of a proper mindset is critical to successful near-zero-fluoroscopy ablation. In this chapter, the authors briefly review LVOT arrhythmias and discuss their approach for mapping and ablating these arrhythmias with zero or minimal use of fluoroscopy.

Anatomy of the Left Ventricular Outflow Tract

The LVOT is a complex anatomical structure with critical implications for mapping and ablation of VAs. It is centrally located within the heart and bounded superiorly by the aortic valve leaflets (**Figure 17.1**). The left coronary aortic valve leaflet is situated most superiorly, while the right coronary leaflet is more anterior and inferior, and the non-coronary aortic valve leaflet is located most inferiorly. The insertion of the aortic leaflets is semilunar in shape, creating triangular extensions of aortic root between the leaflets. The left ventricular ostium (os) is covered by a fibrous membrane through which the aorta and mitral valve extend, known as the aortoventricular membrane.[4] In contrast to the right ventricular outflow tract (RVOT), the LVOT is comprised of both muscular and fibrous regions.[5] The anteroseptal region is comprised of myocardium but also includes the membranous portion

Fluoroscopy Reduction Techniques for Catheter Ablation of Cardiac Arrhythmias. © 2019 Mansour Razminia, Paul C. Zei, eds.
Cardiotext Publishing, ISBN: 978-1-942909-30-9.

of the ventricular septum.[1] The posterior border of the LVOT consists of fibrous tissue that is continuous with the aortomitral continuity (AMC), a fibrous structure with small regions of ventricular myocardium in contact with the left fibrous trigone. The lateral LVOT consists of myocardium and is continuous with the superior border of the left ventricle (LV) in a region known as the left ventricular summit. The LV summit is bounded anteriorly by the left anterior descending artery (LAD) and laterally by the left circumflex artery. It is divided into 2 regions by the great cardiac vein: (1) an inferior region that is more accessible and amenable to catheter ablation via an epicardial approach, and (2) a superior, more inaccessible region lying in close proximity to the proximal portions of the LAD and left circumflex arteries and covered by epicardial fat.[6]

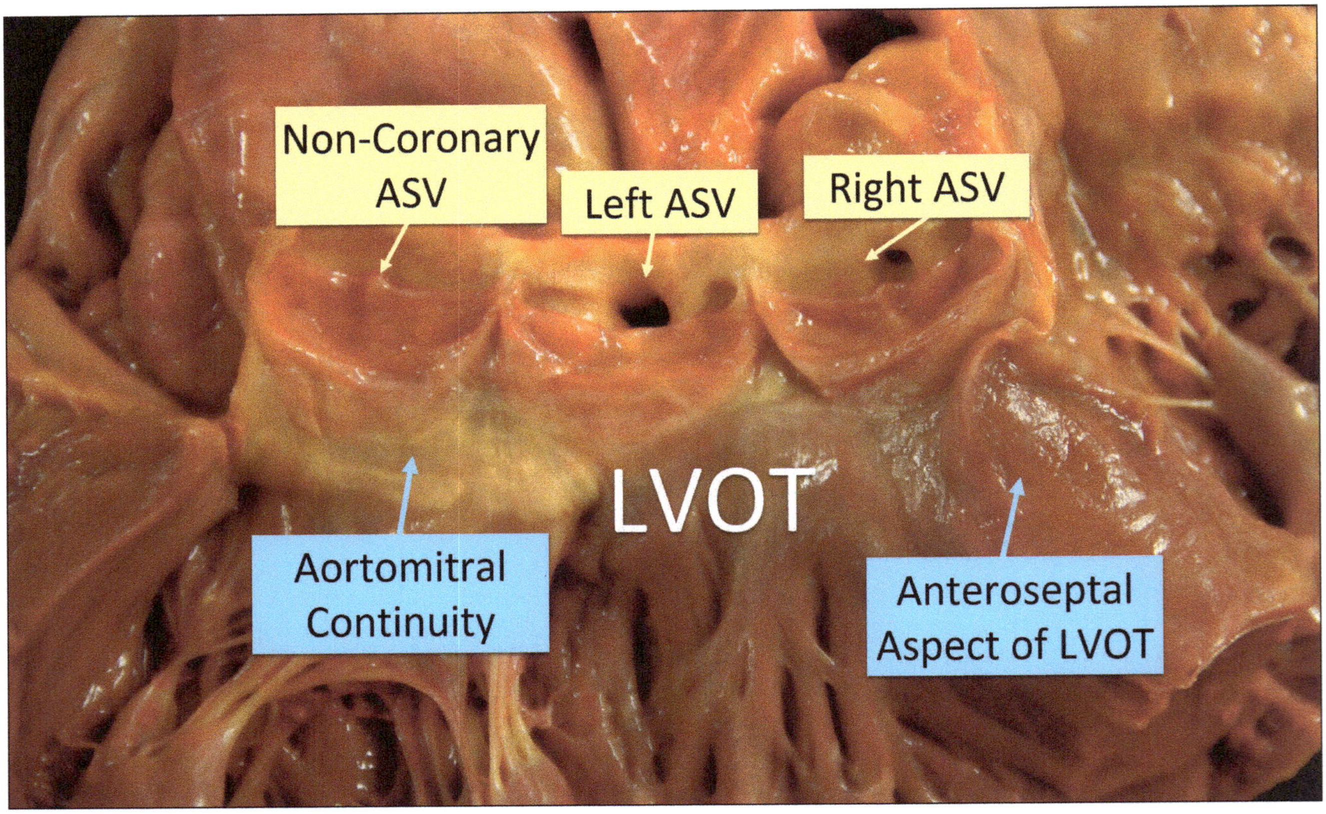

Figure 17.1 Anatomy of the LVOT. Gross anatomy of the LVOT is shown with dissection performed along the aortic root bisecting the right and non-coronary aortic sinuses of Valsalva. The left- and non-coronary aortic sinuses are continuous with the aortomitral continuity which forms the fibrous posterior aspect of the LVOT. The anteroseptal aspect of the LVOT is thicker and is comprised of muscular tissue. ASV: aortic sinus of Valsalva; LVOT: left ventricular outflow tract.

Arrhythmias Arising from the Left Ventricular Outflow Tract

The structural characteristics of each LVOT region generate variability in the incidence of associated arrhythmias. The left coronary aortic sinus of Valsalva (ASV), the right coronary ASV, and the junction between these 2 aortic leaflets are common sources of aortic root arrhythmias.[4] Idiopathic and scar-mediated VAs originating from the AMC have been described.[7] Small sleeves of myocardium within the fibrous tissue in the AMC have been demonstrated as sources of ventricular arrhythmias.[8] It is estimated that 8–11% of left ventricular ostial VAs arise from this region.[4,6] The LV summit is the most common site of idiopathic epicardial VAs originating from the LV.[6] LV summit VAs present a particular challenge for catheter-based ablation due to difficulty in accessing the region in addition to safety concerns given the proximity of the region to the coronary arteries. Multiple approaches are available to target these arrhythmias, which include endocardial ablation, ablation within the coronary venous system and its branches, and epicardial ablation via a percutaneous or surgical approach.[9] Careful mapping of the region and annotation of the coronary arteries and surrounding structures are necessary to safely perform ablation in this region, which has implications for a minimal-fluoroscopy approach. While ablation is ideally performed at the site of earliest VA activation, proximity to a coronary artery or inaccessibility with a catheter may require ablation at remote sites by the left coronary ASV, LV endocardium, or septal RVOT.[9] Finally, while the majority of LVOT VAs are idiopathic, reentrant arrhythmias arising from periaortic scar tissue have also been described.[10] Although patients with these arrhythmias do not have evidence of overt structural heart disease, they have multiple inducible morphologies of VT. Due to the presence of more extensive abnormal substrate as well as possible intramural sources of VAs in these cases, outcomes after ablation are generally less favorable when compared to ablation of idiopathic LVOT VAs.

Zero-Fluoroscopy Approach: Delineation of Left Ventricular Outflow Tract Anatomy

A critical part of a zero-fluoroscopy approach to the mapping and ablation of any arrhythmia is an accurate delineation of the anatomy of interest using appropriate imaging modalities. We have found intracardiac echocardiography (ICE), when used in concert with electroanatomic mapping, to be an indispensable part of non-fluoroscopic ablation. Imaging with ICE can be used to guide transseptal access, track catheter positioning, and monitor for complications. Furthermore, the use of the CARTOSOUND module (Biosense Webster, Irvine, CA) allows creation of 3D ICE-generated contours of cardiac structures that can be fully integrated into the electroanatomic map. The authors use an 8-Fr phased-array ICE catheter (SOUNDSTAR, Biosense Webster). There are several ICE views that are critical for zero-fluoroscopy mapping and ablation of LVOT VAs. First, the individual ASV should be readily identified and traced on the electroanatomic map (**Figure 17.2**A). From the home view, the ICE catheter is deflected anteriorly and advanced into the RV. Clockwise rotation is then applied until the aortic and pulmonic valves are visualized. With slight withdrawal and torque adjustment, the ICE catheter can be positioned to center the aortic valve in short axis. Furthermore, from this view, adjustments can be made to visualize the os of the left main coronary artery and the proximal left anterior descending artery (Figure 17.2B and C). Further clockwise rotation will visualize the aortic root in long axis and can demonstrate the os of the right coronary artery. Slight counterclockwise rotation from the view of the aortic valve allows visualization of the anterior LVOT and AMC (Figure 17.2D). With these views, all of the relevant structures abutting the LVOT including the pulmonary valve leaflets and RVOT can be traced and annotated on the electroanatomic map (Figure 17.2E).

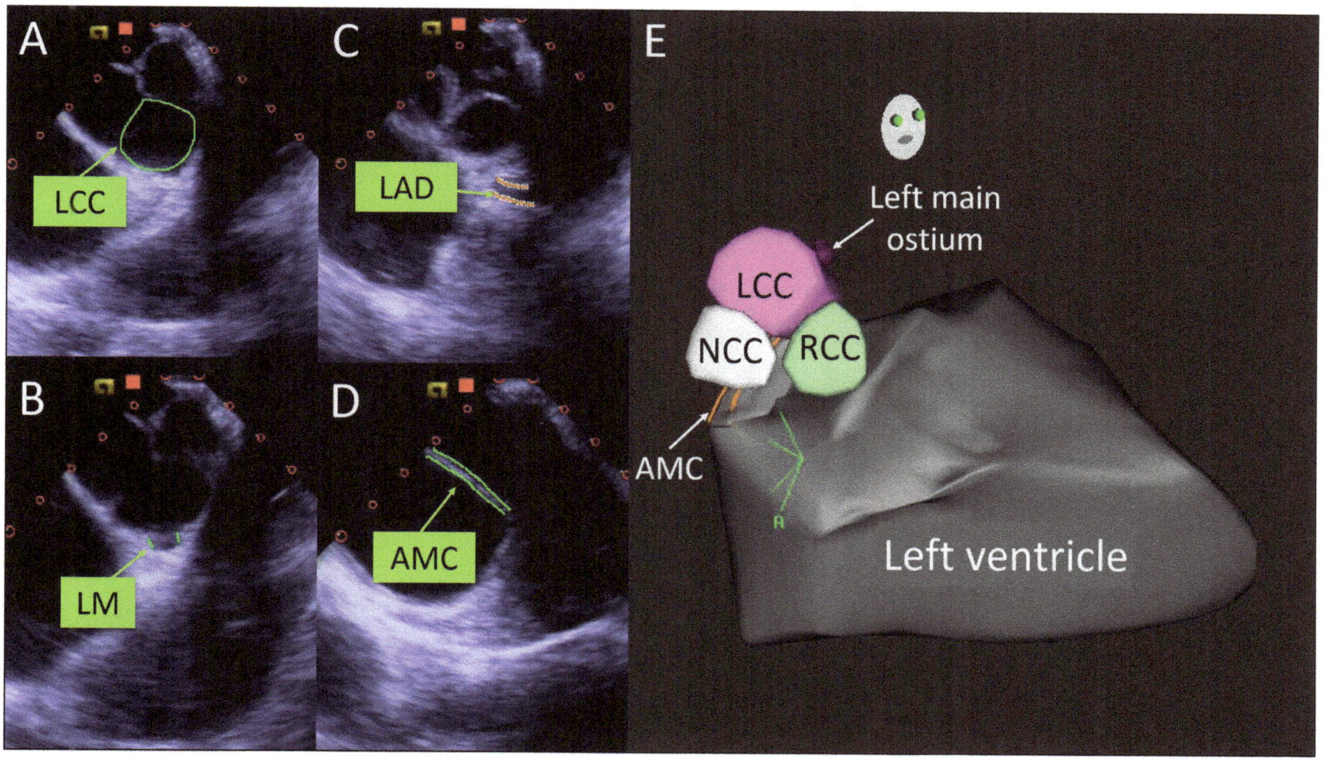

Figure 17.2 Integration of ICE imaging of the LVOT with 3D electroanatomic mapping. ICE images of the components of the LVOT are traced in **green**: **A:** Left coronary aortic sinus of Valsalva. **B:** Ostium of the left main artery. **C:** Proximal left anterior descending artery. **D:** Aortomitral continuity. **E:** ICE-generated contours of the LVOT are integrated into the electroanatomic mapping system (RAO cranial view). The left main ostium is tagged in **purple** and the aortomitral continuity is outlined in **orange**. AMC: aortomitral continuity; LAD: left anterior descending artery; LCC: left coronary cusp; LM: left main artery; NCC: non-coronary cusp; RCC: right coronary cusp.

Once a complete anatomy of the LVOT has been created with ICE, a mapping catheter may be readily advanced into the region and additional anatomy can be added to the existing ICE-generated map. However, it is critical at this juncture to plan what kind of approach will be used to access the LVOT region. Achieving catheter access to the LVOT for mapping and ablation is typically achieved using at least one of the following four methods: (1) retrograde transaortic approach via femoral arterial access, (2) transseptal approach via femoral venous access, (3) epicardial approach via coronary venous access, and (4) epicardial approach via subxiphoid percutaneous access. With appropriate tools and planning, most of these approaches can be performed with minimal or no use of fluoroscopy.

Approach to the LVOT via Retrograde Transaortic Access

Catheter advancement retrogradely through the aortic valve via femoral arterial access offers a direct approach to the LVOT. To start, we always use ultrasound guidance for both arterial and venous access to minimize the risk of groin complications.[11] This also obviates the need for fluoroscopy to confirm vascular access guidewire position. Once arterial access is obtained, a long sheath is placed in the aorta to minimize the risk of catheter-induced aortic plaque embolization. Using ICE, the aortic root and ascending aorta can be imaged through several views and allow confirmation of guidewire placement (**Figures 17.3**A and B). As the ablation catheter is advanced through the long sheath to the ascending aorta and the aortic root, its position can be tracked using the electroanatomic mapping system. Moreover, if a cardiac computed tomography scan is available, an ICE view of the aortic root cutting across the ASV may be used to integrate a CT image of the aortic root into the electroanatomic map (Figure 17.3C). After prolapsing the ablation catheter across the aortic valve into the left ventricle, one can use the ICE contours of the ASV as a marker of the aortic valve plane. Knowledge of the location of the aortic valve plane can help prevent inadvertent withdrawal of the ablation catheter back into the aortic root. Repetitive unnecessary movement of the ablation catheter through the aortic valve leaflets can lead to embolization of aortic valve debris as well as aortic valve damage.

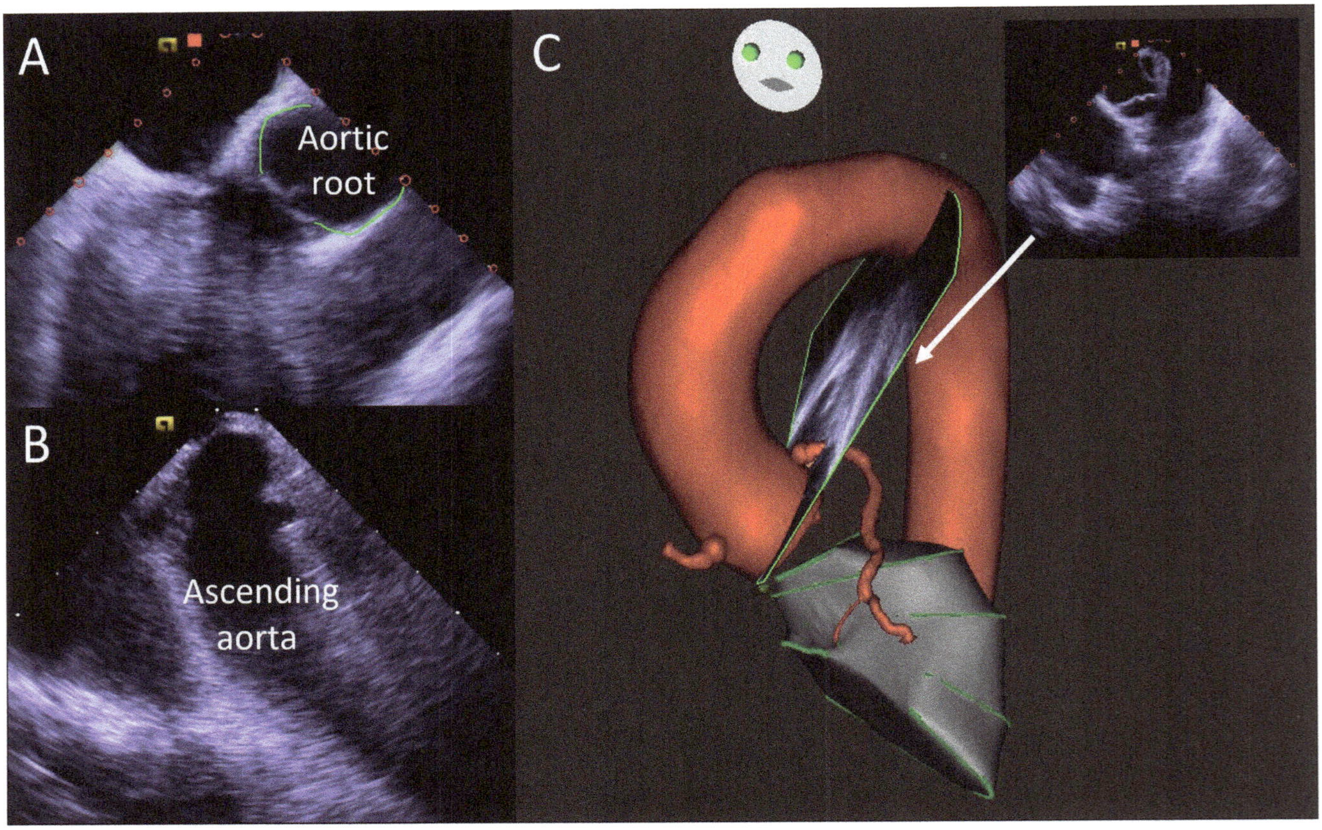

Figure 17.3 Use of integrated intracardiac echocardiographic (ICE) and computed tomographic (CT) imaging to faciliate retrograde transaortic access to the LVOT. **A:** With the ICE probe in the right atrium, the aortic root is traced in **green**. **B:** With the ICE probe in the right ventricle, a long-axis view of the ascending aorta can be obtained. Of note, the ostium of the right coronary artery can also be seen. **C:** With ICE localization of the aortic root cutting through the aortic sinuses of Valsalva (**inset**), a CT scan of the aortic root can be integrated into the electroanatomic map (LAO cranial view). RCA: right coronary artery.

One of the advantages of using the retrograde transaortic approach to the LVOT is that catheter manipulation is usually straightforward and most regions of the LVOT can be reached with little effort. Compared to an anterograde transseptal approach, contact force achieved by a retrograde approach is significantly higher in the basal anteroseptum.[12] However, it should be noted that for some cases, a combined transseptal and transaortic approach may be necessary for optimal mapping of all regions of the LVOT.[13] If using a manual approach, we typically use a contact force-sensing catheter in order to ensure adequate contact and stability to achieve good lesion depth during ablation. This is especially important when targeting epicardial LV summit arrhythmias using an endocardial approach where deep lesions are required. There are potential disadvantages with using a retrograde transaortic approach to LVOT VA ablation. The region of the LVOT directly below the aortic valve leaflets may sometimes be inaccessible to an ablation catheter positioned retrogradely across the aortic valve.[1] In addition, femoral arterial access can increase the risk of groin hematoma, pseudoaneurysm, or arteriovenous fistula formation. Moreover, aortic instrumentation can lead to embolization of clot and plaque. A significant rate (58%) of magnetic resonance imaging-detected silent cerebral emboli was identified in a small series of patients undergoing ablation of left VAs.[14] In all of the cases in that study where cerebral emboli were detected, the retrograde transaortic approach was used. These risks should be considered whether or not a non-fluoroscopic approach is used, given that fluoroscopy alone is unlikely to help decrease the risks of the aforementioned complications.

Approach to the LVOT via Anterograde Transseptal Access

For most LVOT VAs, a transseptal approach yields adequate access for mapping and ablation. In particular, excellent contact force can be achieved with an ablation catheter positioned in the anterior wall of the LVOT using a transseptal approach.[12] An anterograde transseptal approach with a "reversed S-curve" catheter orientation as described by Ouyang and colleagues permits thorough mapping of the LVOT directly below the aortic valve leaflets, which as mentioned earlier, may be inaccessible using a retrograde approach.[1] With the use of ICE, transseptal puncture can be achieved safely and readily without fluoroscopy. The authors favor a more anteriorly and inferiorly directed transseptal puncture (with visualization of the left atrial appendage on the ICE viewing plane) to facilitate catheter manipulation into the LV. Advantages of the transseptal approach include avoidance of femoral arterial puncture and aortic instrumentation. Given the ease of ICE-guided transseptal access, this approach is particularly suitable for non-fluoroscopic mapping and ablation. For these reasons, anterograde transseptal access is a first-line approach in our lab for mapping and ablation of LVOT arrhythmias. An example of an LVOT VA ablated successfully using a transseptal approach with ICE guidance without fluoroscopy is shown in **Figure 17.4**.

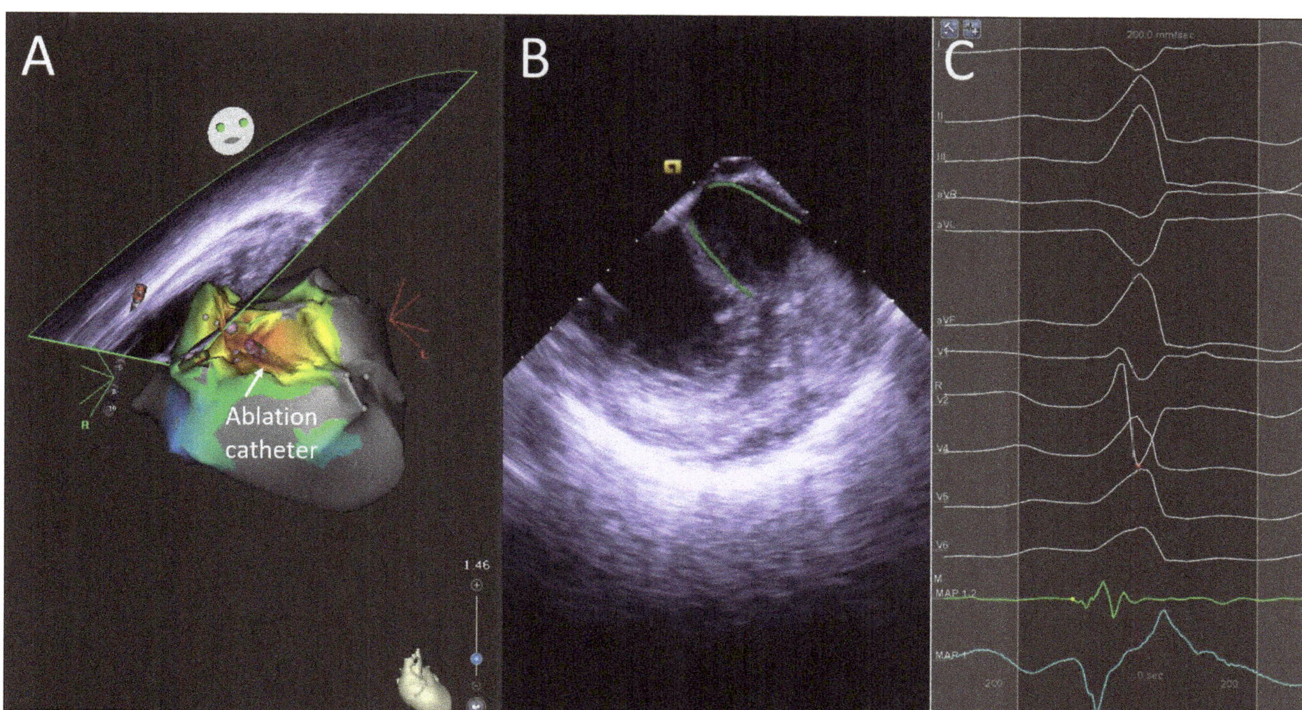

Figure 17.4 Catheter ablation of the LVOT premature ventricular complex (PVC) with zero-fluoroscopy via transseptal approach. **A:** Electroanatomic map of the aortic root from a shallow RAO projection with the His catheter visualized. The viewing sector of intracardiac echocardiography in relation to the map is shown. **B:** The ICE image of the aortic root corresponding to the view in panel A.

Approach to the LVOT via Coronary Venous Access

Mapping and ablation from within the coronary venous system is frequently required for arrhythmias originating from the left ventricular summit, which may be targeted via the great cardiac and anterior interventricular veins. Using electrogram and electroanatomic map guidance, the coronary sinus (CS) can be accessed without using fluoroscopy. A navigation-enabled catheter is advanced to the right atrium, deflected into the right ventricle, and then slowly withdrawn with clockwise torque until it enters the coronary sinus. With the additional use of ICE guidance, CS access is even more straightforward. From a home view, the CS ostium (os) is located using slight clockwise rotation of the ICE catheter, and the os is annotated to provide a visual guide for catheter positioning. Once coronary venous access is obtained, the ablation catheter can often be readily advanced to the junction of the great cardiac vein and anterior interventricular vein. However, depending on the angle of catheter entry into the CS and coronary venous caliber, catheter manipulation can be challenging. If using a manual approach, care must be taken to avoid coronary venous perforation and dissection by careful monitoring of catheter position and contact force. Venography of the coronary venous system may be necessary if difficulty is encountered during catheter advancement into distal coronary sinus.[9] Moreover, mapping of smaller communicating branches of the coronary venous system may be necessary to determine the optimal site of ablation of LV summit arrhythmias.[15] One study used a 2-Fr mapping catheter directed into the communicating vein at the LV summit with CS venogram guidance to identify the site of earliest VA activation. Using the catheter position as a landmark, successful ablation of LV summit VAs via adjacent structures was achieved in 71% of cases. There are currently no data on the use of this technique without fluoroscopy. Using the EnSite NavX mapping system (Abbott, Abbott Park, IL), mapping within smaller branches of the coronary venous system can be feasible using the Vision Wire (Biotronik GmbH, Berlin, Germany). The 0.014-inch guidewire has a polyethylene coating covering all but the distal 15 mm and proximal 30 mm. The proximal tip of the wire can be connected to a recording system using an alligator clamp, enabling recording of unipolar electrograms from the distal tip within the coronary sinus. This technique has been described for mapping the coronary sinus in order to position a coronary sinus lead, but its applicability for mapping of ventricular arrhythmias without fluoroscopy remains to be determined.[16,17]

Approach to the LVOT via Percutaneous Epicardial Access

Some epicardial LVOT arrhythmias arising from the LV summit may require approach from the epicardium due to anatomical constraints from the endocardial surface and within the coronary venous system. Epicardial access for mapping and ablation of ventricular tachycardias was first described by Sosa et al. in 1996.[18] There are currently no data on the use of a zero-fluoroscopy approach to epicardial access. Typically, fluoroscopy is used to allow proper guidance of the needle on its trajectory using an anterior or posterior approach. Although ultrasound-guided pericardiocentesis has been performed with high procedural success and few complications,[19] the absence of an echolucent space of fluid to target during access makes this difficult to achieve. An epicardial access needle with real-time pressure monitoring has recently been evaluated,[20] and its use may reduce complications and radiation exposure. Whether or not this technology can allow safe, non-fluoroscopic epicardial access remains to be determined. Although epicardial mapping is straightforward without fluoroscopy, once epicardial access is obtained, fluoroscopic assessment of the coronary arteries prior to ablation is necessary to avoid iatrogenic coronary injury. Once coronary arterial anatomy has been obtained, use of coronary angiography integration into the electroanatomic mapping system with software such as CARTOUNIVU (Biosense Webster) can eliminate the need for further fluoroscopy during ablation.

Remote Magnetic Navigation and Zero-Fluoroscopy Approach

In our experience, remote magnetic navigation (RMN) guidance can greatly facilitate non-fluoroscopic mapping and ablation, especially for regions such as the LVOT. Using the Stereotaxis Niobe ES magnetic navigation system (Stereotaxis, St. Louis, MO), catheter manipulation to the LVOT via transseptal access is straightforward. Whereas a reverse S-curve has to be created with a manual catheter to allow access to the LVOT, the flexibility of the RMN ablation catheter permits advancement into the area with 0.08–0.1 Tesla magnetic field strength. After an initial downward vector to direct the catheter towards the left ventricular apex, a subsequent upward vector towards the septal aspect of the LVOT with slight catheter withdrawal will readily direct the catheter right under the aortic valve leaflets (**Figure 17.5**). Despite the lack of contact force information from the catheter, the risk of mechanical perforation with RMN mapping is virtually zero. RMN has been shown to substantially reduce fluoroscopy use in ablation of atrial fibrillation,[21] right ventricular outflow tract tachycardia,[22] papillary muscle VA[23] and other ventricular arrhythmias.[24] The flexibility of the RMN catheter is also helpful for navigating the coronary venous system and can readily target arrhythmias arising by the distal great cardiac vein–anterior interventricular vein junction.[25]

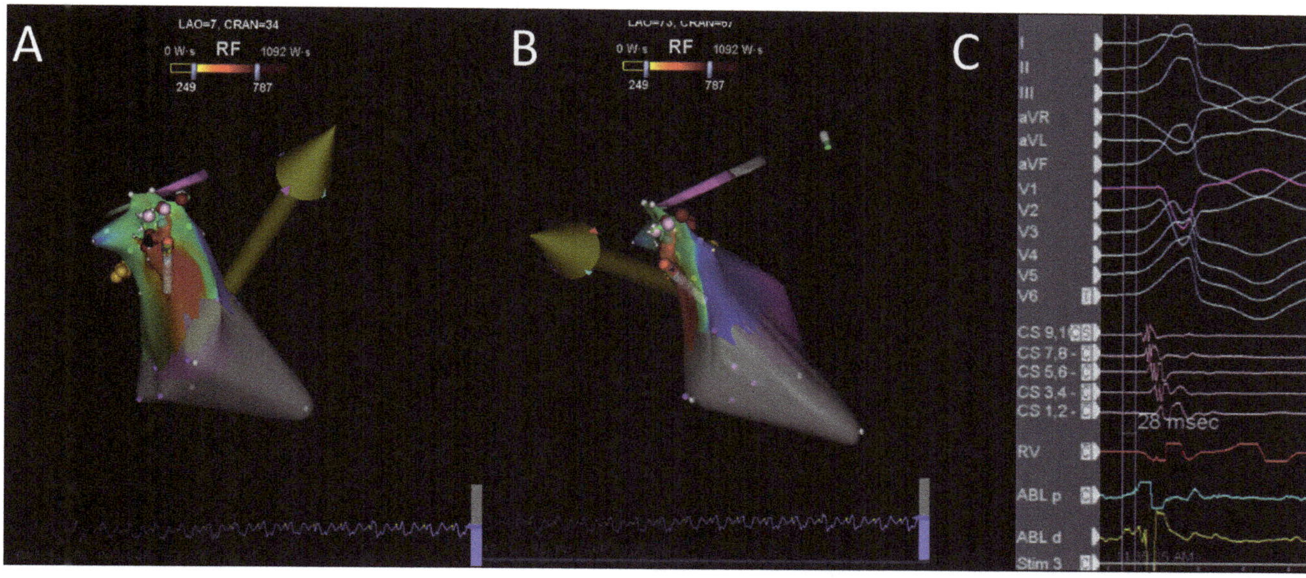

Figure 17.5 Remote magnetic navigation-guided catheter manipulation to the LVOT. Electroanatomic map showing activation timing of a premature ventricular complex (PVC) mapped to the LVOT inferior to the commissure between the left and right coronary cusps. The ablation catheter is positioned at the site of the earliest PVC activation with an upward and anterior RMN vector with shallow LAO an steep LAO views shown in **A** and **B**, respectively. **C:** 12-lead electrocardiogram and intracardiac electrograms showing onset of ablation catheter electrogram preceding the onset of the PVC QRS complex by 28 ms. CS: coronary sinus; RV: right ventricle; ABL p: proximal ablation catheter; ABL d: distal ablation catheter.

Caveats to the Zero-Fluoroscopy Approach to the LVOT

Mapping and ablation of LVOT VAs without fluoroscopy is achievable in most situations, but there are cases in which fluoroscopy remains necessary to adequately and safely guide catheter ablation. Modest use of fluoroscopy may be necessary to visualize a guidewire that does not advance smoothly, safely navigate implanted device leads, guide epicardial access and wire placement, or visualize coronary artery anatomy. For this reason, we maintain availability of fluoroscopy in all procedures and use it in conjunction with non-fluoroscopic methods when needed. With judicious selection of frame rate and appropriate collimation, very low exposure rates are achievable.

Conclusion

The LVOT is a common source of VAs that are readily treated with catheter ablation. In most cases, these procedures can be performed using a zero-fluoroscopy approach that eliminates radiation exposure to the patient and staff and obviates the need for heavy personal protective gear. Use of appropriate tools such as electroanatomic mapping and ICE, together with a mindset to reduce radiation exposure to an as-low-as-reasonably-achievable (ALARA) goal, permits successful zero-fluoroscopy mapping and ablation of LVOT VAs with excellent efficacy and safety.

References

1. Ouyang F, Mathew S, Wu S, et al. Ventricular arrhythmias arising from the left ventricular outflow tract below the aortic sinus cusps: Mapping and catheter ablation via transseptal approach and electrocardiographic characteristics. *Circulation: Arrhythm Electrophysiol.* 2014;7:445–455.
2. Casella M, Dello Russo A, Russo E, et al. X-ray exposure in cardiac electrophysiology: A retrospective analysis in 8150 patients over 7 years of activity in a modern, large-volume laboratory. *J Am Heart Assoc.* 2018;7:e008233.
3. Klein LW, Miller DL, Balter S, et al. Occupational health hazards in the interventional laboratory: Time for a safer environment. *Radiology.* 2009;250:538–544.
4. Yamada T, Litovsky SH, Kay GN. The left ventricular ostium: An anatomic concept relevant to idiopathic ventricular arrhythmias. *Circulation: Arrhythm Electrophysiol.* 2008;1:396–404.
5. Heeger C-H, Hayashi K, Kuck K-H, Ouyang F. Catheter ablation of idiopathic ventricular arrhythmias arising from the cardiac outflow tracts—recent insights and techniques for the successful treatment of common and challenging cases. *Circulation.* 2016;80:1073–1086.
6. Yamada T, McElderry HT, Doppalapudi H, et al. Idiopathic ventricular arrhythmias originating from the left ventricular summit: Anatomic concepts relevant to ablation. *Circ Arrhythm Electrophysiol.* 2010;3:616–623.
7. Steven D, Roberts-Thomson KC, Seiler J, et al. Ventricular tachycardia arising from the aortomitral continuity in structural heart disease: Characteristics and therapeutic considerations for an anatomically challenging area of origin. *Circ Arrhythm Electrophysiol.* 2009;2:660–666.

8. Kumagai K, Fukuda K, Wakayama Y, et al. Electrocardiographic characteristics of the variants of idiopathic left ventricular outflow tract ventricular tachyarrhythmias. *J Cardiovasc Electrophysiol.* 2008; 19(5):495–501.
9. Enriquez A, Malavassi F, Saenz Luis C, et al. How to map and ablate left ventricular summit arrhythmias. *Heart Rhythm.* 2017;14:141–148.
10. Nagashima K, Tedrow UB, Koplan BA, et al. Reentrant ventricular tachycardia originating from the periaortic region in the absence of overt structural heart disease. *Circ Arrhythm Electrophysiol.* 2013;7:99–106.
11. Sobolev M, Shiloh AL, Di Biase L, Slovut DP. Ultrasound-guided cannulation of the femoral vein in electrophysiological procedures: A systematic review and meta-analysis. *Europace.* 2017;19(5):850–855.
12. Tilz RR, Makimoto H, Lin T, et al. In vivo left-ventricular contact force analysis: Comparison of antegrade transseptal with retrograde transaortic mapping strategies and correlation of impedance and electrical amplitude with contact force. *Europace.* 2014;16:1387–1395.
13. Mizuno H, Vergara P, Maccabelli G, et al. Contact force monitoring for cardiac mapping in patients with ventricular tachycardia. *J Cardiovasc Electrophysiol.* 2013;24:519–524.
14. Whitman IR, Gladstone RA, Badhwar N, et al. Brain emboli after left ventricular endocardial ablation: Clinical perspective. *Circulation.* 2017;135:867–877.
15. Komatsu Y, Nogami A, Shinoda Y, et al. Idiopathic ventricular arrhythmias originating from the vicinity of the communicating vein of cardiac venous systems at the left ventricular summit. *Circ Arrhythm Electrophysiol.* 2018;11: e005386.
16. Cock CC, Res JCJ, Hendriks ML, Allaart CP. Usefulness of a pacing guidewire to facilitate left ventricular lead implantation in cardiac resynchronization therapy. *Pacing Clin Electrophysiol.* 2009;32:446–449.
17. Mafi RM, Blaauw Y, Dinh T, et al. Left ventricular lead placement in the latest activated region guided by coronary venous electroanatomic mapping. *Europace.* 2014;17:84–93.
18. Sosa E, Scanavacca M, D'Avila A, Pilleggi E. A new technique to perform epicardial mapping in the electrophysiology laboratory. *J Cardiovasc Electrophysiol.* 1996;7:531–536.
19. Tsang TSM, Enriquez-Sarano M, Freeman WK, et al. Consecutive 1127 therapeutic echocardiographically guided pericardiocenteses: Clinical profile, practice patterns, and outcomes spanning 21 years. *Mayo Clinic Proc.* 2002;77:429–436.
20. Di Biase L, Burkhardt JD, Reddy V, et al. Initial international multicenter human experience with a novel epicardial access needle embedded with a real-time pressure/frequency monitoring to facilitate epicardial access: Feasibility and safety. *Heart Rhythm.* 2017;14(7):981–988.
21. Adragão PP, Cavaco D, Ferreira AM, et al. Safety and long-term outcomes of catheter ablation of atrial fibrillation using magnetic navigation versus manual conventional ablation: A propensity-score analysis. *J Cardiovasc Electrophysiol.* 2016; 27:S11–S16.
22. Zhang F, Yang B, Chen H, et al. Magnetic versus manual catheter navigation for mapping and ablation of right ventricular outflow tract ventricular arrhythmias: A randomized controlled study. *Heart Rhythm.* 2013;10:1178–1183.
23. Bassil G, Liu CF, Markowitz SM, et al. Comparison of robotic magnetic navigation-guided and manual catheter ablation of ventricular arrhythmias arising from the papillary muscles. *EP Europace.* 2018;20:ii5–ii10.
24. Valderrábano M, Dave AS, Báez-Escudero JL, Rami T. Robotic catheter ablation of left ventricular tachycardia: Initial experience. *Heart Rhythm.* 2011;8:1837–1846.
25. Bassil G, Saleh L, Markowitz SM, et al. Outcomes of magnetic navigation-guided catheter ablation of left ventricular summit arrhythmia accessible via the coronary venous system. (Abstract). *J Am Coll Cardiol.* 2017;69:495.

18

How to Perform Papillary Muscle Premature Ventricular Complex Ablation Using No Fluoroscopy

Oliver D'Silva, MD; Hany Demo, MD;
Theodore Wang, MD; Mansour Razminia, MD

Introduction

Ablation of ventricular ectopy originating from the left ventricular papillary muscles poses unique challenges. The complex 3-dimensional (3D) structure of the papillary muscles is often difficult to appreciate using fluoroscopy and a 3D mapping system alone. Furthermore, maintaining catheter stability while mapping and ablating on these mobile structures is another challenge. A non-fluoroscopic approach that involves a high reliance on intracardiac echocardiography (ICE) may actually enhance procedural success, as it allows for a better understanding of the papillary muscle anatomy and for monitoring catheter stability during mapping and ablation.

Procedure

Choice of Access to the Left Ventricle

Ablation of ventricular arrhythmias involving the papillary muscles may be performed via a transseptal or retrograde aortic approach. The retrograde approach may be preferred for the posteromedial papillary muscle (PMPM) and the medial aspect of the anterolateral papillary muscle (ALPM). Transseptal access may be more suitable to address arrhythmias arising from the lateral aspect of the ALPM.[1] When an aortic valve prosthesis or significant atheromatous peripheral vascular or aortic disease is present, a transseptal approach is preferred.

Vascular Access and Creation of Right Atrial Geometry

Percutaneous femoral vascular access is obtained by the modified Seldinger technique guided by vascular ultrasound. If a retrograde approach is planned, an 8-Fr sheath (Input PS, Medtronic, Minneapolis, MN) is placed in the right femoral artery. If a transseptal approach is planned, one 8-Fr sheath is placed in the right femoral vein. In both instances, one 7-Fr sheath (Input PS, Medtronic) is placed in the right femoral vein; one 10-Fr long sheath (Super Arrow-Flex introducer, Teleflex, Morrisville, NC) and another 6-Fr sheath (Input PS, Medtronic) are placed in the left femoral vein. A 9-Fr ICE catheter (ViewFlex, Abbott, Abbott Park, IL) is inserted through the 10-Fr long sheath in the left femoral vein and advanced to the inferior vena cava (IVC) while maintaining an echo free-space at the tip of the transducer as previously described. The ICE catheter is then advanced to the right atrium (RA). An anterior curve is applied to the ICE catheter, and it is then maneuvered across the tricuspid valve into the right ventricle (RV) to evaluate for any baseline pericardial effusion. Baseline images are stored.

A 3D mapping system is essential to the non-fluoroscopic approach; the choice of mapping system is dependent on operator and system availability. In our center, a 6-Fr decapolar catheter (Inquiry, Ten Ten Diagnostic Catheter, Abbott) is inserted into the right femoral vein and advanced to the IVC under the guidance

Fluoroscopy Reduction Techniques for Catheter Ablation of Cardiac Arrhythmias. © 2019 Mansour Razminia, Paul C. Zei, eds.
Cardiotext Publishing, ISBN: 978-1-942909-30-9.

of the electroanatomic mapping (EAM) system (EnSite Velocity, Abbott). Geometry of the IVC is collected as the decapolar catheter is advanced to the IVC. The appearance of electrograms on the distal bipoles of the decapolar catheter indicates when the catheter tip has reached the border of the inferior RA and IVC, as described in Chapter 14. The decapolar catheter is then advanced into the RA and into the SVC. The RA–SVC junction is marked by a loss of electrogram signals on the proximal poles of the decapolar catheter as the catheter enters the SVC. Geometry of the SVC is collected on the EAM system. The decapolar catheter is then withdrawn into the RA. Under ICE and EAM guidance, the decapolar catheter is placed inside the coronary sinus (CS) to serve as a reference for the EAM system.

Transseptal Access to the Left Ventricle

A weight-based heparin bolus is administered prior to the transseptal puncture. The activated clotting time (ACT) is monitored throughout the procedure, and intravenous heparin boluses are administered to target an ACT of 300 to 350 seconds.

From the home view on ICE, clockwise rotation is added to visualize the interatrial septum and the left atrium (LA). Then, a posterior tilt is added, and minimal counterclockwise rotation is applied to visualize the SVC. Next, through the 8-Fr sheath, a 180-cm, 0.032-inch J-wire (fixed-core J-tip guidewire, Medtronic) is advanced inside the SVC under direct visualization of the ICE. The 8-Fr sheath is withdrawn from the body and exchanged for a transseptal sheath-dilator assembly (SL-0, Abbott), which is advanced over the wire into the SVC. The wire is then withdrawn from the body. The RF Transseptal Needle (NRG RF Transseptal Needle, Baylis Medical, Montreal, Canada) is placed in the sheath-dilator assembly. The sheath–dilator assembly is withdrawn minimally to expose the blunt tip of the RF Transseptal Needle. The transseptal assembly is withdrawn into the RA, while tracked on the EAM system and on ICE, until tenting of the interatrial septum is seen on ICE. In contrast to RF ablation of atrial fibrillation, which requires left pulmonary veins visualization on ICE while performing transseptal puncture, a relatively anterior and inferior transseptal puncture is preferred for ablation of ventricular tachycardia. This can be achieved by visualizing the transseptal needle tip on the mid to inferior part of the septum after the ICE catheter is rotated slightly counterclockwise relative to the location of the 2 left-sided pulmonary veins. Hemodynamic pressure monitoring is used to confirm entry into the LA along with direct ICE visualization.

If a standard transseptal needle, rather than an RF Transseptal Needle, is used, the operator will rely solely on ICE to track the sheath-dilator assembly position, without exposing the needle tip, as it is withdrawn from the superior vena cava (SVC) down to the interatrial septum.

Under ICE guidance, a steerable duodecapolar catheter with 2-2-2 spacing (Livewire, Abbott) or an Advisor HD Grid Mapping Catheter, SE (Abbott) may be inserted through the SL-0 transseptal sheath into the LA and then across the mitral valve into the left ventricle (LV) (**Figure 18.1**).

Retrograde Access to the Left Ventricle

A weight-based heparin bolus is administered prior to entering the LV. The ACT is monitored throughout the procedure, and intravenous heparin boluses are administered to target an ACT of 300 to 350 seconds.

A steerable duodecapolar catheter with 2-2-2 spacing (Livewire, Abbott) is inserted through the right femoral arterial sheath. The duodecapolar catheter is advanced retrogradely into the aorta and geometry is continuously collected on EAM. As the catheter approaches the aortic arch, a curve is applied. The desired distal U-curve is confirmed by noting the reversal of the sequence of distal to proximal electrode numbers on EAM. This U-curve is maintained during the advancement of the duodecapolar catheter toward the aortic cusps to avoid dissection of the coronary arteries (**Figure 18.2**). ICE may be used to visualize the duodecapolar catheter as it is prolapsed across the aortic valve. From the home view on ICE, minimal counterclockwise rotation is applied to visualize the long axes of the aortic valve, aorta, and LVOT (**Figure 18.3**).

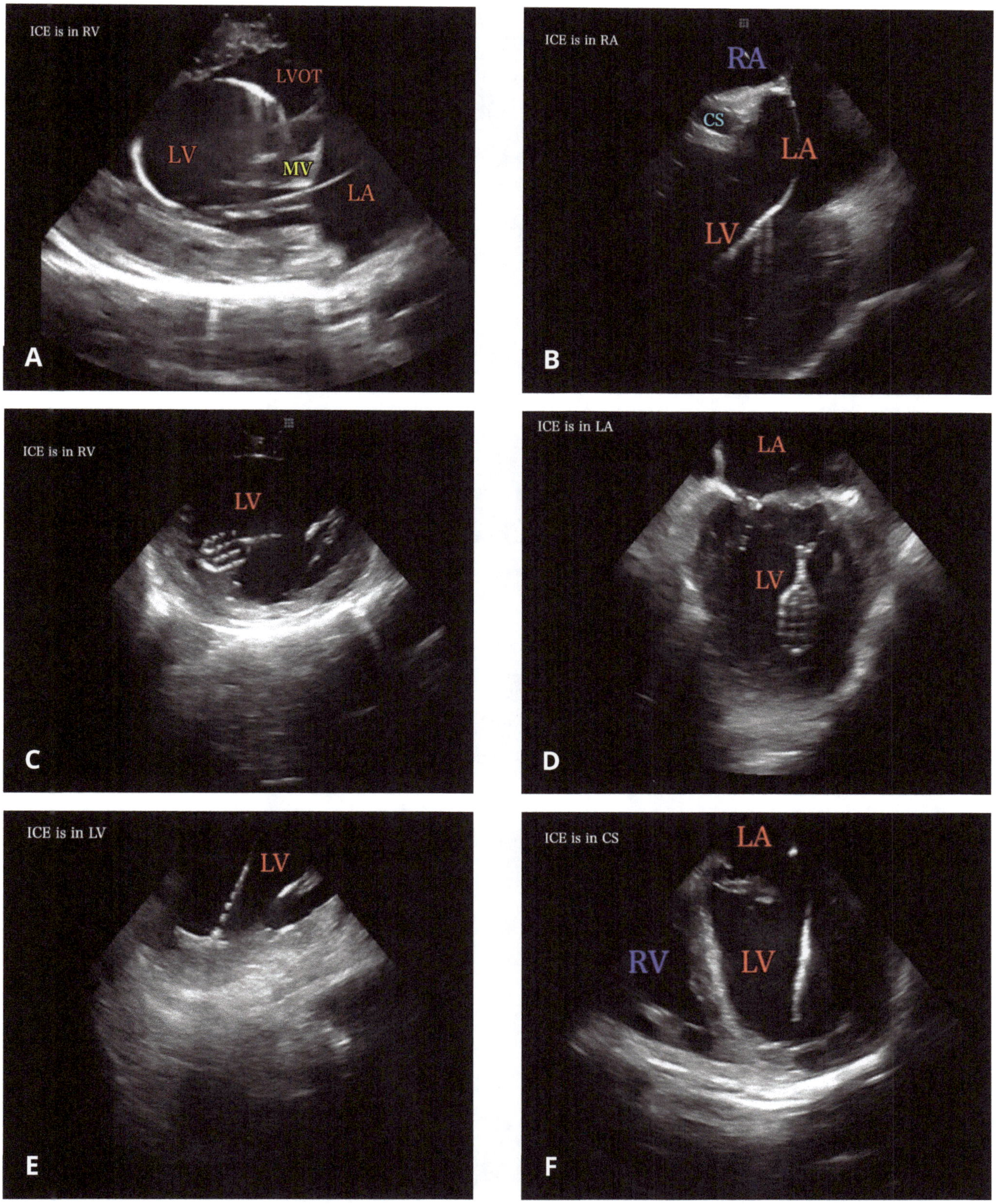

Figure 18.1 **A:** ICE catheter is placed in the RV and showing a steerable duodecapolar mapping catheter with 2-2-2 spacing passing through the SL-0 transseptal sheath and across the mitral valve into the LV. **B:** ICE catheter is placed in the RA and showing the Advisor HD Grid Mapping Catheter, SE, passing through the SL-0 transseptal sheath and across the mitral valve into the LV. **C:** ICE catheter is placed in the RV and showing the Advisor HD Grid Mapping Catheter, SE in the LV via transseptal approach. **D:** ICE catheter is placed in the LA and showing the Advisor HD Grid Mapping Catheter, SE across the mitral valve into the LV. **E:** ICE catheter is placed in the LV and showing the Advisor HD Grid Mapping Catheter, SE in the LV via transseptal approach. **F:** ICE catheter is placed in the coronary sinus and showing the Advisor HD Grid Mapping Catheter, SE across the mitral valve into the LV. ICE: intracardiac echo, RA: right atrium, RV: right ventricle, LA: left atrium, LV: left ventricle, CS: coronary sinus.

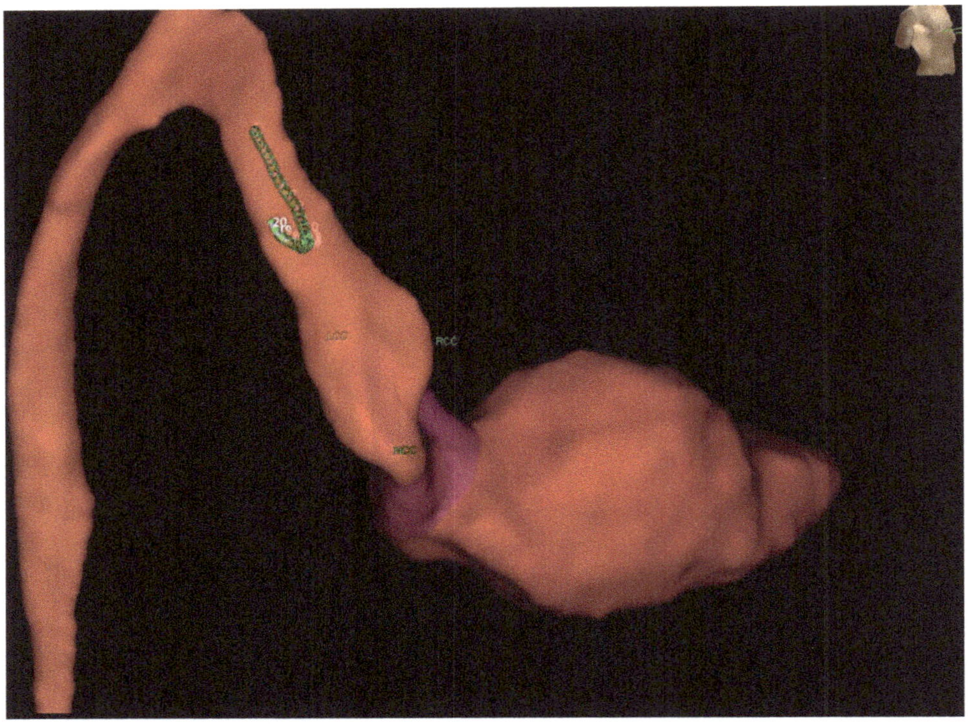

Figure 18.2 A steerable duodecapolar catheter with 2-2-2 spacing is advanced retrogradely into the aorta and geometry is continuously collected on EAM. A distal U-curve is formed in the descending aorta and confirmed by noting the reversal of the sequence of distal to proximal electrode numbers on EAM. This U-curve is maintained during the advancement of the duodecapolar catheter through the aortic valve to avoid dissection of the coronary arteries as well as damaging the valve.

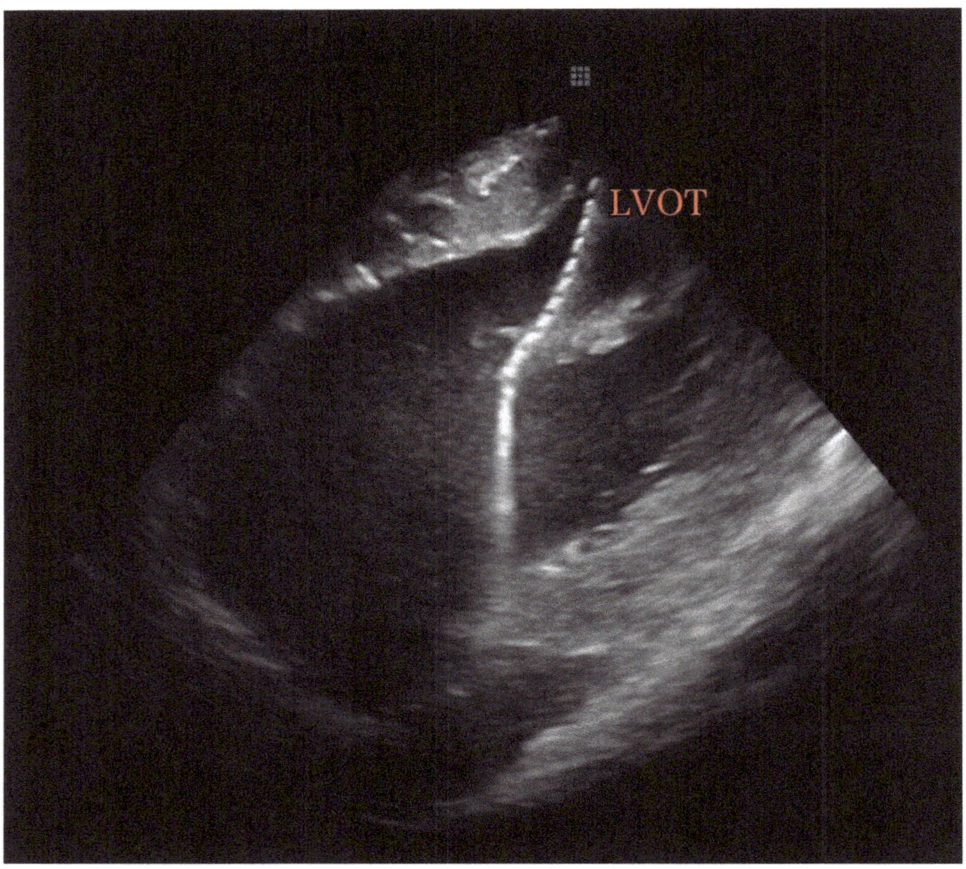

Figure 18.3 ICE visualization of the steerable duodecapolar catheter across the aortic valve into the LV outflow tract (LVOT).

Mapping and Ablation

Whether an antegrade or retrograde approach is used, the ICE catheter should be positioned in the RV to visualize the papillary muscles. From the home view, an anterior curve is applied to the ICE catheter allowing it to be advanced into the RV, and the anterior curve is then removed. The right-left button on the ICE machine is toggled to allow for a view that is similar to the parasternal long-axis transthoracic echocardiographic (TTE) view (**Figure 18.4**).

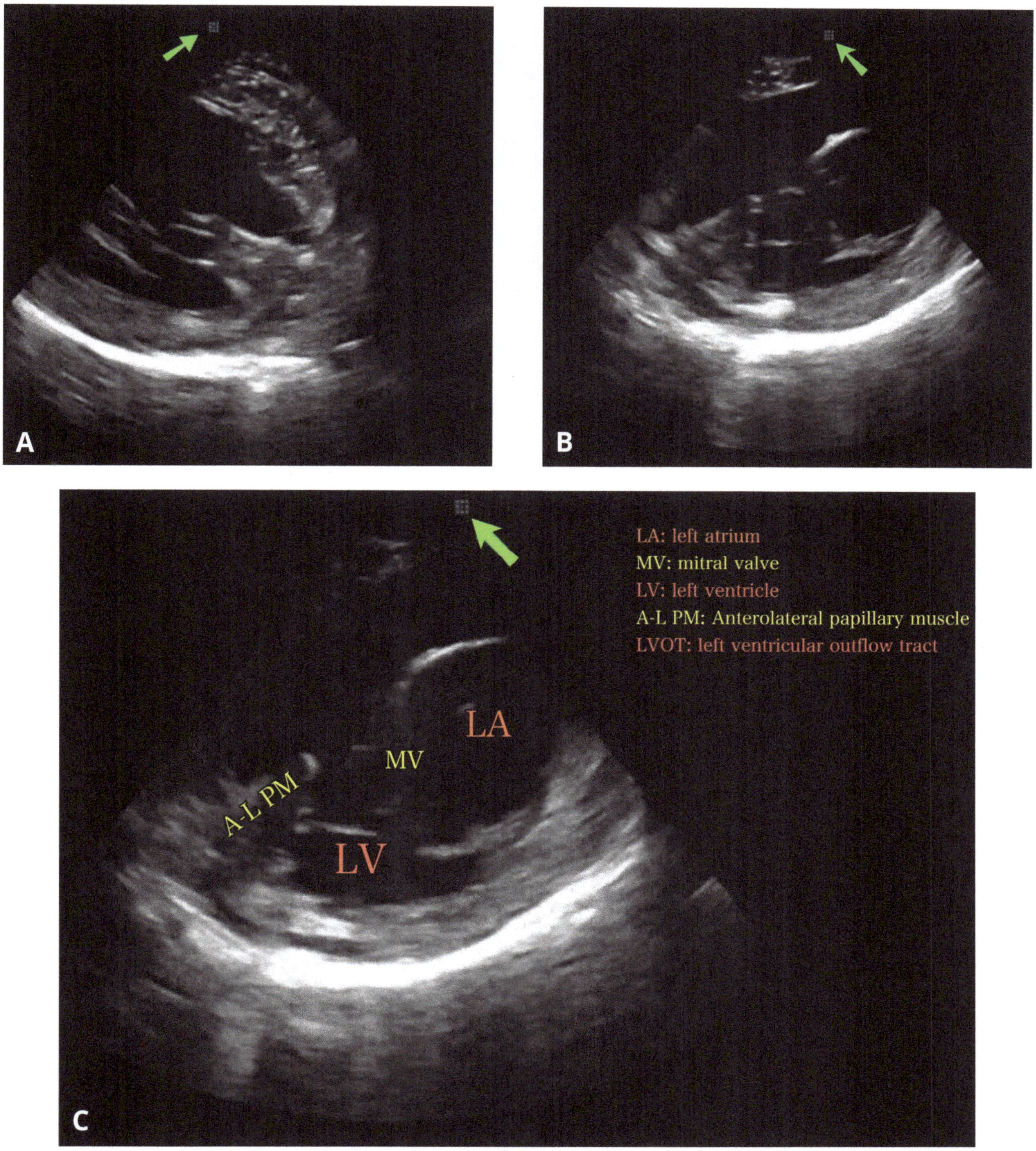

Figure 18.4 **A:** Original ICE orientation. **B:** The right-left button on the ICE machine is toggled to allow for a view that is similar to the parasternal long-axis TTE view. **C:** With changing the ICE orientation, the view becomes similar to the parasternal long-axis view of TTE imaging.

With the ICE catheter in the RV, clockwise rotation is applied resulting in visualization of a long-axis view of the LV and papillary muscles. Initially, more posterior structures are seen, and as more clockwise rotation is applied, more anterior structures are seen. The first papillary muscle seen is the PMPM (**Figure 18.5**); as more clockwise rotation is applied, the ALPM is seen (**Figure 18.6**). If a CARTOSOUND ICE catheter is being used along with the CARTO3 3D mapping system, the anatomic structures seen on ICE may be integrated into the 3D mapping system.

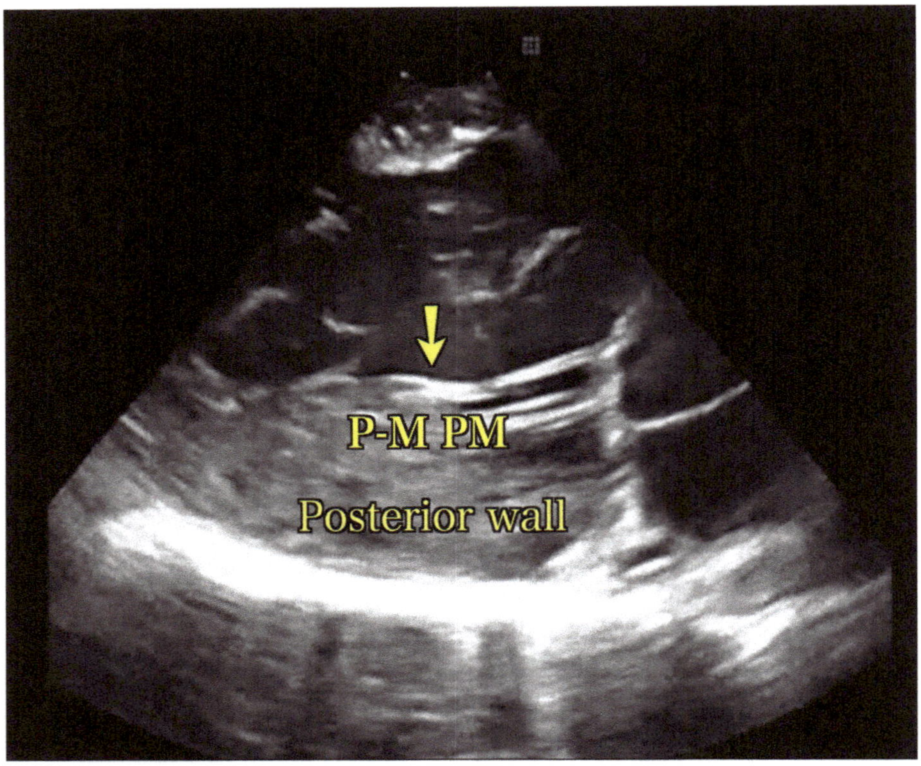

Figure 18.5 Posteromedial papillary muscle is usually the first papillary muscle seen when visualizing from the RV. Relationship to the LV posterior wall can be used to differentiate the 2 papillary muscles on ICE.

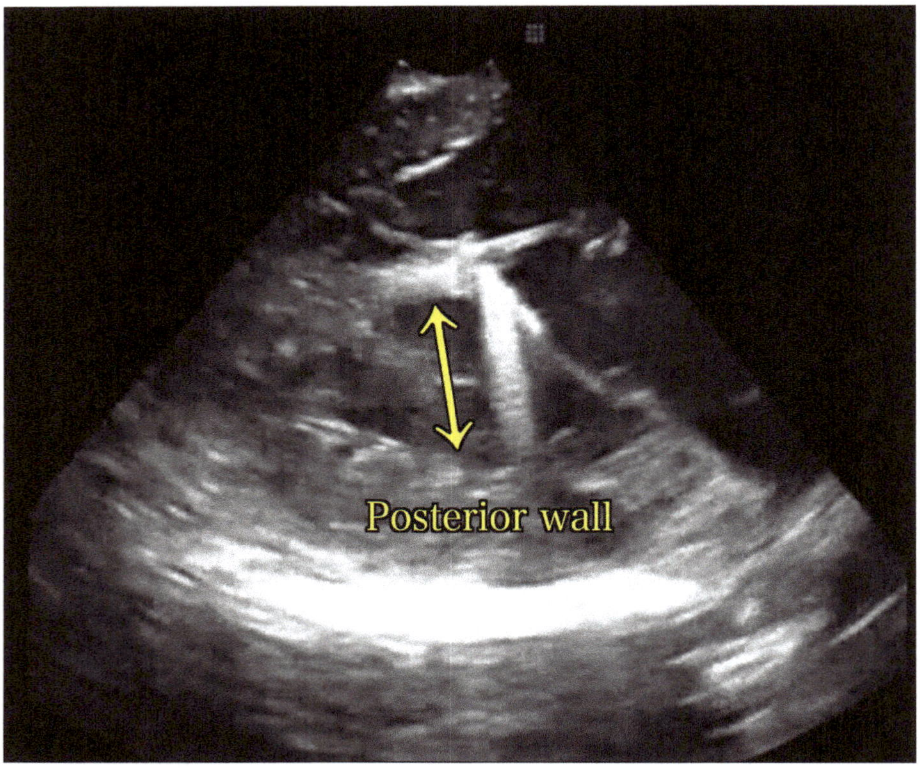

Figure 18.6 The anterolateral papillary muscle on ICE is distant from the LV posterior wall, which differentiates it from the posteromedial papillary muscle.

Activation mapping is performed using the duodecapolar catheter to identify the site of origin of the ventricular ectopy. This location is marked on the EAM and is noted on ICE. At this point, the duodecapolar catheter is withdrawn and exchanged for an 8-Fr irrigated ablation catheter (FlexAbility, Abbott). The method of LV entry for the ablation catheter is the same as for the duodecapolar catheter, whether an antegrade or retrograde approach is used. The ablation catheter is positioned at the site of earliest local ventricular activity. Radiofrequency energy is titrated up to a maximum of 50 W. A successful RF application that results in abatement of ventricular ectopy is continued for at least 60 seconds. During RF applications, the tip of the ablation catheter is continuously monitored for the development of type 2 bubbles, a harbinger of an impending steam pop. Several consolidative lesions are applied near the successful site.

Advantages and Limitations

When compared to traditional ablation using fluoroscopy, fluoroless ablation of ventricular tachyarrhythmias from the papillary muscle offers the key advantage of no harmful radiation being delivered to the patient, EP lab staff, and physicians. Avoiding wearing heavy lead garments may result in reduced orthopedic injuries and disabilities for EP lab staff and physicians. Additionally, pregnant EP lab staff members and members of the anesthesia team may safely assist in the non-fluoroscopic catheter ablation procedure.

By relying heavily on ICE in the fluoroscopy-free technique, the operator gains a better understanding of the complex anatomy of the papillary muscles. Clear visualization of this complex anatomy allows for the ablation catheter to be easily maneuvered around the papillary muscle and chordae tendinae and ensure optimum catheter contact (**Figure 18.7**).

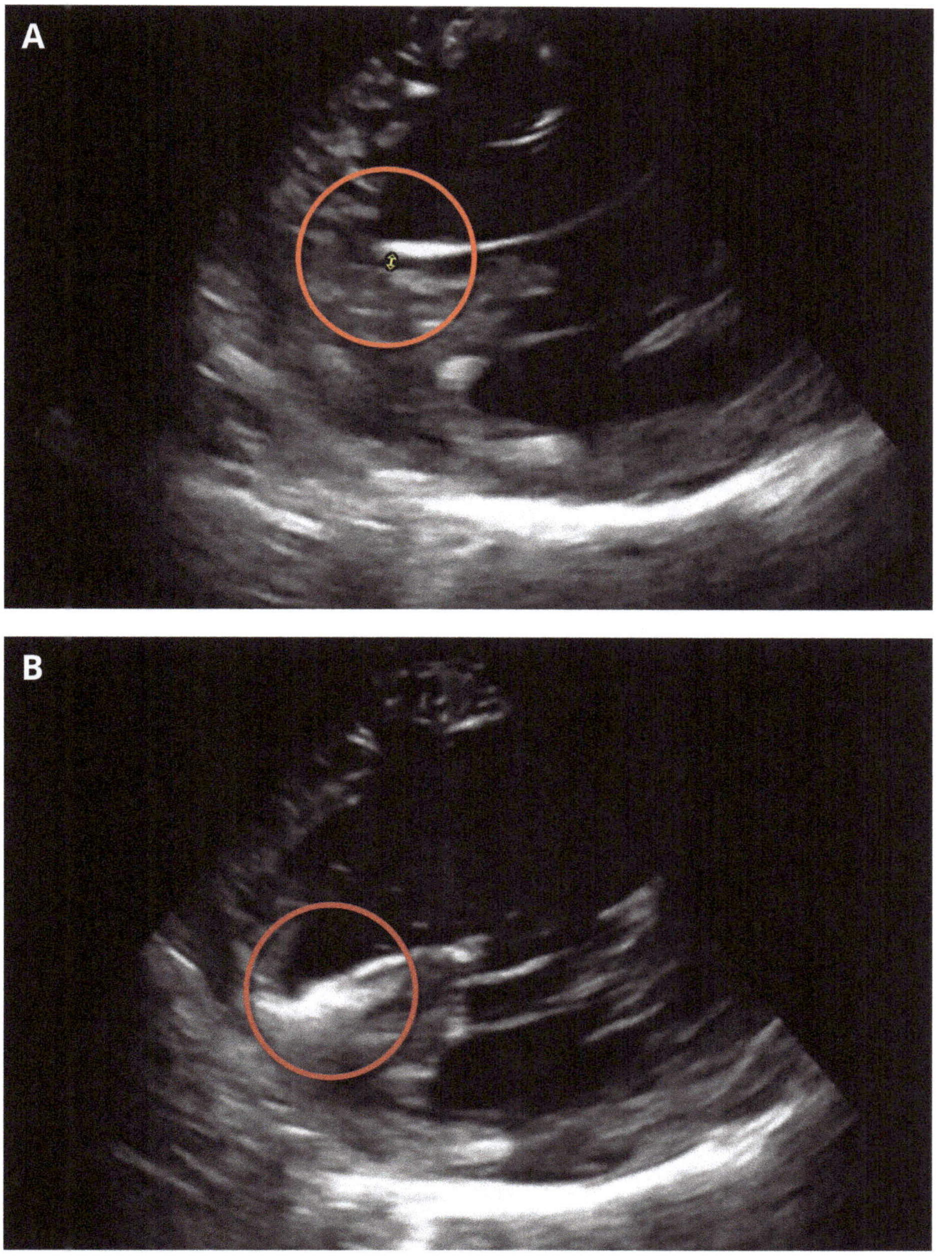

Figure 18.7 **A:** ICE image shows poor catheter contact to the anterolateral papillary muscle during retrograde approach. **B:** Optimum catheter contact is achieved using transseptal approach and confirmed by ICE.

One possible disadvantage of non-fluorscopic ablation of the papillary muscle ventricular tachyarrhythmias is the cost associated with ICE. However, in many labs, this technology is routinely used during catheter ablation procedures. One factor that may be overlooked in assessing the long-term cost effectiveness include avoidance of employee disability due to orthopedic injury related to the use of heavy lead aprons.

Conclusion

The risk that radiation poses to patients and EP staff during catheter ablation procedures is significant, and efforts should be made to try to eliminate unnecessary exposure whenever possible. The non-fluoroscopic technique for ablation of ventricular tachyarrhythmias originating from the papillary muscles can be performed routinely via the use of ICE and the 3D mapping system. This method offers a number of advantages over traditional fluoroscopy-based ablation including facile identification of the complex anatomy of the papillary muscle, safer and easier maneuvering around the papillary muscle due to superior visualization, better monitoring of catheter contact during ablation, avoidance of radiation risks to patient and EP staff members, and the potential for decreased orthopedic injuries for EP lab staff.

Reference

1. Enriquez A, Supple GE, Marchlinski FE, Garcia FC. How to map and ablate papillary muscle ventricular arrhythmias. *Heart Rhythm.* 2017;14(11):1721–1728.

Video Legend

Video 18S Chapter summary and step-by-step procedures by Mansour Razminia. [16:02]

19

How to Perform Ablation of Ischemic and Non-Ischemic Ventricular Tachycardia Using No Fluoroscopy

Amit Thosani, MD

Introduction

Electrophysiologic study (EPS) and ablation of infarct- and noninfarct-related ventricular tachycardia (VT) can be safely and effectively performed with minimal or no fluoroscopy.[1-7] This chapter details methods to integrate the use of vascular ultrasound, intracardiac echocardiography (ICE), 3-dimensional electroanatomic mapping (3D EAM), and intracardiac signal analysis to achieve safe and effective ablation without fluoroscopy. This chapter will detail endocardial mapping and ablation only.

At the time of this writing, epicardial access and ablation is most safely performed with the use of fluoroscopic guidance, though non-fluoroscopic, augmented-reality technology to guide epicardial access has been recently reported and promises to be an area of future development.[8]

Preprocedure Considerations

Infarct- and noninfarct-related VTs encompass a heterogeneous group of arrhythmias requiring detailed clinical analysis prior to EPS. The availability of a 12-lead ECG documenting the tachycardia remains the most useful tool for VT exit-site localization[9] and preprocedure planning, including the operator's decision to target left ventricular VTs from either a retrograde aortic or transseptal approach. Very often, however, 12-lead ECGs of the tachycardia are not available, making induction of the suspected clinical VT during the procedure absolutely essential. Intracardiac electrograms in patients with implantable cardioverter defibrillators (ICDs) are often the only tracings documenting the tachycardia prior to the patient's arrival in the electrophysiology (EP) laboratory. In these cases, near- and far-field ICD electrogram recordings are useful to determine whether the tachycardia induced during either noninvasive programmed stimulation (NIPS) or invasive EPS match the suspected clinical tachycardia(s). In many infarct- and noninfarct-related VT cases, what may begin as a single suspected arrhythmia will result in induction of multiple VT morphologies that often require additional mapping and ablation during the procedure.

A major consideration for all VT ablation remains the patient's clinical and hemodynamic response to sustained VT. Hemodynamically intolerable VT is more likely in the setting of left ventricular (LV) systolic dysfunction in both infarct and noninfarct cases. However, VT that was clinically stable upon presentation may become hemodynamically unstable in the setting of anesthesia administration. Unlike stable VT, hemodynamically unstable VT may require pressor and/or mechanical circulatory support.[10-15] Mechanical support, including percutaneous LV assist devices and extracorporeal membrane oxygenation, are most safely placed with fluoroscopic guidance using standard interventional techniques. Surgically implanted destination or bridge-to-transplant LV assist devices provide effective hemodynamic support during

Fluoroscopy Reduction Techniques for Catheter Ablation of Cardiac Arrhythmias. © 2019 Mansour Razminia, Paul C. Ze , eds.
Cardiotext Publishing, ISBN: 978-1-942909-30-9.

VT ablation[16-18] and are amenable to a low-/zero-fluoroscopic VT ablation strategy.

Capture of VT initiation by 12-lead ECG and telemetry, as well as perturbations in cycle length and response to premature ventricular beats, often help to discern the mechanism of the tachycardia. The suspected arrhythmia mechanism influences the operator's approach to anesthesia during the procedure. While not uniformly true, reentrant scar-related VT is expected to be inducible during the time of EPS, and may be more amenable to general anesthesia from the start of the procedure. This may not be the case with an automatic or triggered rhythms, which may preclude the use of general anesthesia at the start of the case in order to increase the probability of intraprocedural VT induction.

These various considerations are essential to the care of the VT patient. Because each patient and VT case is unique, this chapter will not do justice in detailing each of these various considerations. Furthermore, this chapter will not detail the specific components of EP study, including activation, resetting/entrainment, and pace mapping that have been previously described.[19] Rather, this chapter will discuss in detail the integration of various imaging and mapping techniques common to all infarct and noninfarct VT cases that may be adopted by the operator to reduce or eliminate the use of fluoroscopy without compromising patient safety or procedural efficacy.

Vascular Access

The use of femoral vascular ultrasound is recommended for safely establishing vascular access (Chapter 5). As VT ablation requires the use of intravenous anticoagulation, safe femoral venous and arterial access is an essential first step to preventing femoral vascular bleeding and vessel injury. The use of ultrasound is particularly useful when establishing multiple femoral venous access sites to avoid the femoral artery. Color Doppler imaging allows the operator to avoid femoral arterial side branches that may cross above the femoral vein. Mastery of ultrasound guidance limits the need for fluoroscopically guided femoral vessel access, and in the author's experience, reduces the total time required to achieve safe vascular access.

For a planned retrograde aortic approach, ultrasound is effective for examination of femoral arterial anatomy without fluoroscopy or angiography. Direct ultrasound visualization allows the operator to examine vessel patency, calcification, and optimal puncture site. Perhaps most important, direct ultrasound visualization allows for front wall arterial puncture of the common femoral artery above its bifurcation. Once the arterial access site is certain to be above the femoral bifurcation, vascular closure at the end of the procedure may be performed without the use of fluoroscopy or contrast angiography to confirm arteriotomy location.[20]

Intracardiac Echocardiography and Catheter Placement

Once the operator has made decisions regarding anesthesia (general vs. conscious sedation), VT induction strategy, and LV cavity access approach, catheter placement becomes the next step and one that traditionally has been a driver of intraprocedural fluoroscopy use. ICE (Chapter 2) is a critical next step to improving procedural safety and efficacy and also achieving fluoroscopy reduction.

ICE is useful for delineation of key anatomic structures, integration into 3D EAM (CARTOSOUND, Biosense Webster, Irvine, CA), and catheter placement. ICE catheters may be advanced from the left or right femoral veins, though the author prefers a right femoral venous approach to minimize the risk of venous tortuosity and difficult advancement from the femoral vein into the heart. Venous side branches are often encountered, and gentle catheter resistance may be met during advancement. In this situation, the catheter must not be forced forward but rather retracted and gently advanced, occasionally requiring catheter deflection, until resistance-free passage is achieved. EAM may be used during ICE catheter placement to visualize the catheter tip freely passing from the femoral vein into the inferior vena cava (IVC) and right atrium (RA). The IVC often enters the RA at a slight leftward angle, which must be kept in mind as the catheter is advanced toward the heart.

Once in the RA, the "home view" of the aortic noncoronary and right coronary cusps, septal leaflet of the tricuspid valve, and right ventricular outflow tract (RVOT) is obtained. When using integrated mapping systems, the location of the His bundle can be approximated near the junction of the noncoronary cusp and septal leaflet of the tricuspid valve in this view. This point is marked and used as a midline reference for catheter manipulation during the subsequent steps of the procedure.

Using right anterior oblique (RAO) and left anterior oblique (LAO) EA views with the His bundle site marked, counterclockwise rotation off the septum and anterior flexion of the ICE catheter will yield a view of the tricuspid valve and lateral right ventricle (RV). Using an RAO view, the ICE catheter can then be gently advanced across the tricuspid valve into the RV without fluoroscopy. Anterior flexion is then released as the catheter crosses the tricuspid valve, positioning the catheter within the RVOT (**Figure 19.1**A and **Video 19.1A**).

A survey of the RV free wall, apex, and pericardial space is then performed with slow, gentle clockwise rotation of the ICE catheter. The presence of pericardial fluid at baseline is important to note prior to LV mapping and ablation. Further clockwise rotation allows for visualization of critical LV structures: the posteromedial papillary muscle complex, the endocardial borders and trabeculations of the LV cavity, the anterolateral papillary muscle complex, the mitral valve and associated chordae, the LV outflow tract (LVOT), the aortic valve, coronary cusps, and left main coronary artery (**Figure 19.1**B and **Video 19.1B**). These structures can be traced and incorporated into an EA-integrated imaging platform. Further clockwise rotation allows for a long-axis view of the aortic arch, noncoronary cusp, and right coronary cusp. Careful imaging will allow for visualization of the right coronary artery originating from the right coronary cusp.

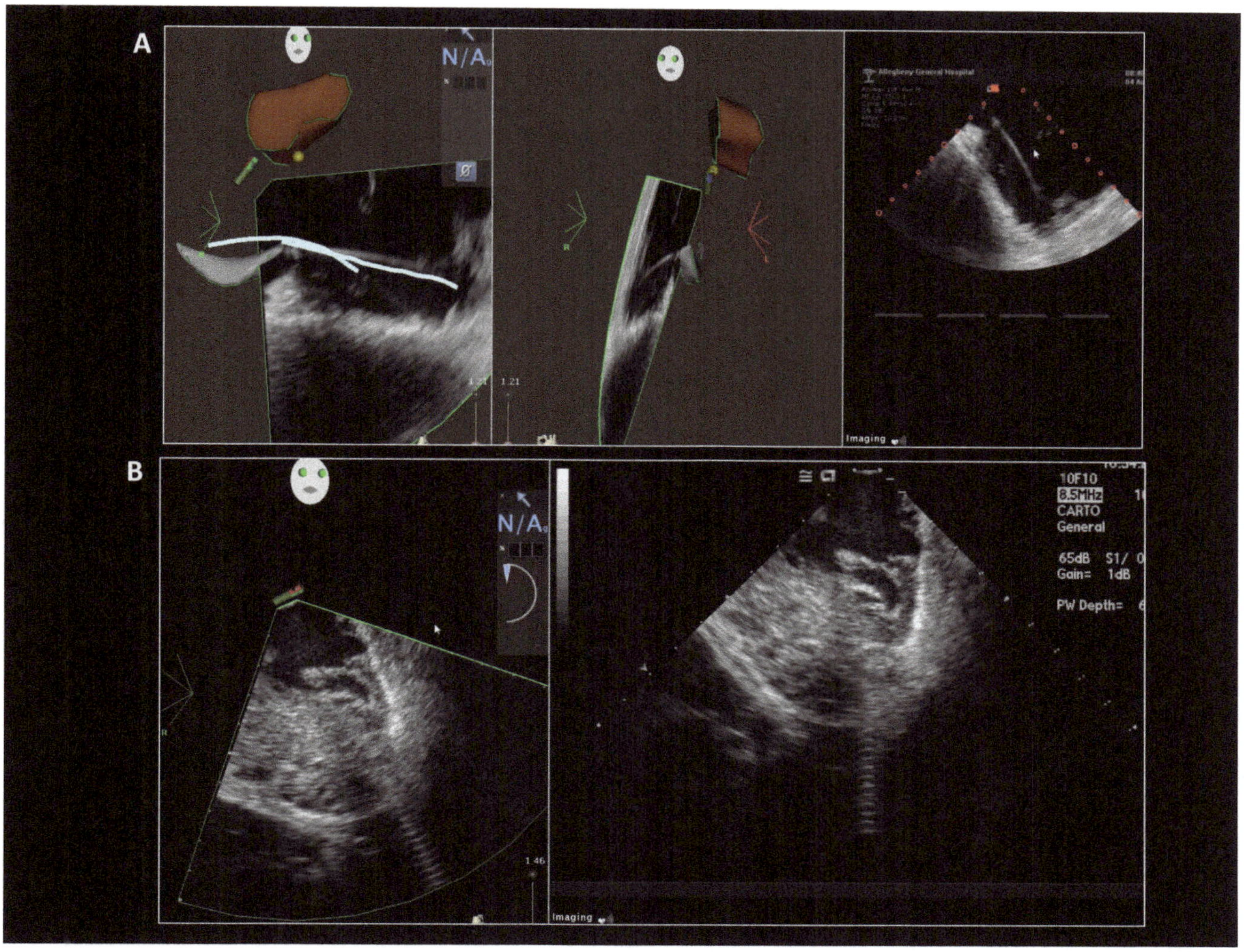

Figure 19.1 Positioning the ICE catheter in the RV without fluoroscopy. **A:** Using RAO and LAO views, the ICE catheter is anterior flexed and counterclockwise rotated gently off the septum. The His bundle position is marked by the **yellow** point. The catheter is then gently advanced across the tricuspid valve into the RV. Anterior flexion of the ICE catheter is then released, positioning it in the RVOT. The RV and RV ICD lead is visualized during this process. **B:** Survey of the LV and LVOT, obtained by slow, clockwise rotation of the ICE catheter from the RVOT position.

Particular attention is paid to existing pacemaker/defibrillator leads. A RA lead can be identified and traced from the superior vena cava (SVC) and high RA into its usual location within or near the RA appendage. Similarly, the course of the RV lead within the RA and crossing the tricuspid valve can be identified and avoided during future catheter manipulation. Coronary sinus (CS) leads can be identified and, if possible, avoided by not placing diagnostic and/or ablation catheters into the CS to prevent lead dislodgement.

Visualizing the RV insertion of any existing RV ICD leads is useful. **Figure 19.2** shows a scar-related VT with a RV apical septal exit site near the insertion of an existing RV ICD lead. EAM and ultrasound guidance were used together to carefully avoid this lead, and the VT was successfully pace mapped, induced, and terminated adjacent to the RV lead insertion site. The RV lead parameters in this case were stable following radiofrequency (RF) ablation.

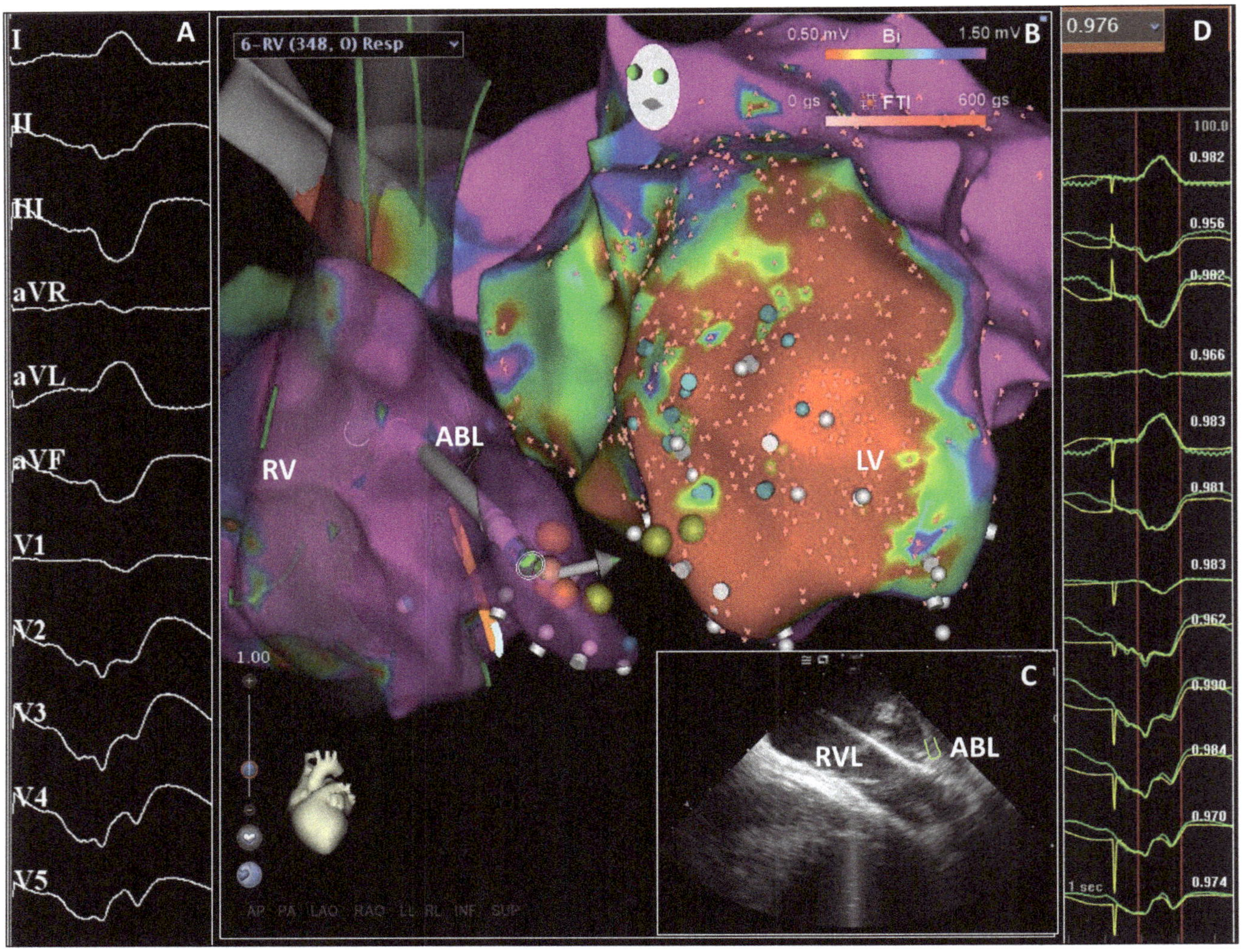

Figure 19.2 Infarct-related VT exiting near the RV ICD lead insertion site. **A:** Left bundle, left superior axis, infarct-related VT. **B**: Detailed EAM of LV apical septal infarction. Pace maps from the LV did not match the clinical VT well. **C:** Ultrasound imaging the RV ICD lead and ablation catheter (**green tip**) in the RV near but avoiding direct contact with the ICD lead. **D:** 98% pace map of the clinical VT on the RV septum near the RV ICD lead. The VT was induced and terminated at this site.
ABL: ablation catheter. LV: left ventricle. RV: right ventricle. RVL: right ventricular ICD lead.

If a retrograde aortic approach is planned for LV access, the author's team routinely notes and marks images of the open aortic valve during ventricular systole in multiple planes for impending advancement of diagnostic mapping and ablation catheters into the LV cavity without fluoroscopy (**Figure 19.3** and **Videos 19.3A–C**).

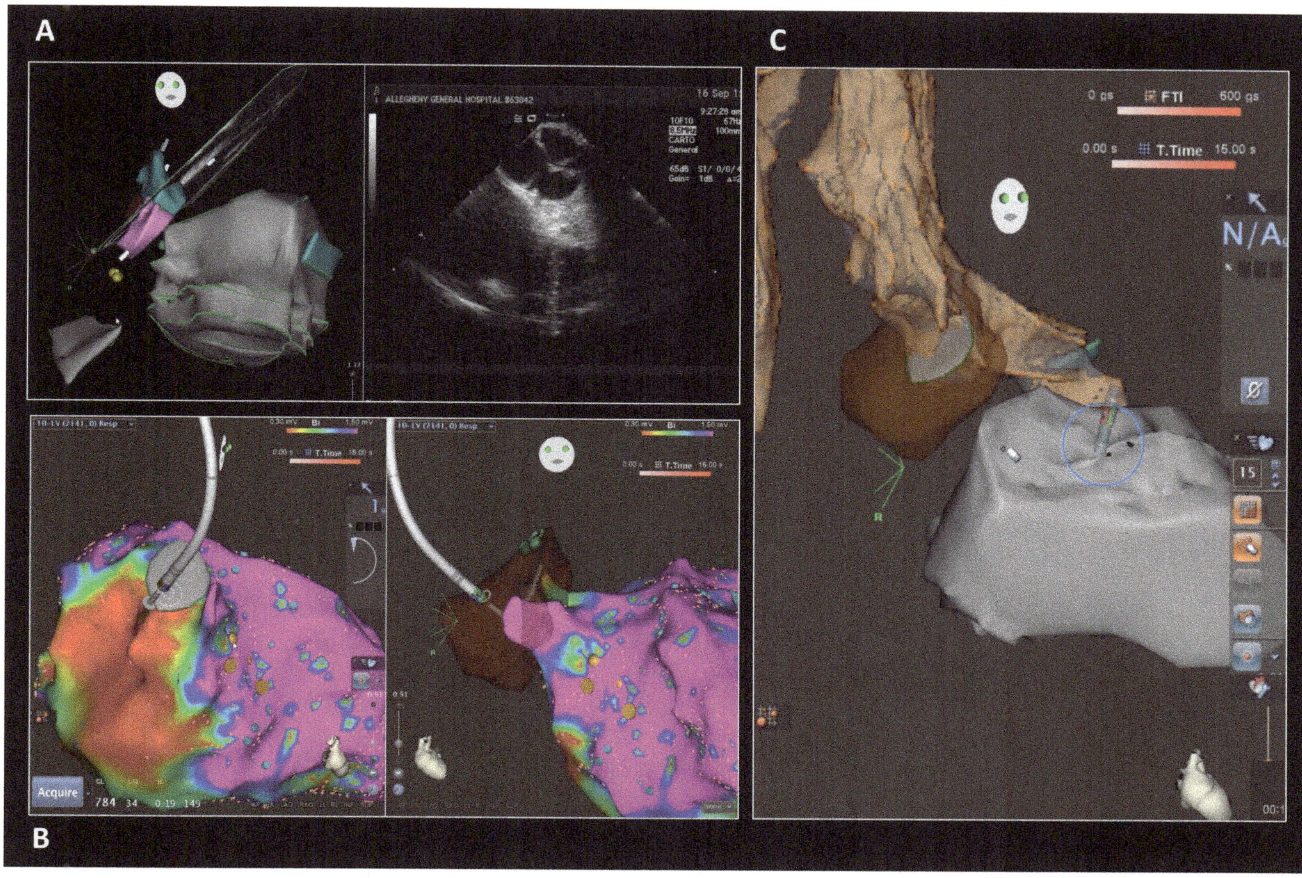

Figure 19.3 Crossing the aortic valve without fluoroscopy. **A:** Tracing the open aortic valve with ICE to guide retrograde access. **B:** Crossing the open aortic valve without fluoroscopy. The **gray circle** denotes the open aortic valve. **C:** Crossing the aortic valve using a multipolar diagnostic catheter without fluoroscopy.

Once ICE imaging, lead identification, and RV, LV, and aortic valve imaging are performed, diagnostic catheter placement is then performed. Catheters may be visualized with EAM systems, and electrograms are used to confirm positioning within the RA and RV chambers.

Retrograde Aortic and Transseptal Left Ventricular Access

In an attempt to minimize fluoroscopy following femoral arterial puncture, the use of stiff guidewires is recommended to allow for delivery of the intravascular sheath through the subcutaneous tissue into the femoral artery with minimal risk of wire kinking or other complications that may require direct fluoroscopic visualization. Stiff wires are preferred to allow enough support to pass through the subcutaneous tissue as well as any potential calcification in the femoral artery (avoided as best as possible after US visualization). The author also favors the use of a long sheath (45 cm or greater) that allows for sheath tip positioning at least within the descending aorta. The location of the sheath tip within the descending aorta allows for resetting of a catheter that may become prolapsed within the aorta during manipulation without having to remove the catheter entirely from the body (as in the case of a short sheath).

Adopters of a lower fluoroscopy approach earlier in the learning process may find it helpful to use short fluoroscopic exposures during wire placement and sheath advancement to become comfortable with the feel required to perform these steps without fluoroscopy. Alternatively, experienced ICE imagers may use appropriate views to identify the wire within the aorta and advancement of a long sheath into the descending aorta.

Transseptal access (Chapter 6) is an effective strategy in many LV VT ablation cases. We prefer the use of a large-curl deflectable sheath (Agilis, Abbott, Abbott Park, IL) with the sheath tip positioned at or past the mitral valve plane to provide catheter support during manipulation within the LV cavity. Due to the frequent presence of intracardiac leads, the author prefers an ICE and EA-guided direct transseptal puncture method rather than a traditional pull-down method from the SVC to the fossa ovalis to avoid interaction with existing leads (**Figure 19.4** and **Videos 19.4A–D**).[21]

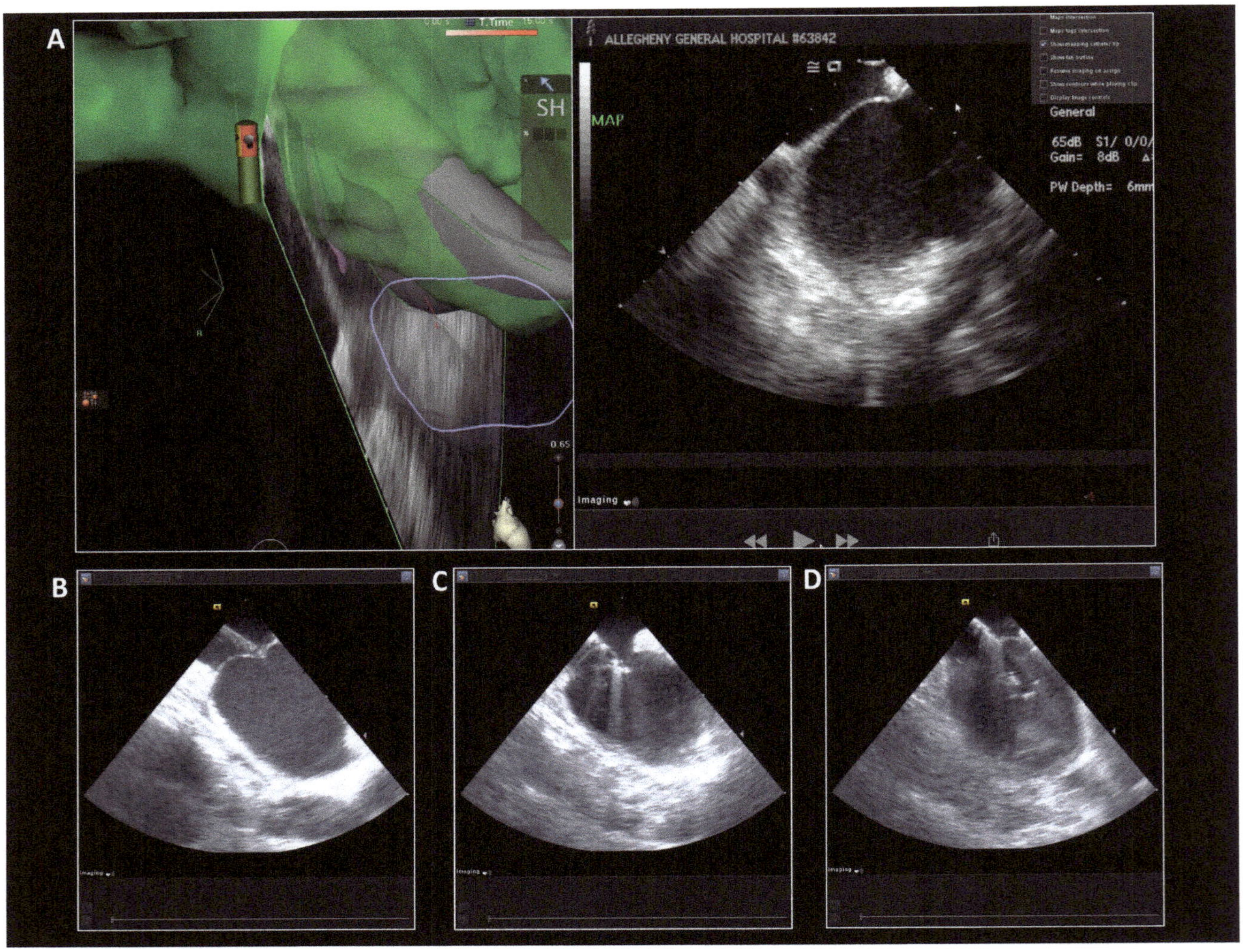

Figure 19.4 Zero-fluoroscopy transseptal puncture using direct sheath delivery method. **A:** The ablation catheter is advanced through a deflectable sheath into the RA, and positioned at the preferred crossing site of the interatrial septum (denoted with **pink line**). The catheter is then withdrawn while holding the sheath in transseptal crossing position. **B:** The transseptal needle and dilator are advanced together; ICE imaging shows opacification of the hollow sheath with the dilator/needle unit. The sheath is then withdrawn and the dilator locked into position. **C:** RF energy is delivered using unipolar cautery for transseptal crossing. The needle tip becomes echogenic and is visualized within the LA. **D:** A J-wire is advanced under ICE guidance into the left superior pulmonary vein, and the sheath advanced across the interatrial septum into the LA. The wire allows for support, especially if the septum is technically challenging to cross. The wire and dilator are then removed.

Ventricular Mapping

EAM systems are essential for detailed 3D ventricular endocardial mapping. Traditional fluoroscopy provides a 2D representation of a 3D chamber. This is partially overcome by using biplane (RAO and LAO) views. EAM allows for 3D representation of the cavity space of each cardiac chamber of interest. Familiar RAO and LAO views can be recreated, in addition to multiple other nontraditional views that are customizable to assist the operator with specific challenges encountered in each case. Specific features of EAM that are useful to improve procedure workflow include catheter tip and shaft visualization, catheter electrode/sheath relationship, multielectrode catheter visualization, contact force measurement, and high-fidelity signal analysis.

In scar-related VT, detailed endocardial voltage mapping is necessary to define areas of normal endocardial voltage, dense scar, and scar border zone. Previously integrated ICE imaging allows for approximation of the various segments of the LV cavity during endocardial catheter manipulation, and well as avoidance of endocardial structures that may impede catheter movement—most commonly, the papillary muscles and mitral valve chordae. Multielectrode catheters are useful for more rapid acquisition of simultaneous voltage recordings of multiple points on the endocardial surface. Catheter spline orientation, sharp near-field bipolar electrogram recordings, and tissue proximity indicator technologies are useful in combination to assure endocardial surface contact and accurate endocardial surface recordings. Multielectrode catheters with smaller interelectrode spacing allow for higher-fidelity recordings and more detailed voltage maps,[22] and are preferred in the author's laboratory (**Figure 19.5**A–C and **Video 19.5A**, **Video 19.5C**). Partial or full endocardial mapping is also achievable with the use of an ablation catheter, in which case catheter tip and shaft visualization, as well as contact force measurements, are useful for precise catheter movement and recording from all segments of the endocardial LV without the use of traditional fluoroscopy. EA visualization and contact force sensing are equally or perhaps more important for activation and entrainment mapping of induced VT prior to RF ablation, as this process often requires reaching specific sites within the suspected critical isthmus quickly and accurately. Contact force recording, in particular, is useful to ensure direct endocardial contact, and eliminates the need for fluoroscopy to achieve the same purpose (Figure 19.5D and **Video 19.5D**).

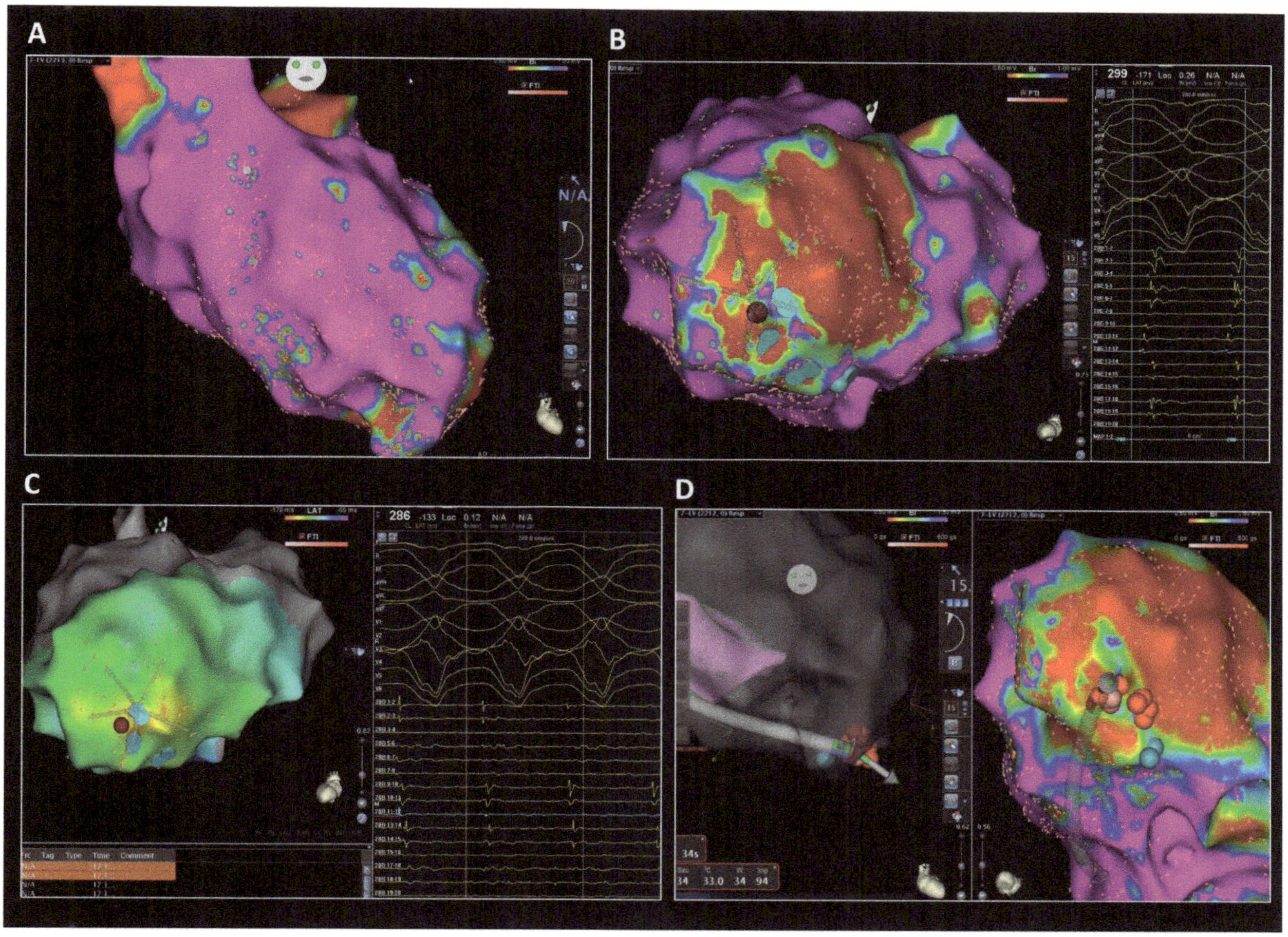

Figure 19.5 Electroanatomic mapping and ablation of scar-related VT in a congenital cardiomyopathy patient. **A:** Voltage map showing dense apical lateral scar. **B:** Multielectrode catheter (Pentaray) with splines flush against endocardial scar. Mid diastolic potentials are recorded during VT. **C:** Activation mapping during VT using multielectrode catheter positioned within and outside of dense scar. **D:** RF ablation with contact force sensing of VT exit site with termination of tachycardia.

The same tools useful for catheter manipulation, mapping, and ablation of scar-related VT are useful for noninfarct-related and idiopathic ventricular tachycardia. **Figure 19.6** details a case a ventricular bigeminy-induced cardiomyopathy. The PVC morphology resembled manifest preexcitation utilizing a posteroseptal accessory pathway and was suspected to originate from the posterior epicardial crux of the LV. EAM, catheter visualization, direct ICE imaging, and unipolar and bipolar signal analysis were used in combination to localize and successfully ablate the frequent PVC from within the coronary sinus without the use of fluoroscopy.

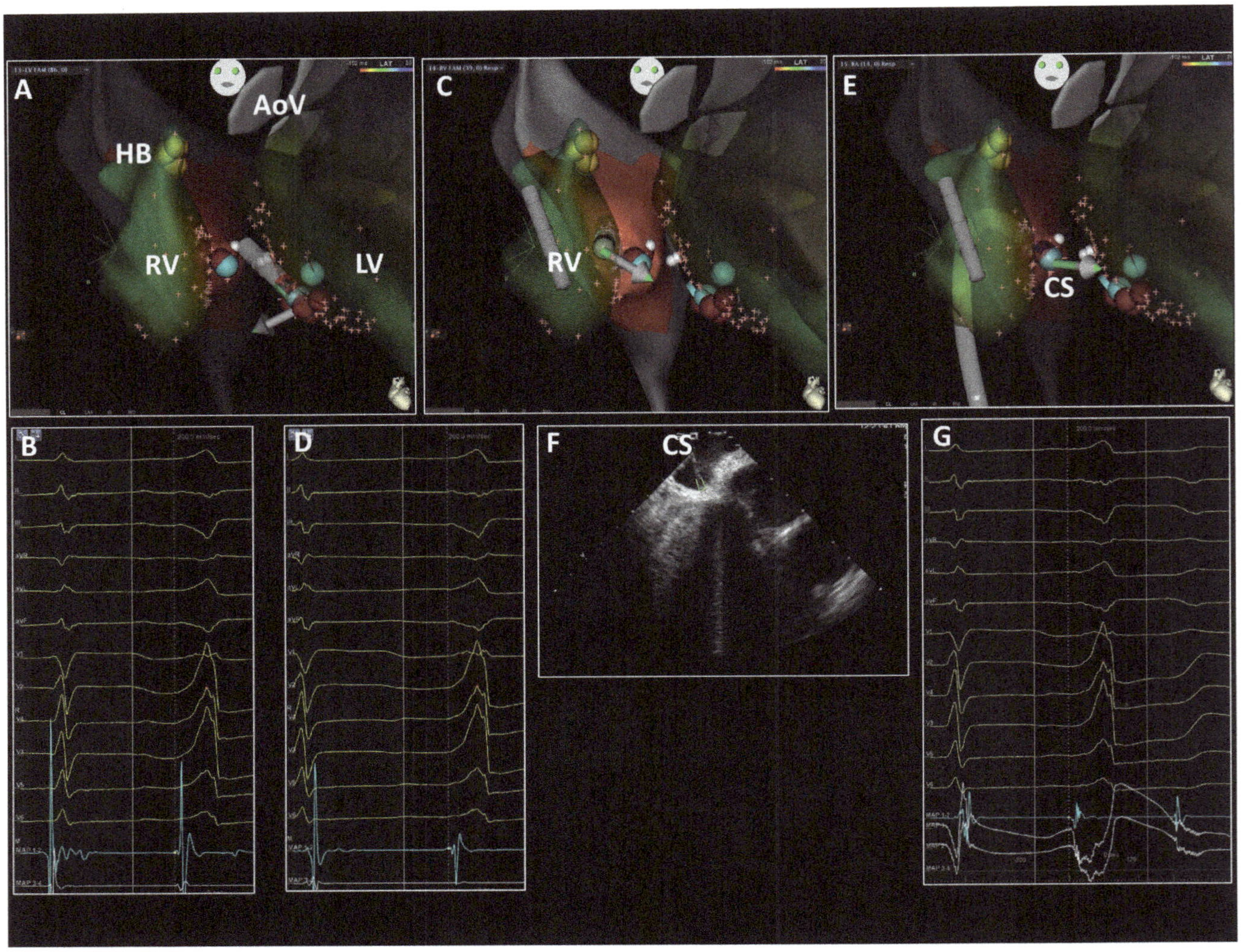

Figure 19.6 Electroanatomic mapping in a PVC-induced cardiomyopathy patient. **A:** Ablation catheter at the LV basal septum following EAM of the structures of interest. Contact force is directed toward the epicardial posterior LV. **B:** Earliest LV bipolar signals on distal ablation catheter (MAP 1-2, **blue**) timed to onset of surface QRS. **C:** Ablation catheter at RV basal septum. **D:** Earliest RV bipolar signals on distal ablation catheter (MAP 1-2, **blue**) timed to onset of surface QRS. **E:** Ablation catheter located within the CS ostium directed toward the epicardial posterior LV. **F:** Intracardiac ultrasound image of ablation catheter tip highlighted in **green** within the CS ostium. **G:** 20 ms presystolic bipolar signals (MAP 1-2, **blue**) and QS unipolar signals (MAP 1: distal unipolar, **white**; MAP 2: proximal unipolar, **white**). The PVC was successfully terminated within the CS, with subsequent resolution of LV systolic dysfunction. AoV: aortic valve. CS: coronary sinus. HB: His bundle. LV: left ventricle. RV: right ventricle.

Conclusion

Achieving a zero-fluoroscopy procedure should never be the primary goal for the treatment of the VT patient. Instead, patient safety, procedural efficacy, and clinical outcome always remain the ultimate objectives. The use of each of the techniques and modalities discussed in this and other chapters allows for fluoroscopy reduction not as the primary goal, but rather a natural consequence of optimizing all the tools currently available during endocardial VT mapping and ablation.

References

1. Razminia M, Manankil MF, Eryazici PL, et al. Nonfluoroscopic catheter ablation of cardiac arrhythmias in adults: feasibility, safety, and efficacy. *J Cardiovasc Electrophysiol.* 2012;23:1078–1086.
2. Cano Ó, Andres A, Osca J, et al. Safety and feasibility of a minimally fluoroscopic approach for ventricular tachycardia ablation in patients with structural heart disease: Influence of the ventricular tachycardia substrate. *Circ Arrhythm Electrophysiol.* 2016;9(2):e003706. doi:10.1161/CIRCEP.115.003706
3. Lamberti F, Di Clemente F, Remoli R, et al. Catheter ablation of idiopathic ventricular tachycardia without the use of fluoroscopy. *Int J Cardiol.* 2015;190:338–343. doi:10.1016/j.ijcard.2015.04.146

4. Von Bergen NH, Bansal S, Gingerich J, et al. Non-fluoroscopic and radiation-limited ablation of ventricular arrhythmias in children and young adults: A case series. *Pediatr Cardiol.* 2011;32:743–747.
5. Giaccardi M, Del Rosso A, Guarnaccia V, et al. Near zero x-ray in arrhythmia ablation using a 3-dimensional electro-anatomic mapping system: a multicenter experience. *Heart Rhythm.* 2016;13(1):150–156. doi:10.1016/j.hrthm.2015.09.003
6. Aryana A, d'Avila A, Heist EK, et al. Remote magnetic navigation to guide endocardial and epicardial catheter mapping of scar-related ventricular tachycardia. *Circulation.* 2007;115(10):1191–200.
7. Skoda J, Arya A, Garcia F, et al. Catheter ablation of ischemic ventricular tachycardia with remote magnetic navigation: STOP-VT Multicenter Trial. *J Cardiovasc Electrophysiol.* 2016;27 Suppl 1:S29–S37. doi:10.1111/jce.12910
8. Ector J, David W, Willems J, De Buck S, et al. An augmented reality approach to epicardial access during catheter ablation procedures (P302). *EP Europace.* 2018;20(1 Suppl):i44.
9. Josephson ME, Horowitz LN, Waxman HL, et al. Sustained ventricular tachycardia: role of the 12-lead electrocardiogram in localizing site of origin. *Circulation.* 1981;64:257–272.
10. Abuissa H, Roshan J, Lim B, Asirvatham SJ. Use of the Impella microaxial blood pump for ablation of hemodynamically unstable ventricular tachycardia. *J Cardiovasc Electrophysiol.* 2010;21(4):458–461. doi:10.1111/j.1540-8167.2009.01673.x
11. Shavelle DM, Clavijo L, Matthews RV. Percutaneous devices to support the left ventricle. *Expert Rev Med Devices.* 2011;8(6):681–694. doi:10.1586/erd.11.50
12. Bunch TJ, Mahapatra S, Reddy YM, Lakkireddy D. The role of percutaneous left ventricular assist devices during ventricular tachycardia ablation. *Europace.* 2012;14(Suppl. 2):ii26–ii32.
13. Bunch TJ, Darby A, May HT, et al. Efficacy and safety of ventricular tachycardia ablation with mechanical circulatory support compared with substrate-based ablation techniques. *Europace.* 2012 May;14(5):709–714. doi:10.1093/europace/eur347
14. Miller MA, Dukkipati SR, Koruth JS, et al. How to perform ventricular tachycardia ablation with a percutaneous left ventricular assist device. *Heart Rhythm.* 2012;9(7):1168–1176. doi:10.1016/j.hrthm.2012.02.005
15. Miller MA, Dukkipati SR, Chinitz JS, et al. Percutaneous hemodynamic support with Impella 2.5 during scar-related ventricular tachycardia ablation (PERMIT 1). *Circ Arrhythm Electrophysiol.* 2013;6(1):151–159. doi:10.1161/CIRCEP.112.975888
16. Cantillon DJ, Bianco C, Wazni OM, et al. Electrophysiologic characteristics and catheter ablation of ventricular tachyarrhythmias among patients with heart failure on ventricular assist device support. *Heart Rhythm.* 2012 Jun;9(6):859–864. doi: 10.1016/j.hrthm.2012.01.018
17. Sacher F, Reichlin T, Zado ES, et al. Characteristics of ventricular tachycardia ablation in patients with continuous flow left ventricular assist devices. *Circ Arrhythm Electrophysiol.* 2015;8(3):592–597. doi:10.1161/CIRCEP.114.002394
18. Moss JD, Flatley EE, Beaser AD, et al. Characterization of ventricular tachycardia after left ventricular assist device implantation as destination therapy: A single-center ablation experience. *JACC Clin Electrophysiol.* 2017;3(12):1412–1424. doi:10.1016/j.jacep.2017.05.012
19. Josephson ME. *Josephson's Clinical Cardiac Electrophysiology: Techniques and Interpretations.* 5th ed. Philadelphia: Lippincott Williams & Wilkins; 2015.
20. Manolis AS, Georgiopoulos G, Stalikas D, Koulouris S. Simplified swift and safe vascular closure device deployment without a local arteriogram: Single center experience in 2074 consecutive patients. *Indian Heart J.* 2016 Jul-Aug;68(4):529–538. doi:10.1016/j.ihj.2015.11.036
21. Baykaner T, Thosani A, Yasmeh B, et al. Safety and efficacy of zero fluoroscopy transseptal puncture (PO02-126). *Heart Rhythm.* 2018;15(5):S232.
22. Tschabrunn CM, Roujol S, Dorman NC, et al. High-resolution mapping of ventricular scar: Comparison between single and multielectrode catheters. *Circ Arrhythm Electrophysiol.* 2016;9(6). pii: e003841. doi:10.1161/CIRCEP.115.003841

Video Legends*

Video 19.1A Zero-fluoroscopy method for crossing the ICE catheter across the tricuspid valve. [00:16]

Video 19.1B LV ICE survey. [00:31]

Video 19.3A Tracing the open aortic valve with ICE to guide retrograde access. [00:12]

Video 19.3B Crossing the aortic valve without fluoroscopy. [00:08]

Video 19.3C Crossing the aortic valve using a multipolar diagnostic catheter without fluoroscopy. [00:15]

Video 19.4A Use of the ablation catheter to position a sheath at the preferred site of transeptal crossing. [00:13]

Video 19.4B Advancement of needle and dilator into the sheath at the site of transeptal crossing. [00:04]

Video 19.4C RF energy applied to the needle to cross the interatrial septum. [00:04]

Video 19.4D J-wire is advanced into the left superior pulmonary vein under ICE guidance. [00:04]

Video 19.5A EA LV map in a congenital cardiomyopathy patient. [00:07]

Video 19.5C Activation mapping during VT using a multielectrode catheter. [00:28]

Video 19.5D RF ablation with contact force sensing at site of VT termination. [00:07]

*Video numbering corresponds to the figure numbers.

Section 5

Special Populations

20

How to Perform Catheter Ablation During Pregnancy: Special Considerations

John D. Ferguson, MBChB, MD

Introduction

Cardiac arrhythmias are a recognized but uncommon complication of normal pregnancy. The majority of symptomatic cardiac rhythm disturbances are benign, with sinus tachycardia[1] being the most common; atrial premature contractions (APCs) occur in up to 50% of normal pregnancies, with APC burdens greater than 100/day occurring in up to 7% of symptomatic patients.[2] Fortunately, clinically significant tachyarrhythmias are rare during normal pregnancy. Supraventricular tachycardia (SVT) is the most common sustained arrhythmia with a reported incidence of 13 to 24 per 1000 pregnancies.[3] Atrial fibrillation, atrial flutter, and ventricular tachycardia (VT) can occur but are infrequent. Arrhythmias are significantly more frequent in patients with a history of arrhythmias prior to pregnancy or with structural heart disease.[4] Many patients with symptomatic tachyarrhythmia have been successfully managed medically. However, antiarrhythmic drug therapy must be carefully directed to avoid risk to fetal life and development; adverse maternal and fetal events can occur with recurrent or refractory symptoms. Indeed, fetal risks, including prematurity, respiratory distress syndrome, small size, and congenital heart diseases, occurred in 20% of pregnancies complicated by maternal arrhythmia in a large series of women treated medically with antiarrhythmic drugs.[4]

Although catheter ablation for recurrent SVT is now widely regarded as the therapy of choice in nonpregnant patients, there has been a reticence to perform ablation during pregnancy. The risks of an invasive procedure and radiation exposure present unique challenges in this patient cohort. Recent advances in fluoroscopy reduction techniques have helped minimize the radiation exposure during catheter ablation. Such techniques could lower the threshold to perform ablation in pregnant women and thus avoid potentially harmful medications.

Radiation Risk to the Developing Fetus

A major concern relating to catheter ablation is the risk of x-ray fluoroscopy to both the mother and, of particular importance, the developing fetus. Ablation should preferably be delayed until at least the second trimester. There are many potential adverse effects of radiation on the developing fetus, including congenital deterministic effects: fetal death, intrauterine growth restriction, major organ malformations, cognitive deficits, and microcephaly. Deterministic effects are predictable and typically occur at a threshold exposure, and their severity is directly related to radiation dose and time of exposure. The majority of deterministic effects of radiation occur prior to 17 weeks' gestation at fetal doses of ionizing radiation greater than 200 mGy.[5] Stochastic effects also occur; these effects

Fluoroscopy Reduction Techniques for Catheter Ablation of Cardiac Arrhythmias. © 2019 Mansour Razminia, Paul C. Zei, eds. Cardiotext Publishing, ISBN: 978-1-942909-30-9.

are probabilistic, occurring more frequently with greater exposure, but their severity is not related to exposure. This risk does increase with dose, but the lifetime risk is still quite low, with a lifetime attributable cancer risk of 2% with exposure of 50 mGy at greater than 15 weeks of gestation.[6] Case-control studies have suggested that antenatal exposure of as little as 10 mGy may increase risk of childhood cancer.[7] Doses described here are in milli-Grays, which is a measurement of radiation at a point in space; absorbed radiation is expressed in Sieverts or rems. A typical catheter ablation procedure results in ~8.3 mSv/h to an adult patient[8]; but fetal absorption would be expected to be less than that for the mother. The doses of radiation from the cases described here relate more directly to the mother, as the beam would be directed toward the chest and not the abdomen. Abdominal shielding of the mother, extending completely around the gravid abdomen, may limit but not eliminate fetal radiation exposure. This method was utilized in the majority of published studies. Radiation dosing to the shielded, gravid abdomen with fluoroscopy has been studied directly in pregnant vascular surgeons, with average fetal exposure below the limit of detection by dosimetry.[9]

Patient Selection

The American Heart Association/American College of Cardiology guidelines support catheter ablation as a IIB indication in recurrent, highly symptomatic, drug-refractory SVT in pregnant patients past the first trimester.[10,11] These guidelines emphasize the importance of fluoroscopy reduction or elimination techniques using electroanatomical techniques or intracardiac ultrasound. Importantly, lead shielding of the gravid abdomen does not reliably shield the fetus given that most exposure is from radiation scatter.

Procedural Considerations

Care for the gravid patient presents unique safety concerns and technical challenges to the electrophysiologist and the EP laboratory staff. Collaboration with an experienced obstetrics and anesthesia team is necessary to ensure safety of the mother and fetus. The choice of anesthesia care should be individualized to the unique clinical situation prioritizing maternal and fetal safety. Managed anesthesia care limits anesthetic exposure and may improve inducibility of the clinical tachycardia. General anesthesia may improve maternal airway and hemodynamic control and also may increase catheter stability. Any potential risks of general anesthesia would need to be weighed against the implicit maternal risk of prolonging or failing to complete a necessary invasive procedure.

For the ablation procedure, the patient should be positioned in the left lateral tilt position rather than supine to avoid aortocaval compression by the gravid uterus. Rapid pacing and time in tachycardia should be minimized to avoid hypotension. Cases should be streamlined in terms of time and equipment provided that safety and efficacy is not compromised.

In some cases, fetal cardiotocography is employed for intraprocedural fetal monitoring.[12] In general, continuous fetal monitoring should be considered, particularly when emergent cesarean delivery may be an option at a gestational age of 24 weeks or more. Potentially correctable changes in the fetal heart rate pattern in response to changes in the maternal physiologic condition might be identified; for example, fetal heart rate decelerations in response to hypotension that may resolve after augmentation of the blood pressure. The decision to deliver the baby in response to critical changes in the fetal heart rate pattern would depend on the gestational age, the stability of the mother at that point in the ablation procedure, and most important, the wishes of the patient as determined in preprocedure counseling by the obstetrical and neonatal consultants. Fetal monitoring in nonviable pregnancies (earlier than 23–24 weeks) is more controversial, as emergent delivery is not an option, and in general, obstetricians would not advocate for avoiding or not completing treatment of a serious maternal illness at a gestational age when the fetus is not viable.

Venous access is generally via the transfemoral route, but uterine compression can present a challenge to advancing catheters. In one study, catheter ablation was done entirely via the internal jugular routes to avoid femoral access.[13]

Intraprocedural Medications

It is important to consider what medications may be required during the procedure, especially for sedation and analgesia. Common drugs used in catheter ablation procedure and their risks during pregnancy are presented below (**Table 20.1**). With all medications, it is important to balance the potential fetal risk of using a medication against the risks to the mother and fetus of withholding a medication to treat a serious maternal medical condition. In general, the fetal risk is lower after organogenesis is completed, usually by the 10th week of gestation. Pregnancy is a period of heightened risk for venous thromboembolism, with a risk 4–5 times higher than a nonpregnant woman. Prolonged immobilization, obesity, and tobacco smoking further increase this risk. Special consideration should be given with regard to intraprocedural anticoagulation to reduce the risk of thromboembolic complications.

Table 20.1 Common antiarrhythmic or periprocedural drugs and effects, either definite or possible, on fetal life and development.

Drug	Pregnancy Classification	Adverse Effects
Midazolam	D	Congenital malformations not increased; potential for neonatal abstinence with prolonged maternal use
Lorazepam	D	Low teratogenic potential; may cause neonatal sedation or respiratory depression if used near term; potential for neonatal abstinence with prolonged maternal use
Fentanyl	C	Embryo toxicity observed in rats; neonatal respiratory depression may occur if used near delivery
Lidocaine	B	Doses <30 mg/kg
Heparin	C	Does not cross placenta; not associated with teratogenesis or fetal loss
Isoproterenol	C	27% crosses placenta, affects uterine contraction. Associated with embryo loss and congenital abnormalities in animals; limited human use has not confirmed this effect
Adenosine	C	No reports of adverse effects
Esmolol	C	Acute administration likely safe
Metoprolol	C	Not associated with congenital abnormalities; possible increased risk of fetal growth restriction with chronic maternal use of beta-blockers
Verapamil	C	Developmental abnormalities, fetal loss in animals; no human reports of birth defects
Ibutilide	C	Teratogenic and embryocidal in animals; no human data available
Amiodarone	D	Congenital goiter and hypo- or hyperthyroidism
Diltiazem	C	Possible teratogenic effects in animals with limited human data
Digoxin	C	Serum levels unreliable; no increased risk of adverse fetal effects
Procainamide	C	Unknown

PREGNANCY class **A:** Evidence of safety, **B:** No evidence of risk, **C:** Unknown risk, **D:** Evidence of risk, **X:** Evidence of risk, contraindicated.

Cardiopulmonary Resuscitation during Pregnancy

Should cardiac arrest occur during the electrophysiology procedure, resuscitation, including shock therapy and advanced cardiac life support drugs, should be used as in the nonpregnant patient. Cardiopulmonary resuscitation (CPR) should be modified in patients at more than 20 weeks of gestation. The gravid uterus can compress the inferior vena cava, impeding venous return and reducing cardiac output during CPR. To avoid this, pregnant patients should be positioned either with a left lateral tilt of 10–30 degrees or supine with a second responder manually displacing the gravid uterus leftward to further reduce aortocaval compression.[14] There are reports that direct-current shock can produce premature uterine contraction. In a near-term pregnancy, it is generally recommended to consider emergency cesarean after 4–5 minutes of CPR in order to improve the effectiveness of chest compressions and improve venous return from the lower extremities. This intervention may also rescue the fetus from a dying mother.

Non-Fluoroscopic Ablation during Pregnancy

Over recent years, evolving technologies have facilitated significant reduction or even complete elimination of x-ray exposure during catheter ablation. These techniques are described in detail elsewhere in this book. Most data regarding fluoroscopy-reduction techniques comes from supraventricular tachycardia ablation in nonpregnant patients, but there is a growing number of studies reporting catheter ablation in pregnant women.[15]

We identified 20 published reports describing 41 pregnant patients undergoing catheter ablation (**Table 20.2**). All were retrospective reports, with the largest case series involving 11 patients. In the majority of reported cases, patients presented with SVT: 6 patients with atrial tachycardia, 7 with atrioventricular reciprocating tachycardia (AVRT), 4 with atrioventricular nodal reentrant tachycardia (AVNRT), 1 with atrial flutter and atrial fibrillation, and 3 with persistent junctional reciprocating tachycardia. Only 4 patients had ventricular tachycardia: 1 with RVOT tachycardia, 2 with PVCs, and 1 with arrhythmogenic right ventricular dysplasia (ARVD). The mean age of patients was 29 years (range: 16–50), with ablation performed at a mean gestational age of 25 (range: 10–38) weeks. The most common indication for ablation was recurrent symptomatic palpitations refractory to medical therapy. Syncope, congestive heart failure, LV systolic dysfunction, and cardiac arrest prompting ablation were less common indications for ablation. Reduced left ventricular systolic function was present in 9 patients.

Table 20.2 Characteristics of individual patients from included reports.

Ref.	Author and Date	Patients	Tachycardia Mechanism	Maternal Age (years)	Gestation (weeks)	Fluoroscopy Time (sec)/Dose	Mapping
18	Gras 1992	1	AFL, AF	27	22	NR	No
19	Dominguez 1999	1	R AP	31	20	70 (NR)	No
16	Bombelli 2003	3	AVNRT, LL AP, R AP	27–32	29–30	408 (1.2 mGy) – 1176 (5.2 mGy)	No
20	Pagad 2004	1	RAT	24	26	240 (NR)	No
21	Kanjwal 2005	1	LL AP	32	22	457 (NR)	No
22	Berruezo 2007	1	RAT (RAA)	30	30	481 (0.25 mGy)	No
33	Szumowski 2006	1	LL AP	22	12	109 (0.1 mGy)	No
23	Bongiorni 2008	1	AVNRT	32	10	0	ICE
12	Szumowski 2008	9	RAT (2), PJRT (3), AVNRT (1), LL AP (3)	24–31	12–38	0–120 (NR)	Yes
24	Manjaly 2011	1	R AP (CS OS)	33	15	0	NavX
25	Wu 2011	1	RAT (RAA)	32	14	55 (<0.1 mGy)	NavX
26	Ferguson 2011	1	LAT	20	27	0	NavX/ICE
27	Stec 2013	1	RV VT	26	23	90 (0.1 mGy)	CARTO
28	Clark 2014	1	AVNRT	27	22	0	NavX
29	Hogarth 2014	1	RVOT VT	36	31	60 (9.9 mGy)	NavX
30	Leiria 2014	1	LL AP	33	26	0	NavX
31	Zuberi 2014	1	RAT	48	30	0	NavX
17	Yang 2014	2	AT (2)	30–32	17–21	360 (15.1 mGy)	NavX
32	Bigelow 2015	1	AVNRT	27	22	0	NavX
13	Kozluk 2017	11	WPW (3), AVNRT (2), PJRT (1), AT (3), PVC (2)	15–50	16–32	0	CARTO, NavX

The majority of cases used radiofrequency energy, and 2 utilized cryoablation. All were reported as successful. There were no reported arrhythmia recurrences or repeat ablation procedures during the index pregnancy. Total procedural times were only reported for 15 patients; in the largest series, procedural time averaged 56 minutes with a standard deviation of 8 minutes; the longest reported procedure was 186 minutes. None of the studies reported time in tachycardia during the electrophysiology study and ablation. Fluoroscopic guidance was used in the majority of cases, and total fluoroscopy time was reported in 20 of 27 cases. Unfortunately, direct radiation dosing was only reported in 8 cases in which fluoroscopic guidance was used. In 1 case, almost 30 minutes of fluoroscopy was used. Less than 9 minutes of fluoroscopy (28–516 seconds), with a mean fluoroscopy time of 141 seconds, was used in the other cases where fluoroscopy was used and times reported. Non-fluoroscopic techniques with no reported radiation were used in 18/41 cases, all of which occurred after 2007.

Few maternal or fetal problems were reported. Periprocedural obstetric care was not described in detail in most cases; fetal heart rate monitoring and cardiotocography was used in a minority of patients. Likewise, procedural use of anesthesia and sedation was not uniformly discussed with the exception of one case that explicitly involved no anesthesia or sedatives. The reported cases ultimately resulted in the successful delivery of 29 infants, as 2 pregnancies involved twins. In terms of reported obstetric complications, there was one reported instance of microcephaly diagnosed at 4 months of age.[16] Additionally, one case was associated with the development of maternal preeclampsia and placental abruption, necessitating early cesarean delivery at 27 weeks, 5 weeks after successful ablation. The neonate developed retinopathy of prematurity but was otherwise in good health.[12] In another case, a 32-year-old woman presented with pulmonary edema at 21 weeks of gestation and incessant atrial tachycardia at 160 bpm. She underwent successful right atrial tachycardia ablation but without heparin. She decompensated immediately postprocedure, requiring ventilation. The mother made a good recovery, but her baby spontaneously aborted.[17]

Conclusion

Current guidelines support catheter ablation as a IIB indication in drug-refractory, poorly tolerated SVT in pregnant patients past the second trimester.[1,12] In the published reports, the majority of pregnant patients had life-threatening or medically refractory arrhythmia as the indication for ablation. Pregnant patients with a single episode of non-life-threatening SVT should not be considered for catheter ablation. However, given current technological advances and the increasing reports of ablation being performed with little or no fluoroscopy, it is likely that the threshold for catheter ablation in pregnant patients will fall. In fact, in patients with recurrent symptoms, catheter ablation may now be considered prior to the use of antiarrhythmic drugs, most of which have suboptimal efficacy and potential toxicity. Catheter ablation should be avoided in the first trimester and may be more challenging in advanced stages of the third trimester. In the absence of clear guidelines, such a decision will depend on the EP service available at the institution. The decision should be made using a multidisciplinary approach with a careful and well-documented risk benefit discussion with the patient.

References

1. Li JM, Nguyen C, Joglar JA, Hamdan MH, Page RL. Frequency and outcome of arrhythmias complicating admission during pregnancy: Experience from a high-volume and ethnically-diverse obstetric service. *Clin Cardiol.* 2008;31(11):538–541.
2. Shotan A, Ostrzega E, Mehra A, Johnson JV, Elkayam U. Incidence of arrhythmias in normal pregnancy and relation to palpitations, dizziness, and syncope. *Am J Cardiol.* 1997;79(8):1061–1064.
3. Robins K, Lyons G. Supraventricular tachycardia in pregnancy. *Br J Anaesth.* 2004;92(1):140–143.
4. Silversides CK, Harris L, Haberer K, Sermer M, Colman JM, Siu SC. Recurrence rates of arrhythmias during pregnancy in women with previous tachyarrhythmia and impact on fetal and neonatal outcomes. *Am J Cardiol.* 2006;97(8):1206–1212.
5. ACOG Committee on Obstetric Practice. ACOG Committee Opinion. Number 299, September 2004 (replaces No. 158, September 1995). Guidelines for diagnostic imaging during pregnancy. *Obstet Gynecol.* 2004;104(3):647–651.
6. National Council on Radiation Protection and Measurements (NCRP). Considerations regarding the unintended radiation exposure of the embryo, fetus or nursing child. *NCRP Commentary* 1994;9.
7. Doll R, Wakeford R. Risk of childhood cancer from fetal irradiation. *Br J Radiol.* 1997;70:130–139.
8. Perisinakis K, Damilakis J, Theocharopoulos N, Manios E, Vardas P, Gourtsoyiannis N. Accurate assessment of patient effective radiation dose and associated detriment risk from radiofrequency catheter ablation procedures. *Circulation* 2001;104(1):58–62.
9. Chandra V, Dorsey C, Reed AB, Shaw P, Banghart D, Zhou W. Monitoring of fetal radiation exposure during pregnancy. *J Vasc Surg.* 2013 Sep;58(3):710–714.
10. Page RL, Joglar JA, Caldwell MA, et al. 2015 ACC/AHA/HRS guideline for the management of adult patients with supraventricular tachycardia: A report of the American College of Cardiology/American Heart Association Task Force on Clinical Practice Guidelines and the Heart Rhythm Society. *Heart Rhythm.* 2016;13:e136–e221.
11. European Society of Gynecology (ESG), Association for European Paediatric Cardiology (AEPC), German Society for Gender Medicine (DGesGM), Regitz-Zagrosek V, Blomstrom Lundqvist C, Borghi C, et al. ESC Guidelines on the management of cardiovascular diseases during pregnancy: The Task Force on the Management of Cardiovascular Diseases during Pregnancy of the European Society of Cardiology (ESC). *Eur Heart J.* 2011;32(24):3147–3197.
12. Szumowski Ł, Szufladowicz E, Orczykowski M, et al. Ablation of severe drug-resistant tachyarrhythmia during pregnancy. *J Cardiovasc Electrophysiol.* 2010;21(8):877–882.
13. Kozluk E, Piatkowska A, Kiliszek M, et al. Catheter ablation of cardiac arrhythmias in pregnancy without fluoroscopy: A case control retrospective study. *Adv Clin Exp Med.* 2017;26(1):129–134.
14. Lavonas EJ, Drennan IR, Gabrielli A, Heffner AC, et al. Part 10: Special Circumstances of Resuscitation: 2015 American Heart Association Guidelines Update for Cardiopulmonary Resuscitation and Emergency Cardiovascular Care. *Circulation.* 2015;132[suppl 2]:S501–S518.
15. Driver K, Chisholm CA, Darby AE, Malhotra R, DiMarco JP, Ferguson JD. Catheter ablation of arrhythmia during pregnancy. *J Cardiovasc Electrophysiol.* 2015;26(6):698–702.
16. Bombelli F, Lagona F, Salvati A, Catalfamo L, Ferrari AG, Pappone C. Radiofrequency catheter ablation in drug refractory maternal supraventricular tachycardias in advanced pregnancy. *Obstet Gynecol.* 2003;102(5 Pt 2):1171–1173.
17. Yang P, Park J, Pak H. Radiofrequency catheter ablation of incessant atrial tachycardia in pregnant women with minimal radiation exposure: Lessons from two case studies. *J Cardiol Cases.* 2014;9:213–216.

18. Gras D, Mabo P, Kermarrec A, Bazin P, Varin C, Daubert C. Radiofrequency ablation of atrioventricular conduction during the 5th month of pregnancy. *Arch Malad Coeur Vaiss.* 1992;85(12):1873–1877.
19. Dominguez A, Iturralde P, Hermosillo AG, Colin L, Kershenovich S, Garrido LM. Successful radiofrequency ablation of an accessory pathway during pregnancy. *Pacing Clin Electrophysiol.* 1999;22(1 Pt 1):131–134.
20. Pagad SV, Barmade AB, Toal SC, Vora AM, Lokhandwala YY. 'Rescue' radiofrequency ablation for atrial tachycardia presenting as cardiomyopathy in pregnancy. *Indian Heart J.* 2004;56(3):245–247.
21. Kanjwal Y, Kosinski D, Kanj M, Thomas W, Grubb B. Successful radiofrequency catheter ablation of left lateral accessory pathway using transseptal approach during pregnancy. *J Interv Card Electrophysiol.* 2005 Sep;13(3):239–242.
22. Berruezo A, Diez GR, Berne P, Esteban M, Mont L, Brugada J. Low exposure radiation with conventional guided radiofrequency catheter ablation in pregnant women. *Pacing Clin Electrophysiol.* 2007;30(10):1299–1302.
23. Bongiorni MG, Di Cori A, Soldati E, et al. Radiofrequency catheter ablation of atrioventricular nodal reciprocating tachycardia using intracardiac echocardiography in pregnancy. *Europace* 2008;10(8):1018–1021.
24. Manjaly ZR, Sachdev B, Webb T, Rajappan K. Ablation of arrhythmia in pregnancy can be done safely when necessary. *Eur J Obstet Gynecol Reprod Biol.* 2011;157(1):116–117.
25. Wu H, Ling LH, Lee G, Kistler PM. Successful catheter ablation of incessant atrial tachycardia in pregnancy using three-dimensional electroanatomical mapping with minimal radiation. *Intern Med J.* 2012;42(6):709–712.
26. Ferguson JD, Helms A, Mangrum JM, DiMarco JP. Ablation of incessant left atrial tachycardia without fluoroscopy in a pregnant woman. *J Cardiovasc Electrophysiol.* 2011;22(3):346–349.
27. Stec S, Krynski T, Baran J, Kulakowski P. "Rescue" ablation of electrical storm in arrhythmogenic right ventricular cardiomyopathy in pregnancy. *BMC Cardiovasc Disord.* 2013;58(13):1471–2261.
28. Clark JM, Bigelow AM, Crane SS, Khoury FR. Catheter ablation of supraventricular tachycardia without fluoroscopy during pregnancy. *Obstet Gynecol.* 2014;123 Suppl 1:44S–45S.
29. Hogarth AJ, Graham LN. Normal heart ventricular tachycardia associated with pregnancy: Successful treatment with catheter ablation. *Indian Pacing Electrophysiol J.* 2014; 14(2):79–82.
30. Leiria TLL, Pires LM, Kruse ML, de Lima GG. Supraventricular tachycardia and syncope during pregnancy: A case for catheter ablation without fluoroscopy. *Portug J Cardiol.* 2014;pii: S0870-2551(14)00253-4.
31. Zuberi Z, Silberbauer J, Murgatroyd F. Successful non-fluoroscopic radiofrequency ablation of incessant atrial tachycardia in a high risk twin pregnancy. *Indian Pacing Electrophysiol J.* 2014;14(1):26–31.
32. Bigelow, AM, Crane, SS, Khoury F, Clark, JM. Catheter ablation of supraventricular tachycardia without fluoroscopy during pregnancy. *Obstet Gynecol.* 2015;125:1338–1341.
33. Szumowski Ł, Walczak F, Dangel J, et al. Ablation of atypical, fast atrio-ventricular nodal tachycardia in a pregnant woman–a case report. *Kardiol Pol.* 2006;64(2):221–224.

21

How to Perform Catheter Ablation in the Pediatric Population Using No Fluoroscopy

Nicholas H. Von Bergen, MD; Ian H. Law, MD

Introduction

Pediatric electrophysiologists have played an important role in the advancement towards radiation-free procedures. The first article published about non-fluoroscopic procedures was reported by a pediatric electrophysiologist, who demonstrated the feasibility of radiation-free ablation of right-sided manifest accessory pathways using a single catheter and an early 3D mapping system.[1] Around the time of this 2002 publication, the average fluoroscopy time for all SVT procedures was 47 ± 40 minutes, highlighting the significant achievement of a radiation-free procedure in this era of fluoroscopic-guided catheterizations.[2]

A few years later, the radiation reduction movement was advanced by pediatric electrophysiologists publishing a report on the ability to perform full electrophysiology (EP) studies without any radiation use,[3,4] including more complex substrates such as ventricular tachycardia.[5]

The interest in pursuing radiation-free procedures for this group, as witnessed by the relatively large number of pediatric-centered "radiation-free" research projects and publications, stems in large part from the added risks of radiation use in pediatric patients in comparison to adults. In particular, children are at increased risk for radiation-induced injuries both secondary to their longer lifespan as well as an increased susceptibility to radiation.[6-9] This is highlighted by the estimated at 0.08%–0.1% estimated lifetime risk of developing fatal cancer in various diagnostic and therapeutic pediatric and adult catheterization studies and radiofrequency ablation procedures, calculated based on radiation exposure levels in the early 2000s.[10-12] This is especially relevant for pediatric patients with congenital heart disease due to the potential for multiple catheterizations, and the association with radiation injury and long-lasting chromosomal damage.[13,14] This increased risk for radiation exposure is further exacerbated by the lack of fluoroscopy equipment specifically designed for pediatric patients, unintentionally resulting in inadequate shielding, collimating, or inadvertent overexposure due to "adult" settings.

Due to the concerns of radiation injury to both patients and providers, the As Low As Reasonably Achievable (ALARA) principle is considered the gold standard for radiation safety. With current technology, the goal should be to advance the ALARA to its logical conclusion: procedures without the use of any radiation. Nevertheless, there continue to be challenges to performing radiation-free procedures in pediatric patients. This is most often due to the patient's smaller size, which may limit the ability to have adequate surface area on the skin to place necessary 3D mapping equipment, or anatomic or vascular size concerns, which may limit the ability to use techniques that could eliminate the use of radiation.

In this chapter, the authors will discuss some basic techniques for performing radiation-free procedures as well as the advantages and disadvantages of these techniques to eliminate fluoroscopy in pediatric patients. Fortunately, as the approach to performing non-fluoroscopic procedures in

Fluoroscopy Reduction Techniques for Catheter Ablation of Cardiac Arrhythmias. © 2019 Mansour Razminia, Paul C. Zei, eds. Cardiotext Publishing, ISBN: 978-1-942909-30-9.

the pediatric population is similar to that in adults, the discussion will center upon alterations in the typical radiation reduction process as opposed to reviewing the complete approach as done in prior chapters. As well, some basic considerations for a radiation-free procedure in patients with congenital heart disease are discussed.

Adjustments to the Non-Fluoroscopic Approach in Children

3D Mapping Systems

Current 3D mapping systems utilize a variety of mechanisms to 3-dimensionally localize the catheters within the patient's vascular system. Though systems generally incorporate magnetic and/or impedance-based catheter localization systems, all systems utilize skin patches placed on the patient's body surface (typically around the chest and/or back) to assist with catheter localization. Unfortunately, with the limited surface area and the need for defibrillation pads and ECG leads, some of the pediatric patients may be too small to have adequate skin area for these patches without patch modification. Though variations exist between systems, most patches will function appropriately with some modification to decrease their "footprint" on the patient's chest.

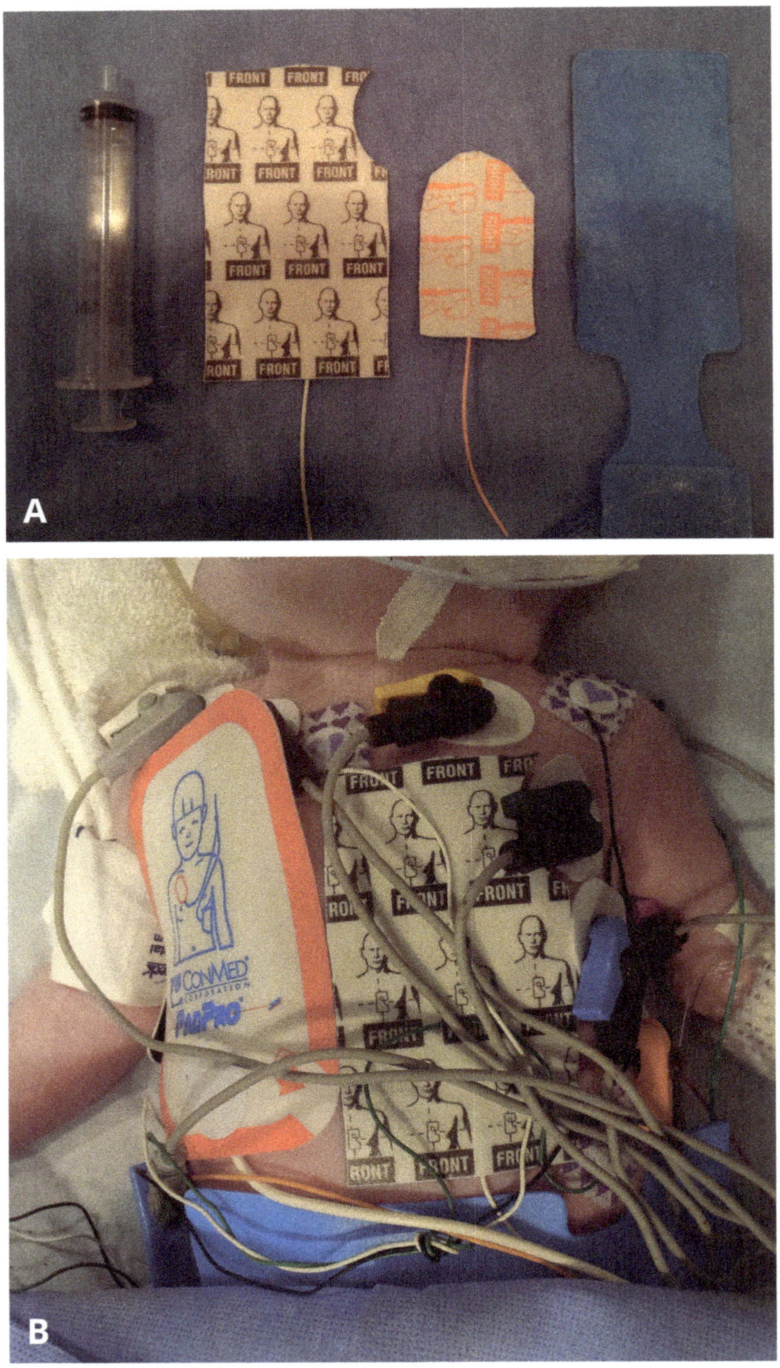

Figure 21.1 Modified EnSite grounding patches to allow attachment in a 4-kg infant with tachycardia-induced cardiomyopathy. **A:** Note the size of 2 of the chest patches and the grounding pad in comparison to a 10 mL syringe. **B:** The chest of a 4-kg infant with modified patches, electrodes, grounding and R2 pads. (Reprinted with permission from Von Bergen NH, Lozier J, Law IH. Three-dimensional mapping system modification to allow a near fluoroless ablation of atrial ectopic tachycardia in an infant with tachycardia induced heart failure. *J Innov Card Rhythm Manag.* 2013;4,1127–1132.)

The surface patches typically contain a conductive portion that connects to a central wire system. From the authors' personal experience, the reference patches function adequately as long as they are not trimmed to the point of wire exposure and patches on alternate sides of the body are kept at approximately the same size, as small as a circular electrode near 3 cm in diameter. An example of modified EnSite patches (Abbott, Abbott Park, IL) is shown in **Figure 21.1**. As specific modifications may be required by different 3D mapping systems, it is recommended that patch alterations be discussed with representatives from the 3D mapping device manufacturer. Fortunately, the need to modify the surface patches is lessening, as smaller size patches continue to be developed for newer versions of the 3D mapping systems.

Transesophageal Echocardiogram in Children

Transesophageal echocardiograms (TEE) during electrophysiology procedures were described as early as 1991.[15] As catheterization technology, 3D mapping systems and imaging systems have improved, TEE was one of the first adjuvant systems electrophysiologists adopted to avoid the use of radiation altogether.[16] Though most commonly used for transseptal puncture, the indications for use overlap with intracardiac echocardiography (ICE). TEE may be used for evaluation of coronary arteries, higher-risk ablation sites, confirmation of catheter contact, evaluating anatomic characteristics of ablation sites, and for cardiac function and/or effusion evaluation. It should be noted that there are both adult and pediatric TEE probes, with smaller lumen sizes and less rigid shafts among pediatric probes. As discussed in other chapters, the practice for transseptal puncture with TEE is similar to when using ICE and can allow accurate needle tip identification. TEE can also be an excellent guide for some of the complex congenital heart disease interventions, such as during a transbaffle puncture or catheter manipulation in a complex heart (**Figure 21.2**).

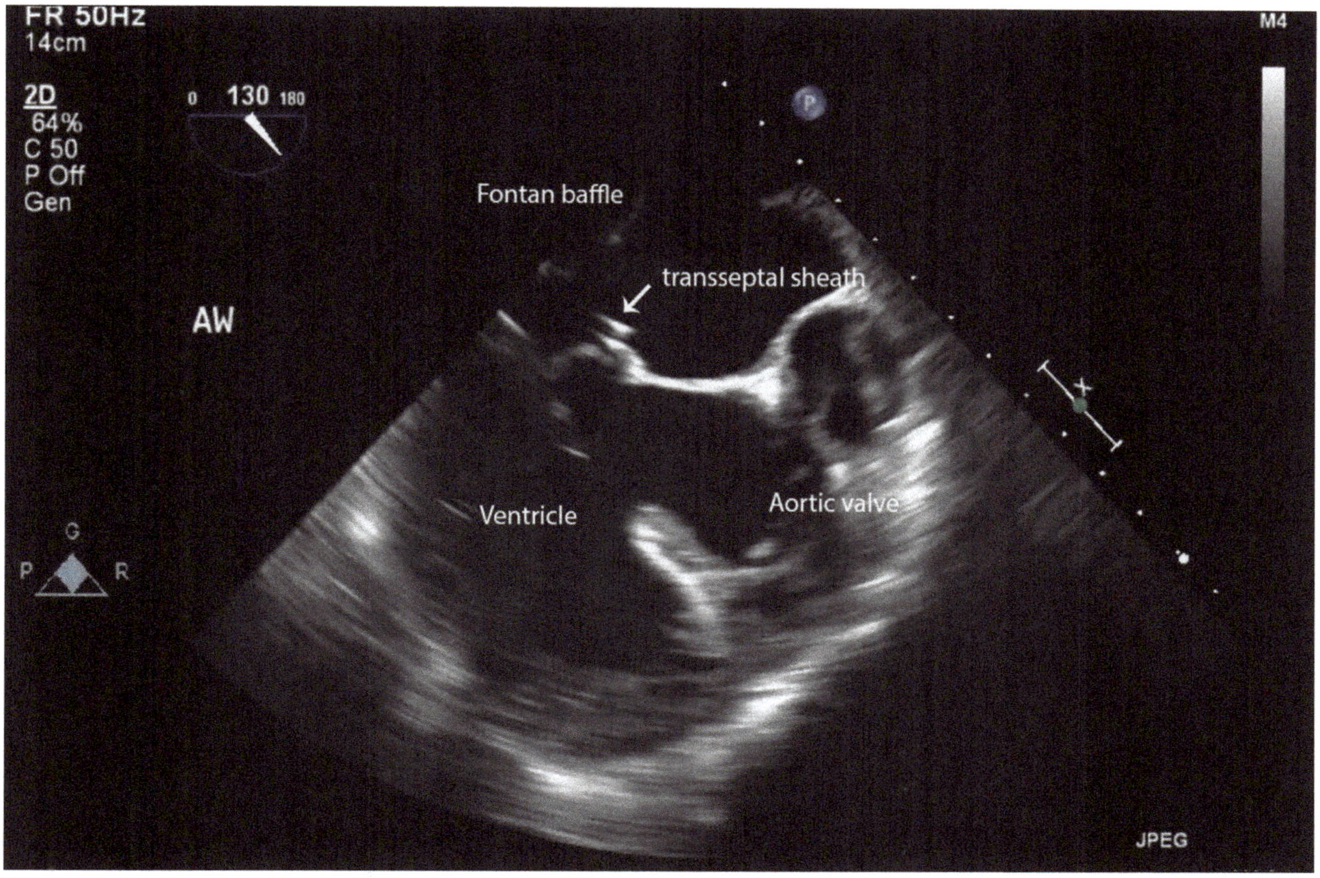

Figure 21.2 A TEE image after TEE-guided transbaffle puncture in a patient with a single ventricle, dextrocardia, atrioventricular nodal reentrant tachycardia, and intra-atrial reentrant tachycardia who is post Fontan procedure. The transseptal sheath is labeled in the pulmonary venous atrium helping confirm sheath location.

A significant disadvantage of TEE use in interventional procedures is the need for an additional provider to obtain the images, which could potentially lengthen the procedural time. Although the use of TEE is not without risks, in general, the risk of a major TEE-related complication is well less than 1%; risk of minor injury such as abrasions or dysphasia is relatively common.[17,18] Some complications, such as esophageal injury, may not be identified until after the patient has left the hospital.

In general, TEEs are contraindicated in patients with active upper GI bleeds or esophageal pathology such as tracheoesophageal fistula repair. Complication risks appear be slightly higher in younger patients, likely due to their smaller size, and the probe may cause airway or mediastinal structure compression in particularly small patients. Nevertheless, it may add value and safety, especially for less experienced transseptal operators.[19–21]

Intracardiac Echocardiography

As the size of intracardiac ultrasound catheters become smaller, and as the price decreases, ICE will likely be increasingly utilized in pediatric patients. However, currently the smallest ICE probes are 8–10 Fr and require a separate femoral venous entry site. Again, size constraints limit the desire for many pediatric electrophysiologists to utilize ICE in younger patients. Nevertheless, it can work well in patients with adequate vessel size, allowing the elimination of radiation for transseptal access, coronary cusp ablations, and other procedures traditionally requiring radiation (**Figure 21.3**).[22,23]

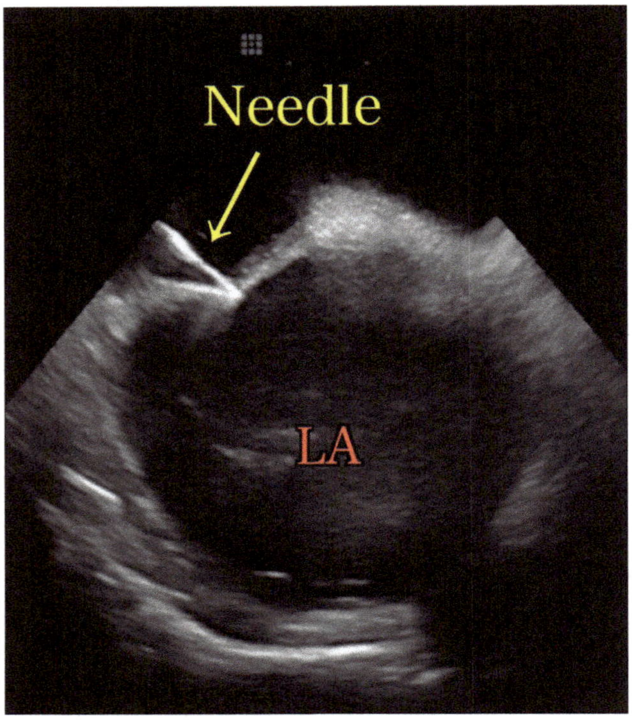

Figure 21.3 An ICE image showing a transseptal needle tip engaging the atrial septum during transseptal puncture.

Many pediatric electrophysiologists would choose a TEE or small amounts of radiation over ICE in those less than 10 to 12 years of age due to the size of the ICE catheter and the risk for vessel damage. However, interventional cardiologists have used ICE in pediatric patients 6 years and younger.[24,25] In very small patients and infants the ICE probe may be used in the esophagus, similar to a TEE. Although imaging via this route is occasionally suboptimal, the imaging has been reported to be sufficient in many cases.[26] In patients with congenital heart disease, ICE and systems that integrate ICE imaging with the 3D map such as CARTOSOUND (Biosense Webster, Irvine, CA) may be especially helpful (**Figure 21.4**).[27,28] Though children may have vascular size limitations that may preclude the use of ICE, the technique for ICE imaging does not differ significantly in children than in adults. Therefore, please refer to the prior chapters for details regarding ICE technique for these procedures.

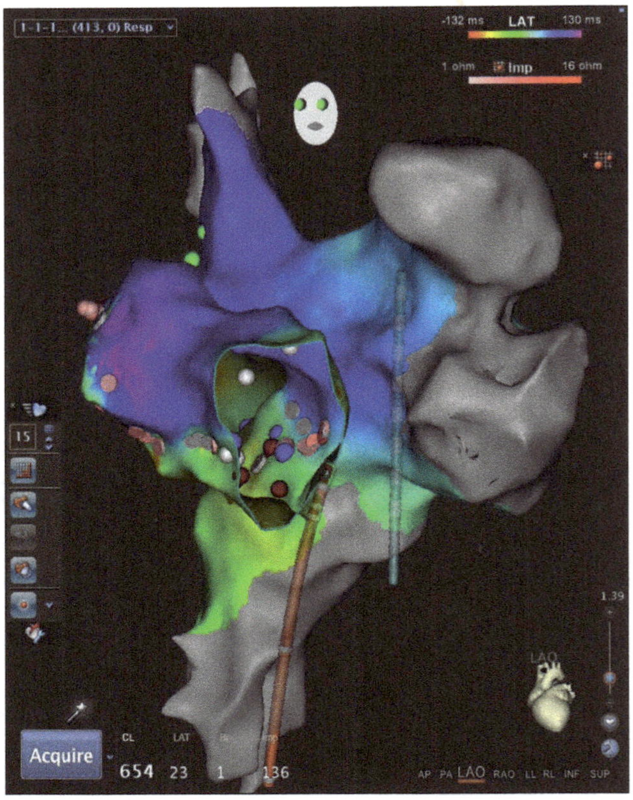

Figure 21.4 A CARTO image of the atria of a patient with D-transposition of the great arteries post Mustard procedure. The SVC and IVC are baffled to the left ventricle. The geometry was obtained with both catheter-guided acquisition as well as with CARTOSOUND, an ultrasound-guided geometry acquisition. A catheter is visualized in the esophagus. (Courtesy of David Bradley, MD.)

Radiation-Free Transseptal Puncture Techniques

The approach to the transseptal puncture in pediatric patients is generally very similar to that for adult patients. However, young patients may be more likely to have a patent foramen ovale, which may or may not be well visualized on a prior transthoracic echocardiogram. Therefore, our practice is to probe for transseptal access prior to attempting a transseptal puncture. After creating right atrial geometry and confirmation of a left-sided arrhythmia, any steerable electrophysiology catheter can be used to probe the atrial septum. At times, crossing the foramen ovale can be achieved by engaging the septum at the site of the fossa ovalis and rotating the catheter slightly posterior with slight pressure. In the authors' experience, using this technique enabled the operator to access the left heart in 27% of pediatric and young adult patients without the need for transseptal puncture.[29] That said, due to the angle and location of the foramen ovale, accessing the left atrium through a patent foramen ovale may make access of the left posterior septum more difficult. This can be easily overcome with the use of a steerable long sheath.

In most 3D mapping systems, attaching an alligator clip to the transseptal needle, or to the back of a wire (such as the SafeSept wire) during the transseptal puncture, will allow 3D localization of a unipolar signal at the site of the tip of the needle/wire on the premade geometry. This can also assist with transseptal puncture localization[29] (**Figure 21.5**).

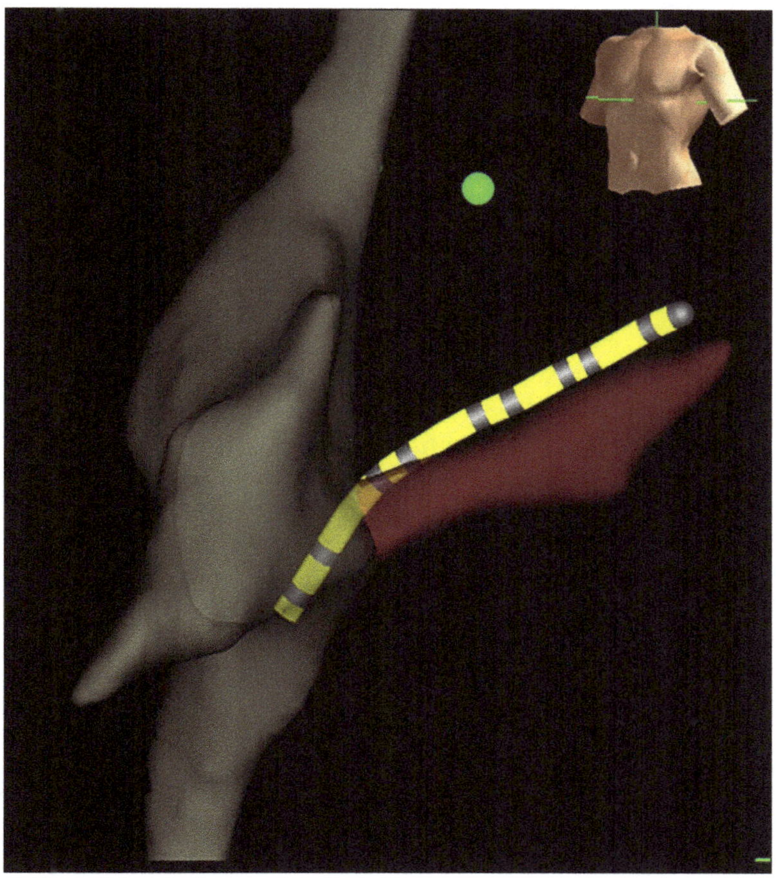

Figure 21.5 Transseptal needle tip localization utilizing 3D EnSite NavX. A right atrial and coronary sinus (CS) geometry has been created and is viewed in a LAO position. The **yellow** catheter is within the CS. A transseptal puncture was preformed while localizing the transseptal needle tip (**green sphere**) with an alligator clip attached proximal end of the needle. This can allow 3D visualization of the needle tip on the premade geometry. (Reprinted with permission from Von Bergen NH, Lozier J, Law IH. Three-dimensional mapping system modification to allow a near fluoroless ablation of atrial ectopic tachycardia in an infant with tachycardia induced heart failure. *J Innov Card Rhythm Manag.* 2013;4,1127–1132.)

Previous studies have shown subacute cognitive decline and the potential for microthrombi correlated with longer left atrial dwell times.[30,31] Therefore, as soon as the necessary ablation lesions are placed, the left-sided catheters are removed to the right atrium. During catheter removal from the left side, the 3D mapping system is used to mark the site of transseptal access for reaccess if necessary. This technique has allowed us to decrease the length of anticoagulation and potentially decrease the risk of left-sided thrombi. When required, the authors have been able to re-access the left atrium through the the patients' marked transseptal site without the need for a repeat transseptal puncture (**Figure 21.6**).[32]

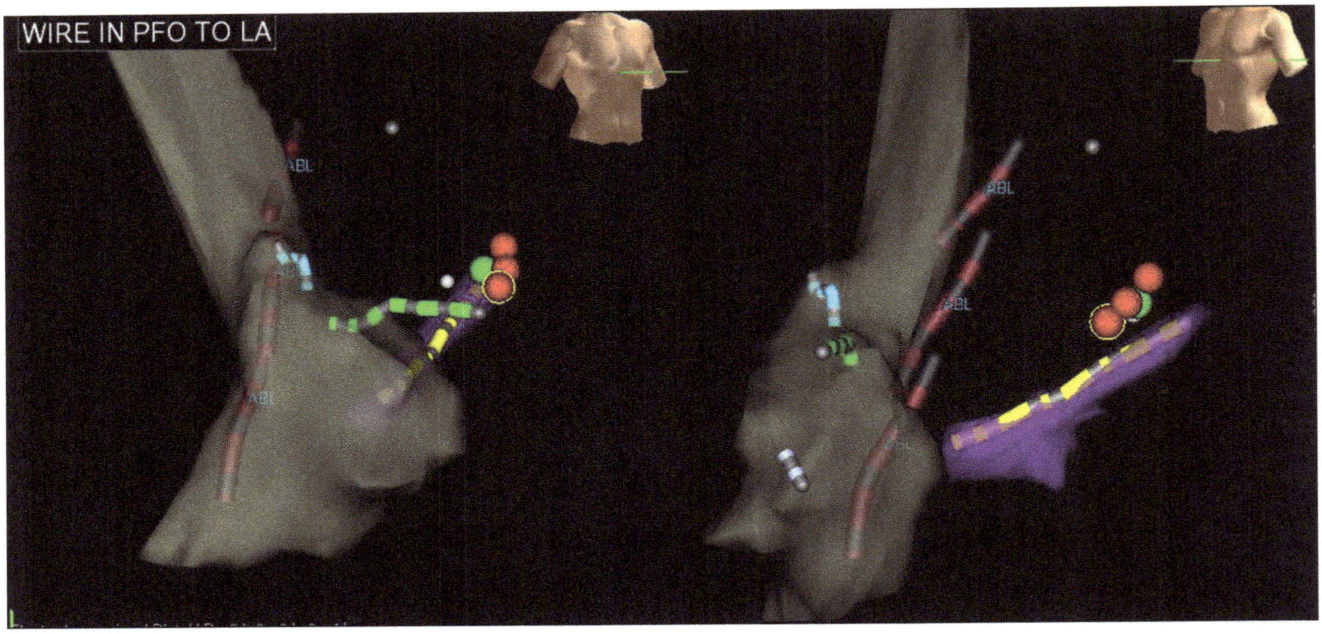

Figure 21.6 The right atrial and CS geometry after the ablation of a left-sided pathway. A wire was passed through the PFO while being monitored by a unipolar reference (**grey sphere** represents the tip of the wire at the time of transseptal passage). This allowed passage of a catheter/sheath transseptal though the PFO without radiation. Immediately after ablation, the ablation catheter was removed from the LA and the PFO was marked by shadowing the ablation catheter to mark the LA access site (**shadowed red ablation catheter images**) in case reaccess was required. A CS (**yellow**) and combined His/RV catheter (**green/grey**) are also seen. The **red** and **green spheres** represent the ablation sites.

Radiation-Free Approach to Patients with Congenital Heart Disease (CHD)

Performing radiation-free procedures in patients with congenital heart disease can be challenging. Patients with congenital heart disease may have unusual anatomy, significant scar, increased calcification of the native and non-native tissue, or vascular obstruction or occlusion (**Figure 21.7**), and they may require access through non-traditional vessels (i.e., hepatic vessels). Given this, radiation is a tool that should be considered when necessary to confirm the catheter/needle location and recommend using small amounts of radiation when it may improve procedural safety or effectiveness. However, given the potential need for multiple catheterizations and other radiologic diagnostic and interventional procedures, patients with congenital heart disease are likely at the highest risk for long-term exposure to radiation therapy, further reinforcing the need for advancing radiation-free techniques.[9-11]

Due to the wide variation of anatomy and electrophysiology concerns in patients with congenital heart disease, it is difficult to recommend specific protocols to avoid radiation for these procedures. It is extremely important to have a firm understanding of the anatomy of each specific type of heart disease as well as the typical arrhythmias and arrhythmia locations associated with a congenital heart defect and surgical procedures. Because of these concerns, it is recommended that any complex CHD procedure be done with the assistance of an electrophysiologist trained in CHD.

Even with operators experienced with CHD and an understanding of the arrhythmia substrate and knowledge of likely ablation sites, this population requires substantial preprocedural planning. We recommend evaluating prior surgical notes, previous studies (e.g., CT, MRI, or prior EP studies) and reviewing noninvasive electrophysiologic testing. An understanding of vascular access to the heart is also very important. This preparation can guide physicians to incorporate the necessary techniques and technology to minimize or eliminate the need for fluoroscopy.

In many cases, physicians may need to be creative in determining the most appropriate vascular access to the heart, as nontraditional access sites may be required or desired for effective ablation. Transesophageal electrophysiology catheters can be very helpful when access is limited as this can allow left atrial pacing and recording. Also, internal jugular, brachial, subclavian, or hepatic venous access can be considered.

In patients with complex congenital heart disease, TEE and/or ICE can be a useful adjunct and occasionally necessary for complex access issues. The CARTOSOUND, which can build geometry while also displaying an ICE image may be especially valuable due to its ability to provide mapping and real-time visualization.[28] Additionally, MRI or CT images can be "merged" into the 3D geometry, allowing pre-procedural geometry creation, which can then be used during the procedure itself (**Figure 21.8**).

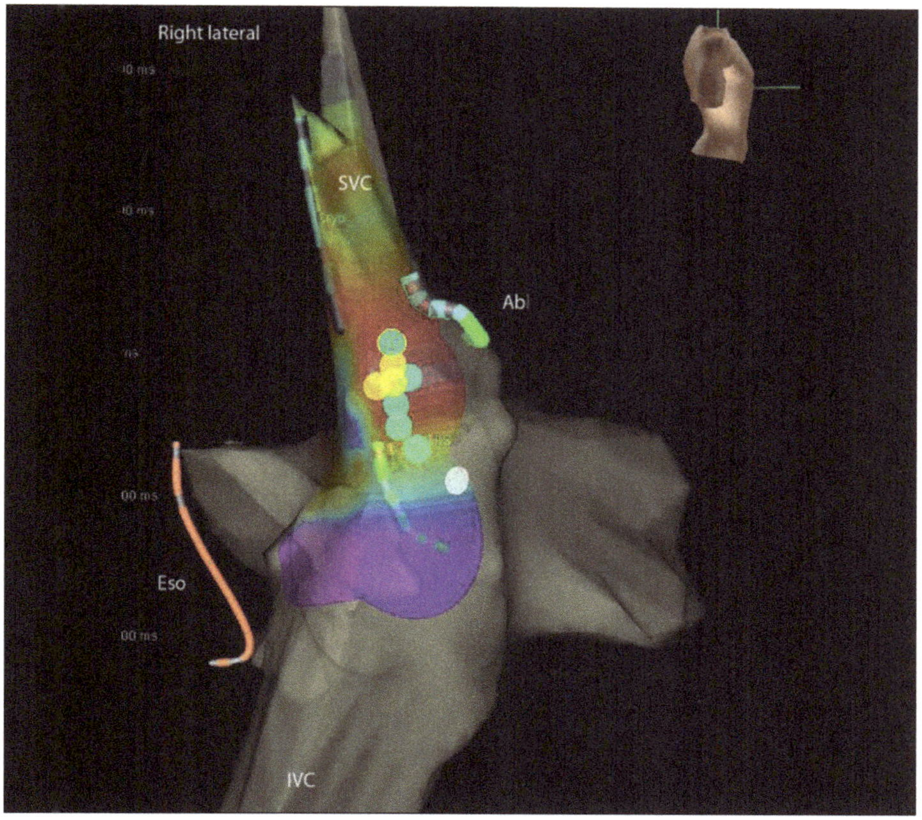

Figure 21.7 A right lateral view of a 3D map of the right atrium in a teenager with D-transposition of the great arteries with obstructed femoral venous access. Catheters were placed via the esophagus, right internal jugular and right brachial vein. The patient had an atrial ectopic tachycardia in close proximity to the sinus node and phrenic nerve, which was ablated with cryotherapy. (Reprinted with permission from Kemmet CK, Maginot KM, Teelin, T, Von Bergen NH. Complex 3D mapping in a young adult with D-TGA, atrial tachycardia, and limited venous access. *J Innov Card Rhythm Manag.* 2012;3,637–641.)

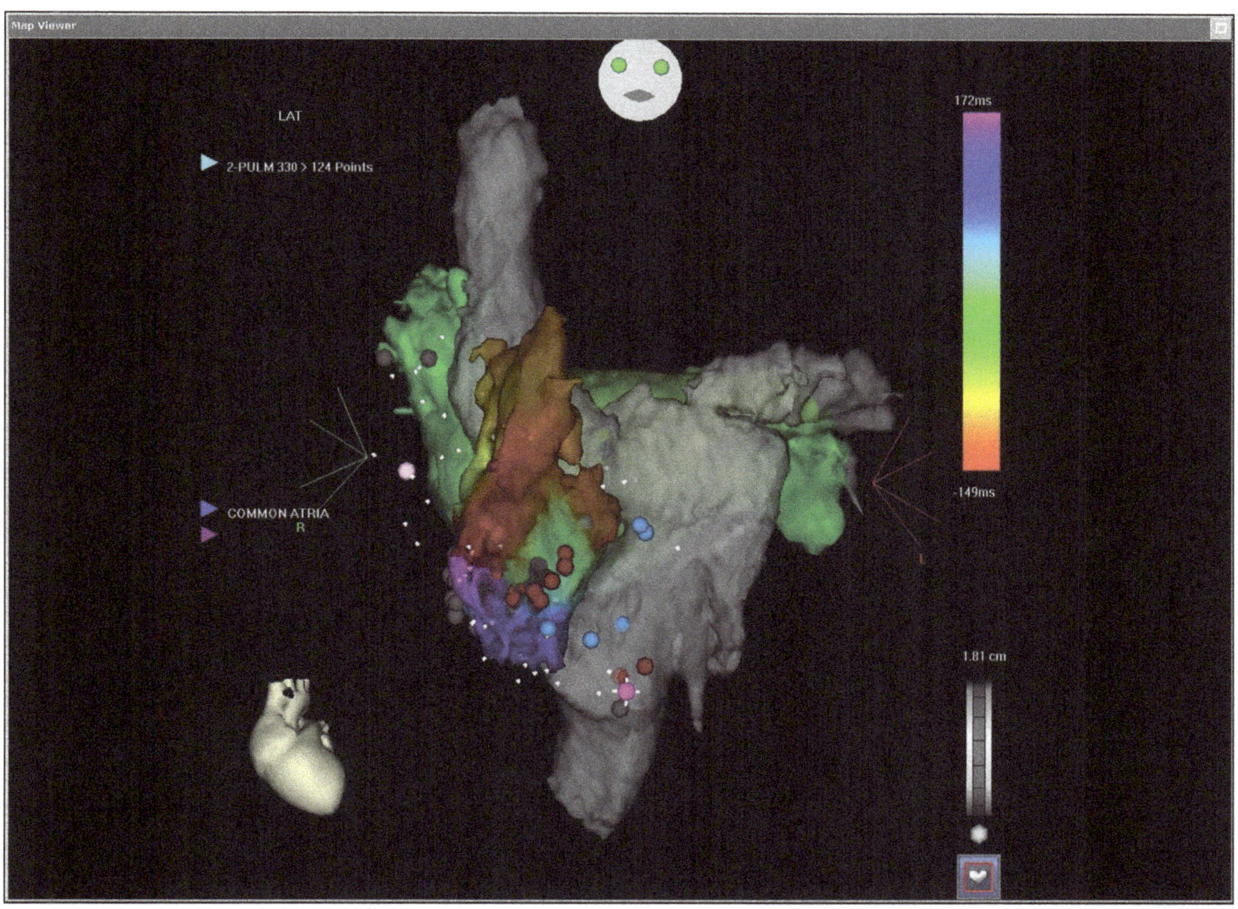

Figure 21.8 MRI images were merged with CARTO to allow geometry acquisition in a patient with D-transposition of the great arteries post Mustard procedure. (Courtesy of David Bradley, MD.)

Patients who have undergone an atrial switch or a Fontan procedure may require a transbaffle/transconduit puncture. In these patients, the type of baffle material should be determined if possible, as these baffles can be derived from pericardium, or polytetrafluoroethylene (Gore-Tex). In patients with polytetrafluorethylene material, the puncture may require substantial effort and additional equipment such as radiofrequency needles and angiography balloons. Due to location of the conduit in patients with the Fontan procedure, it can be challenging to obtain purchase at the ideal baffle site, and the needle can slide along the conduit. If a transbaffle leak is present, this may be utilized, and if not, a snare to stabilize the needle has been described.[33] Fortunately, transbaffle punctures are generally more easily approached in those with an atrial switch, as an anterior angulation of the needle, ~180 degrees from the typical transseptal approach, usually allows a successful puncture of the inferior portion of the right atrial baffle. With a steerable sheath, this can provide access to the tricuspid valve/inferior vena cava isthmus, a common site for intra-atrial reentrant tachycardia in the population. Again, use of ICE, TEE, and some fluoroscopy may be required. In especially challenging cases, alternative approaches may need to be considered to avoid the thicker material.

Conclusion

Safely accomplishing radiation-free procedures in the pediatric and/or congenital heart disease population requires slightly different considerations than when performing procedures in the standard adult patient. This chapter discusses the approach for radiation-free procedures as it relates to radiation risk, patient size, and congenital abnormalities in these unique populations.

References

1. Drago F, Silvetti MS, Di Pino A, Grutter G, Bevilacqua M, Leibovich S. Exclusion of fluoroscopy during ablation treatment of right accessory pathway in children. *J Cardiovasc Electrophysiol.* 2002;13(8):778–782.
2. Kugler JD, Danford DA, Houston K, Felix G. Radiofrequency catheter ablation for paroxysmal supraventricular tachycardia in children and adolescents without structural heart disease. Pediatric EP Society, Radiofrequency Catheter Ablation Registry. *Am J Cardiol.* 1997;80(11):1438–1443.
3. Smith G, Clark JM. Elimination of fluoroscopy use in a pediatric electrophysiology laboratory utilizing three-dimensional mapping. *Pacing Clin Electrophysiol.* 2007;30(4):510–518.
4. Tuzcu V. A non-fluoroscopic approach for electrophysiology and catheter ablation procedures using a three-dimensional navigation system. *Pacing Clin Electrophysiol.* 2007;30(4):519–525.
5. Von Bergen NH, Bansal S, Gingerich J, Law IH. Nonfluoroscopic and radiation-limited ablation of ventricular arrhythmias in children and young adults: A case series. *Pediatric Cardiol.* 2011.
6. Clay MA, Campbell RM, Strieper M, Frias PA, Stevens M, Mahle WT. Long-term risk of fatal malignancy following pediatric radiofrequency ablation. *Am J Cardiol.* 2008;102(7):913–915.
7. Justino H. The ALARA concept in pediatric cardiac catheterization: Techniques and tactics for managing radiation dose. *Pediatric Radiol.* 2006;36 Suppl 2:146–153.
8. Limacher MC, Douglas PS, Germano G, et al. ACC expert consensus document. Radiation safety in the practice of cardiology. American College of Cardiology. *J Am Coll Cardiol.* 1998;31(4):892–913.
9. Wagner LK. Minimizing radiation injury and neoplastic effects during pediatric fluoroscopy: What should we know? *Pediatric Radiol.* 2006;36 Suppl 2:141–145.
10. Bacher K, Bogaert E, Lapere R, De Wolf D, Thierens H. Patient-specific dose and radiation risk estimation in pediatric cardiac catheterization. *Circulation.* 2005;111(1):83–89.
11. McFadden SL, Mooney RB, Shepherd PH. X-ray dose and associated risks from radiofrequency catheter ablation procedures. *Br J Radiol.* 2002;75(891):253–265.
12. National Research Council (U.S.). Committee to Assess Health Risks from Exposure to Low Level of Ionizing Radiation. Health risks from exposure to low levels of ionizing radiation: BEIR VII Phase 2. Washington, D.C.: National Academies Press; 2006.
13. Ait-Ali L, Andreassi MG, Foffa I, Spadoni I, Vano E, Picano E. Cumulative patient effective dose and acute radiation-induced chromosomal DNA damage in children with congenital heart disease. *Heart.* 2010;96(4):269–274.
14. Andreassi MG, Ait-Ali L, Botto N, Manfredi S, Mottola G, Picano E. Cardiac catheterization and long-term chromosomal damage in children with congenital heart disease. *Eur Heart J.* 2006;27(22):2703–2708.
15. Goldman AP, Irwin JM, Glover MU, Mick W. Transesophageal echocardiography to improve positioning of radiofrequency ablation catheters in left-sided Wolff-Parkinson-White syndrome. *Pacing Clin Electrophysiol.* 1991;14(8):1245–1250.
16. Clark J, Bockoven JR, Lane J, Patel CR, Smith G. Use of three-dimensional catheter guidance and trans-esophageal echocardiography to eliminate fluoroscopy in catheter ablation of left-sided accessory pathways. *Pacing Clin Electrophysiol.* 2008;31(3):283–289.
17. Muhiudeen-Russell IA, Miller-Hance WC, Silverman NH. Unrecognized esophageal perforation in a neonate during transesophageal echocardiography. *J Am Soc Echocardiogr.* 2001;14(7):747–749.
18. Lennon MJ, Gibbs NM, Weightman WM, Leber J, Ee HC, Yusoff IF. Transesophageal echocardiography-related gastrointestinal complications in cardiac surgical patients. *J Cardiothorac Vasc Anesth.* 2005;19(2):141–145.
19. Bayrak F, Chierchia GB, Namdar M, et al. Added value of transoesophageal echocardiography during transseptal puncture performed by inexperienced operators. *Europace.* 2012;14(5):661–665.
20. Stevenson JG, Sorensen GK. Proper probe size for pediatric transesophageal echocardiography. *Am J Cardiol.* 1993;72(5):491–492.

21. Hilberath JN, Oakes DA, Shernan SK, Bulwer BE, D'Ambra MN, Eltzschig HK. Safety of Transesophageal Echocardiography. *J Am Soc Echocardiogr.* 2010;23(11): 1115–1127.
22. Proietti R, Rivera S, Dussault C, et al. Intracardiac echo-facilitated 3D electroanatomical mapping of ventricular arrhythmias from the papillary muscles: Assessing the 'fourth dimension' during ablation. *Europace.* 2017;19(1): 21–28.
23. Clark BC, Sumihara K, Berul CI, Moak JP. Off the pedal: Fluoroless transseptal puncture in pediatric supraventricular tachycardia ablation. *Pacing Clin Electrophysiol.* 2017;40(11):1254–1259.
24. Hijazi Z, Wang Z, Cao Q, Koenig P, Waight D, Lang R. Transcatheter closure of atrial septal defects and patent foramen ovale under intracardiac echocardiographic guidance: Feasibility and comparison with transesophageal echocardiography. *Catheter Cardiovasc Interv.* 2001;52(2):194–199.
25. Patel A, Cao QL, Koenig PR, Hijazi ZM. Intracardiac echocardiography to guide closure of atrial septal defects in children less than 15 kilograms. *Catheter Cardiovasc Interv.* 2006;68(2):287–291.
26. Watanabe S, Yoshida Y, Suzuki T, Nakamura Y. Successful catheter ablation using real-time ultrasound-assisted 3-D electroanatomical mapping system for atrioventricular accessory pathway in a 1-year-old girl with criss-cross heart. *Heart Rhythm Case Rep.* 2016;2(4): 351–355.
27. den Uijl DW, Blom NA, Wijnmaalen AP, Bax JJ, Schalij MJ, Zeppenfeld K. Real-time integration of intracardiac echocardiography to facilitate atrial tachycardia ablation in a patient with a Senning baffle. *Circ Arrhythm Electrophysiol.* 2009;2(5):e28–30.
28. Kean AC, Gelehrter SK, Shetty I, Dick M, 2nd, Bradley DJ. Experience with CARTOSOUND for arrhythmia ablation in pediatric and congenital heart disease patients. *J Interv Card Electrophysiol.* 2010;29(2):139–145.
29. Knoedel C, Dexter BC, Lampe J, law IH, Von Bergen NH. Utilizing 3D NavX for transseptal puncture as an additional safeguard: A case series. *J Innov Cardi Rhythm Mgt.* 2016;7:4.
30. Gaita F, Leclercq JF, Schumacher B, et al. Incidence of silent cerebral thromboembolic lesions after atrial fibrillation ablation may change according to technology used: Comparison of irrigated radiofrequency, multipolar nonirrigated catheter and cryoballoon. *J Cardiovasc Electrophysiol.* 2011;22(9):961–968.
31. Medi C, Evered L, Silbert B, et al. Subtle post-procedural cognitive dysfunction after atrial fibrillation ablation. *J Am Coll Cardiol.* 2013;62(6):531–539.
32. Unnithan AG, Dexter BC, Law IH, Von Bergen NH. Limiting left-sided catheter dwelling time using 3-D NavX to mark and reaccess the left atrium via prior transseptal puncture site. *J Interv Card Electrophysiol.* 2014;40(2): 125–128.
33. Uhm JS, Kim NK, Kim TH, Joung B, Pak HN, Lee MH. How to perform transconduit and transbaffle puncture in patients who have previously undergone the Fontan or Mustard operation. *Heart Rhythm.* 2018;15(1):145–150.

Author Disclosures

Amin Al-Ahmad – No relevant disclosures.

Dan Alyesh – No disclosures.

Martin Borlich – No conflicts to declare.

Kristen Breedlove – No disclosures.

Jim W. Cheung – Received consulting fees from Biosense Webster.

John Clark – No disclosures.

Nicholas J. Costa – No relevant disclosures.

Hany Demo – Abbott: consultant; Medtronic: consultant.

Oliver D'Silva – No disclosures.

Jason T. Engel – No relevant disclosures.

Carola Gianni – No relevant disclosures.

Rodney P. Horton – No relevant disclosures.

Christopher I. Jones – No disclosures.

Ian H. Law – No disclosures.

Raman L. Mitra – Biosense Webster: a moderate consultant.

Carlos Monreal – No relevant disclosures.

Gustavo X. Morales – Biosense Webster: research funds, consulting agreement; Boston Scientific: research funds.

Andrea Natale – No relevant disclosures.

José Osorio – Biosense Webster: research grants, consulting; Boston Scientific: research grants, consulting.

Mansour Razminia – Abbott: consultant; Medtronic: consultant.

Clayton Robison – No relevant disclosures.

Zachary J. Rosenblatt – No relevant disclosures.

José Mauricio Sánchez – No current disclosures.

Saurabh Shah –Biotronik: research funding.

Robin Singh – No relevant disclosures.

Philipp Sommer – A member of the Abbott and Biosense Webster physician board and received research funding.

Sri Sundaram – No relevant disclosures.

Amit Thosani – Research support and modest consulting with Biosense Webster.

Roderick Tung – No disclosures.

Nicholas H. Von Bergen – No relevant disclosures.

Theodore Wang – No disclosures.

Cameron Willoughby – Received consulting fees from Abbott in 2018.

Paul C. Zei – Biosense Webster: research support, consultant, advisory board; Abbott: consultant; Boehringer Ingleheim: expert witness; Affera: consultant.

Index

D

E

F

H

I

J

CPSIA information can be obtained
at www.ICGtesting.com
Printed in the USA
BVHW020808090422
633352BV00002BA/3

9 781942 909309